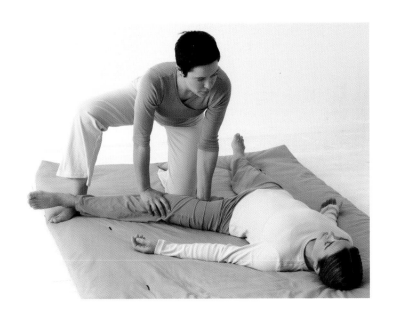

thai massage and shiatsu body work

for health and well-being

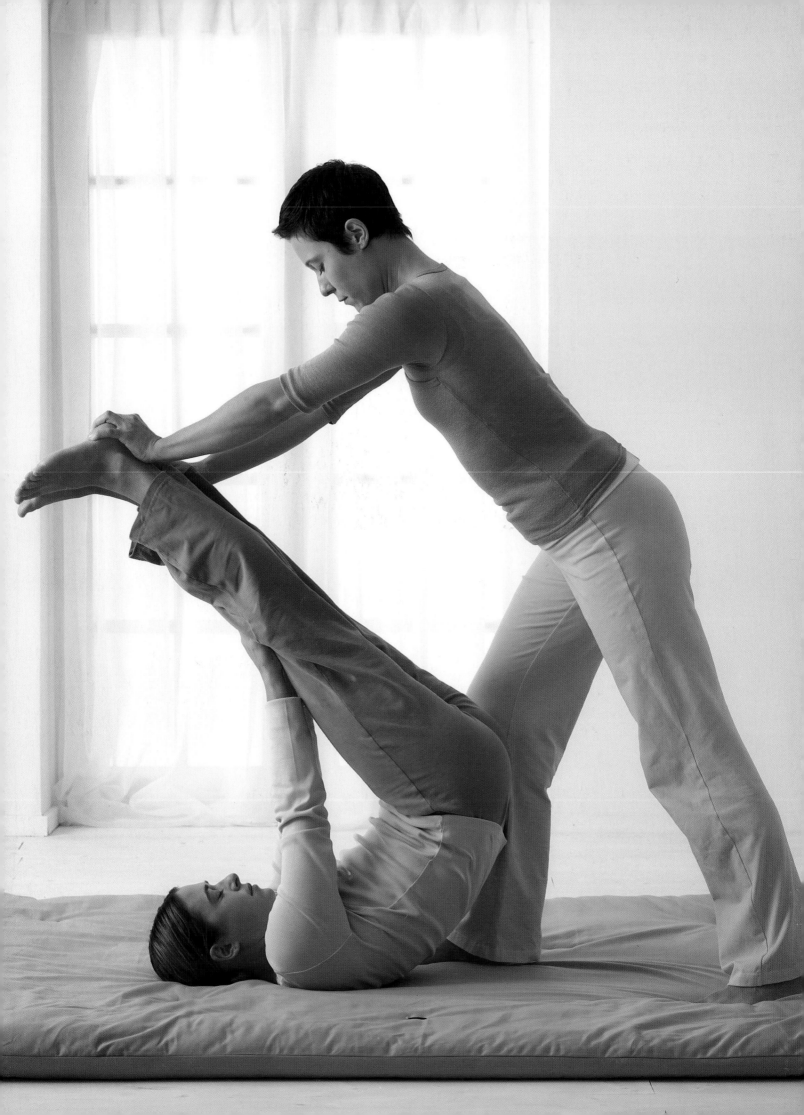

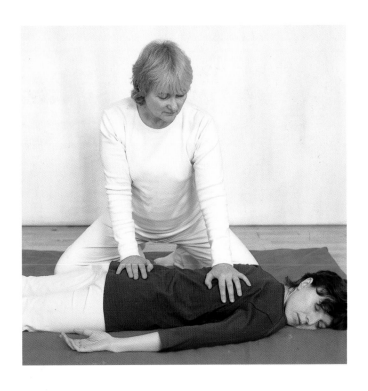

thai massage and shiatsu body work
for health and well-being

A fully illustrated step-by-step guide to the art of healing and relaxation through two powerful Eastern massage techniques, with over 800 colour photographs

Nicky Smith and Hilary Totah

Photography by Paul Bricknell and Clare Park

LORENZ BOOKS

This edition is published by Lorenz Books, an imprint of Anness Publishing Ltd, Hermes House, 88–89 Blackfriars Road, London SE1 8HA; tel. 020 7401 2077; fax 020 7633 9499

www.lorenzbooks.com; www.annesspublishing.com

If you like the images in this book and would like to investigate using them for publishing, promotions or advertising, please visit our website www.practicalpictures.com for more information.

UK agent: The Manning Partnership Ltd; tel. 01225 478444; fax 01225 478440; sales@manning-partnership.co.uk

UK distributor: Grantham Book Services Ltd; tel. 01476 541080; fax 01476 541061; orders@gbs.tbs-ltd.co.uk

North American agent/distributor: National Book Network; tel. 301 459 3366; fax 301 429 5746; www.nbnbooks.com

Australian agent/distributor: Pan Macmillan Australia; tel. 1300 135 113; fax 1300 135 103; customer.service@macmillan.com.au

New Zealand agent/distributor: David Bateman Ltd; tel. (09) 415 7664; fax (09) 415 8892

Publisher Joanna Lorenz
Senior Managing Editor Conor Kilgallon
Project Editors Ann Kay and Emma Clegg
Editorial Reader Penelope Goodare
Designers Lisa Tai and Jane Coney
Photography Paul Bricknell and Clare Park
Illustrator Sam Elmhurst
Production Controller Steve Lang

Dedication

Asokananda, the leading Western practitioner of traditional thai yoga whose words are featured on pages 6–8, died in 2005 after a short illness from cancer. His lifelong commitment to Thai massage and the influence of his work will continue to flourish and grow through the teachers he has supported and through the work of his school and the Sunshine Network. He will be remembered with love.

Ethical trading policy

At Anness Publishing we believe that business should be conducted in an ethical and ecologically sustainable way, with respect for the environment and a proper regard to the replacement of the natural resources we employ.

As a publisher, we use a lot of wood pulp to make high-quality paper for printing, and that wood commonly comes from spruce trees. We are therefore currently growing more than 500,000 trees in two Scottish forest plantations near Aberdeen – Berrymoss (130 hectares/320 acres) and West Touxhill (125 hectares/305 acres). The forests we manage contain twice the number of trees employed each year in paper-making for our books.

Because of this ongoing ecological investment programme, our customers have the reassurance of knowing that a tree is being cultivated on your behalf to naturally replace the materials used to make the book you are holding. Our forestry programme is run in accordance with the UK Woodland Assurance Scheme (UKWAS) and will be certified by the internationally recognized Forest Stewardship Council (FSC). The FSC is a non-government organization dedicated to promoting responsible management of the world's forests. Certification ensures forests are managed in an environmentally sustainable and socially responsible basis. For further information about this scheme, go to www.annesspublishing.com/trees

© Anness Publishing Ltd 2007

A CIP catalogue record for this book is available from the British Library.

Previously published in two separate volumes, *Thai Massage* and *Shiatsu*.

The author and publishers have made every effort to ensure that all instructions contained within this book are accurate and safe, and cannot accept liability for any resulting injury, damage or loss to persons or property, however it may arise. If you do have any special needs or problems, consult your doctor or a physiotherapist. This book cannot replace medical consultation and should be used in conjunction with professional advice. You should not attempt Thai massage or Shiatsu without training from a properly qualified practitioner.

contents

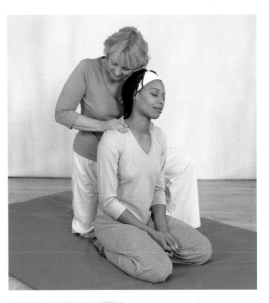

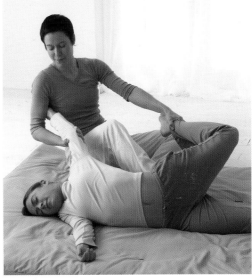

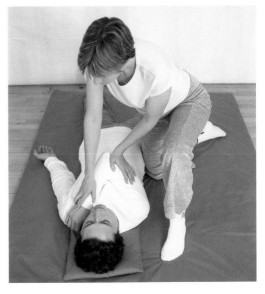

Thai Massage: an introduction by Asokananda

Nicky Smith has put her heart into creating an authentic and thorough introduction to Thai massage, a fascinating form of energy balancing, which was barely known outside Thailand just a few short years ago. As well as producing an authoritative and accessible guide, she has also stayed true to the spirit of tradition, and offers us a refreshingly unique and personal perspective that makes this so much more than simply an instructional manual.

Nicky Smith has been studying with me for several years, with great enthusiasm. She is now one of my senior authorized teachers and she has a profound understanding of the healing power of her work, an understanding that she shares here with the readers of this book. I am sure that the approach she has taken will prove to be a real inspiration for anyone wanting to learn more about a tradition that has only become popular worldwide very recently.

Traditional Thai massage, or Thai yoga massage as it is often called, is a unique and powerful massage therapy. It combines acupressure, energy balancing, stretching and applied yoga exercises. As well as improving flexibility, relaxation and energy levels, a Thai massage can relieve headaches, asthma, constipation and frozen shoulder, improve flexibility for those who enjoy sports, help recovery after a heart attack or stroke, and provide exercise for the disabled – to mention only a few possibilities.

Below and opposite Givers of Thai massage need to learn to work with both sensitivity and grace, to enable their partners to open up their bodies freely and completely.

Asokananda

Born Harald Brust, in Germany, Asokananda was arguably the leading Western teacher of Traditional Thai Yoga Massage. He researched and taught Thai massage, yoga and *vipassana* meditation for over 15 years and personally trained and authorized some of the most established teachers of Thai massage currently practising in the West. After 1978, Asokananda spent most of his time in Asia, studying meditation, yoga and Thai massage with a succession of masters. He also spent some time as a Buddhist monk in Sri Lanka.

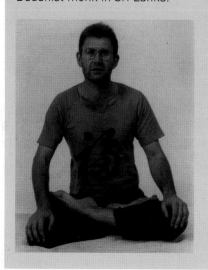

Left Asokananda, author of this foreword and leading teacher of Thai massage (1958–2005).

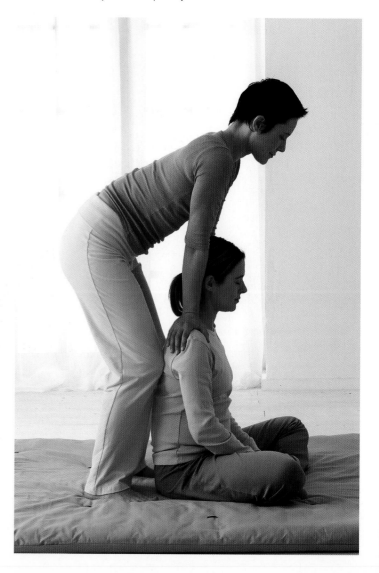

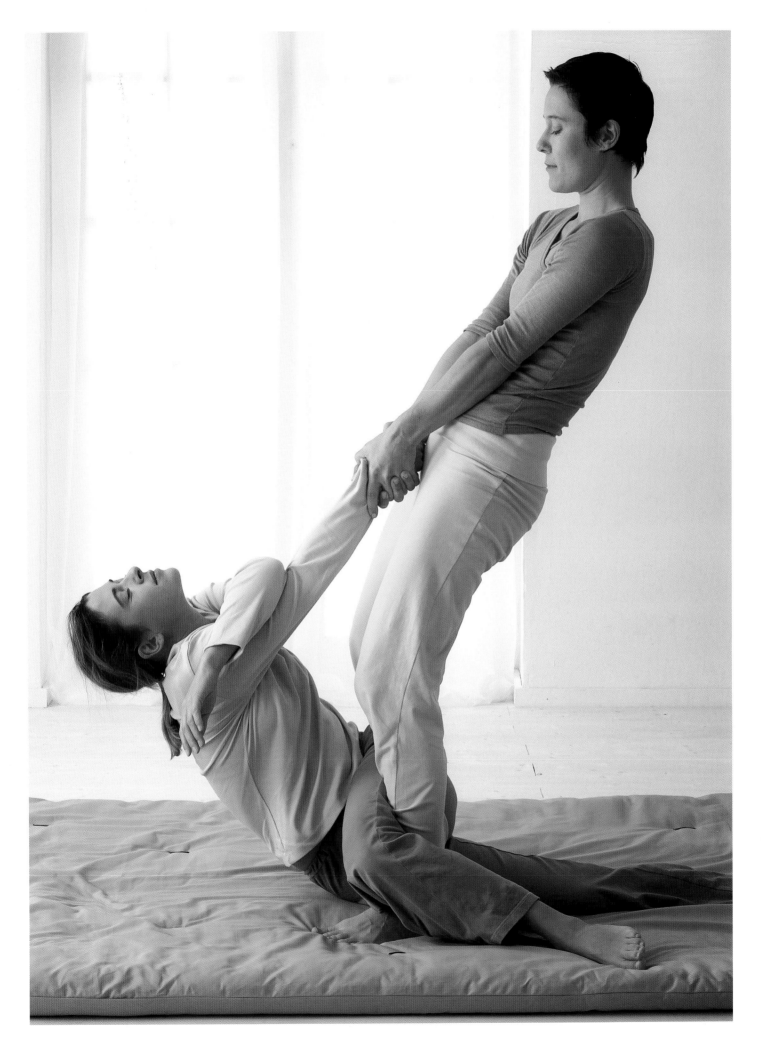

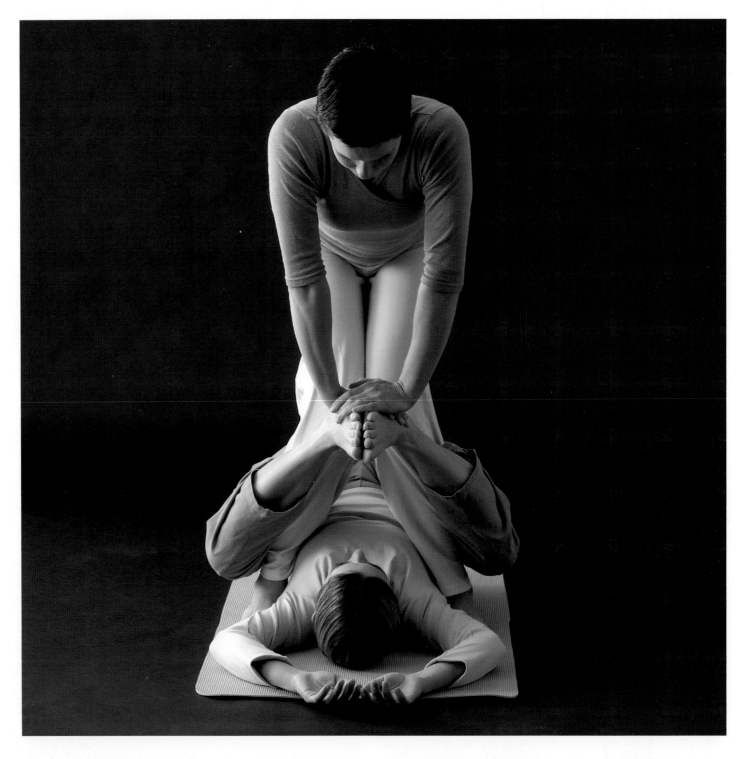

Above It is extremely important that the giver and receiver of a Thai massage treatment maintain good communication throughout, especially during the deeper stretches.

Thai massage therapists work with everyone from performance athletes to office workers and those seeking to find greater calm and improve their energy levels. In offering relief for such a wide range of current health issues, this art is as useful and valid for our age as it has been for thousands of years. I am convinced that the current increase in popularity of Thai yoga massage will continue with more and more people experiencing the balancing benefits of a whole body Thai massage.

THE PERFECT GROUNDING

With growing popularity will come an increasing need for quality training, and the section on Thai massage that follows is the perfect guide. It offers a detailed outline of everything you will need to get started and to find your way into the heart and spirit of the art. Nicky follows the traditional structure, doesn't alter principles in order to "Westernize", and finds a language that is easy for anyone to follow. The instructions are both thorough and clear. Thai massage has found a dedicated advocate in Nicky Smith and her comprehensive guide is a testimony to her love for this fascinating branch of Ayurvedic bodywork.

Shiatsu: an introduction by Saul Goodman

Since its introduction to the Western world in the 1950s, Shiatsu has become widely recognized as one of the most effective body, mind and spirit therapies. The name comes from *shi*, meaning finger, and *atsu*, meaning pressure. Shiatsu has its roots in the traditions of China and Japan and it incorporates the principles of traditional Eastern medicine and the deeper concepts of chi – the life force.

Shiatsu is recognized by many doctors throughout the world as an effective treatment for various ailments. It is widely used in pre- and post-surgical care, and for pain and physical relief in serious illness and trauma. Trials are also in progress to ascertain the benefits to long-term health conditions, such as arthritis, migraine and digestive problems.

Many psychologists see Shiatsu as an indispensable component in the treatment of emotional and behavioural problems. Shiatsu's growing therapeutic reputation has attracted many people with conditions varying from physical ailments to emotional and psychological difficulties.

Shiatsu has demonstrated more than just a strong therapeutic quality. It has repeatedly shown an enigmatic ability to bring people of all backgrounds together over positive common interests such as growth, well-being and harmony. In the last 25 years a global network of practitioners has organically formed, and is now reaching out throughout the whole world. This network has become a motivating voice in the pursuit of healthy and balanced living

Below Shiatsu practitioners throughout the world follow the same course of assessment, diagnosis and treatment.

Saul's biography

The Shiatsu specialist Saul Goodman is the founder and director of the International School of Shiatsu, a group of independent Shiatsu schools located in the United States, Switzerland, Italy, Austria, Belgium, Germany, Spain, Portugal and Croatia. He has been practising and teaching Shiatsu and bodywork since 1977.

Saul's unique style of teaching blends the experience of energetics with Western physiology and science. He has inspired many people throughout the world to discover the benefits of practising Shiastu. His first book, *The Book of Shiatsu*, was published in 1986. His other books include

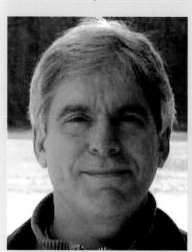

Shiatsu/Shin Tai exploring a form of bodywork known as Shin Tai, *Life Force Recovery*, and *Light Body Activation*. He is based near Philadelphia in the USA.

Left Saul Goodman is an international Shiatsu teacher widely recognized for his inspirational teaching methods.

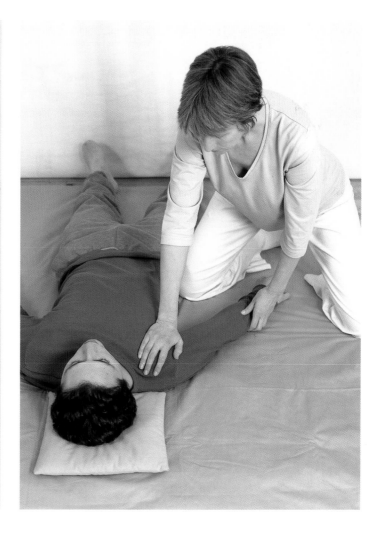

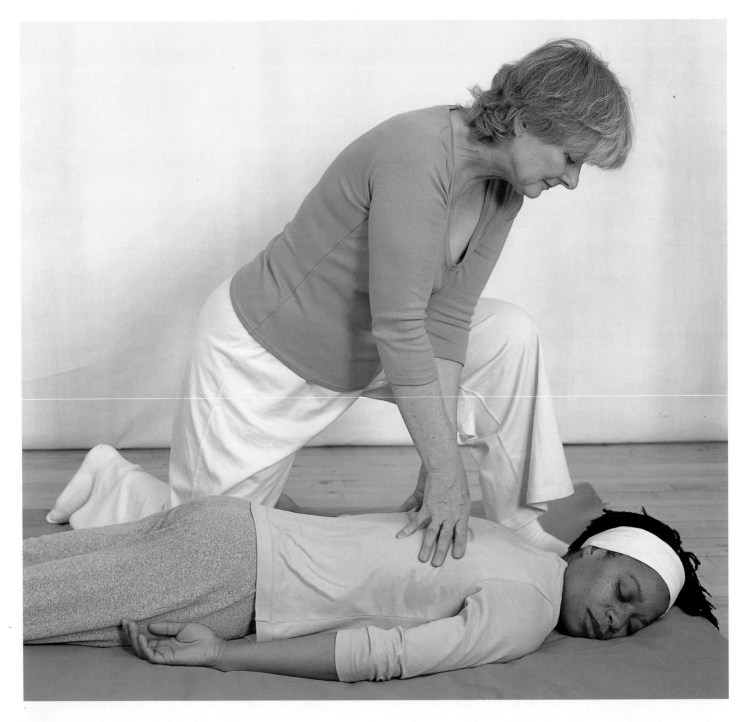

Above and opposite Shiatsu relaxes the body and mind and attempts to unlock and bring into balance the energies of the body, encouraging harmony, good health and well-being.

for individuals, families and organizations. Shiatsu has now become a cornerstone of expanding awareness, influencing positive cultural change for the future.

In recent years, due to licensing and professional scrutiny, a large number of Shiatsu practitioners have moved in a more technical and conceptual direction. This is an important factor in creating an interface with the medical and public healthcare communities.

At the same time, no matter how much is explained and analysed intellectually about Shiatsu, the real power of this work lies in its original simplicity. Essentially, this is the

hand, as an extension of the heart, touching another person with care and empathy. This interaction has an almost magical ability to restore a sense of well-being, no matter what the explanation about how and why it works.

This guide, written by one of my oldest Shiatsu friends, Hilary Totah, gives a fresh and clear perspective about the foundation and practice of Shiatsu. It maintains a strong connection to Shiatsu's essential simplicity. It is a great beginning for aspiring students, and a good reference for practitioners and teachers. It is written by a person who has a great deal of life experience as a mother, Shiatsu practitioner, school director and author.

Hilary has persistently strived to give her skills generously to the world around her and through this guide she makes another valuable contribution.

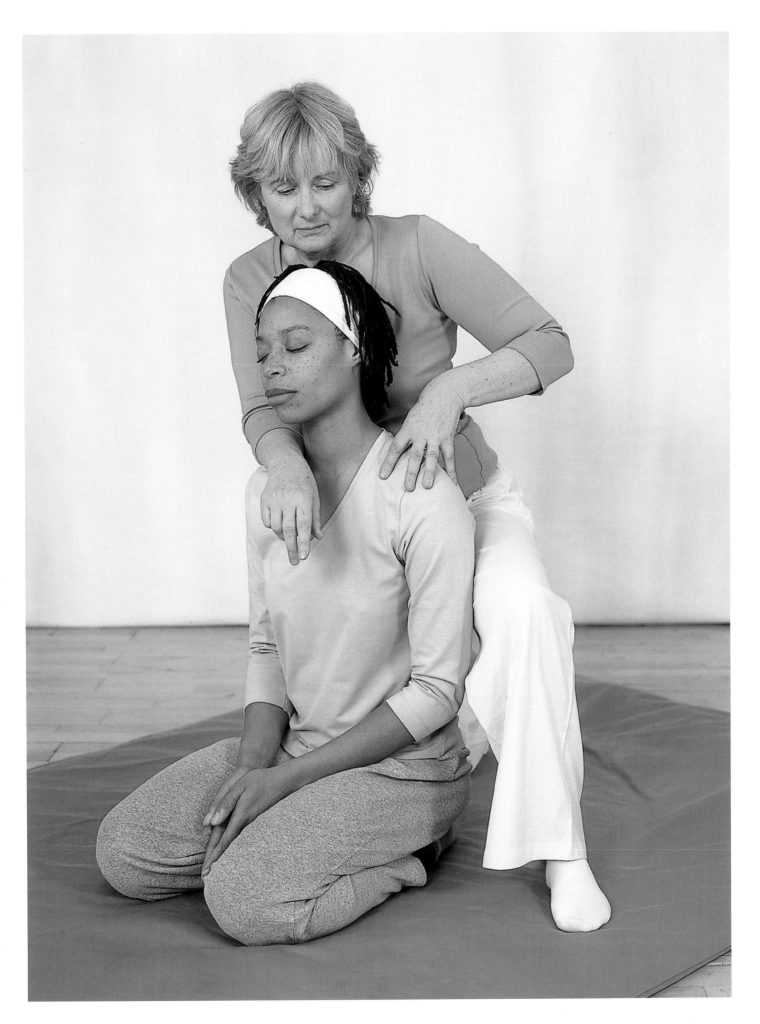

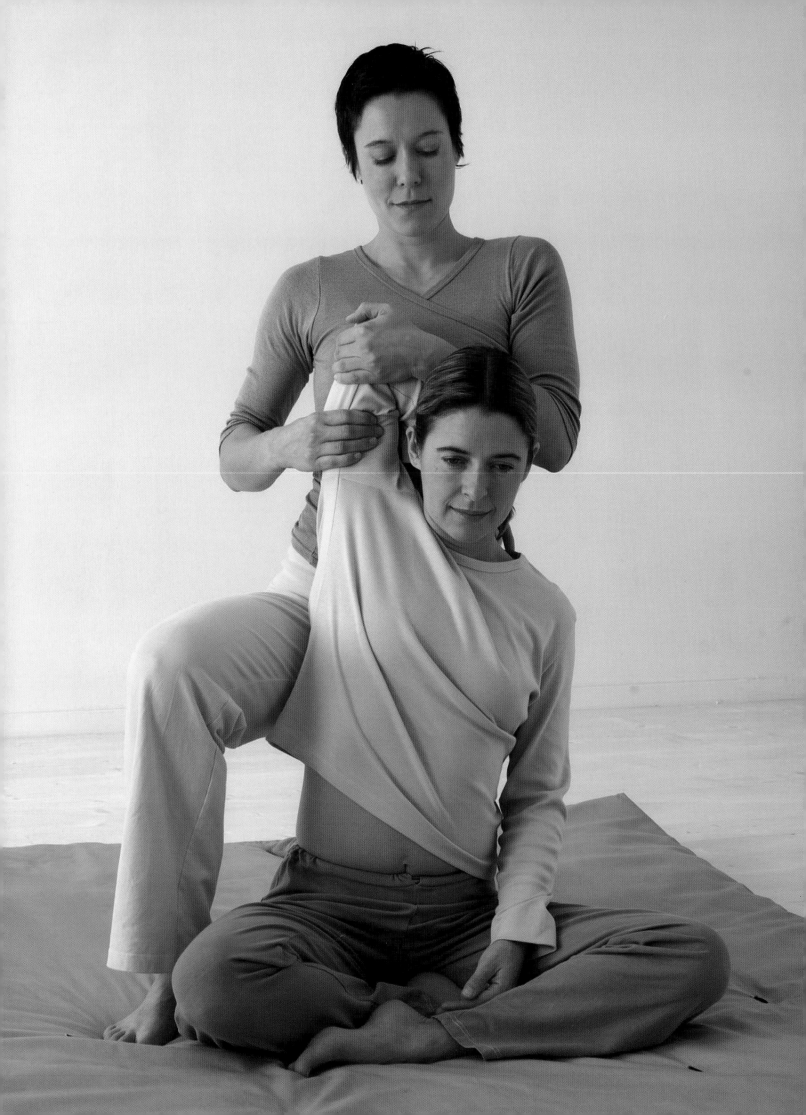

Thai Massage

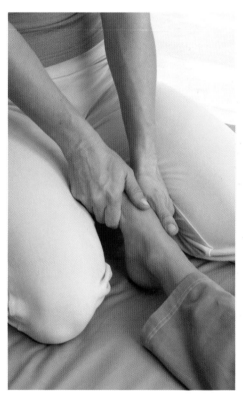
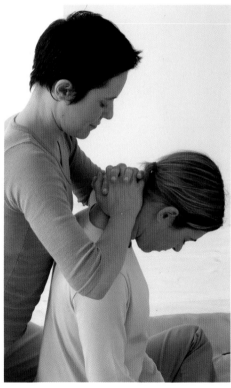
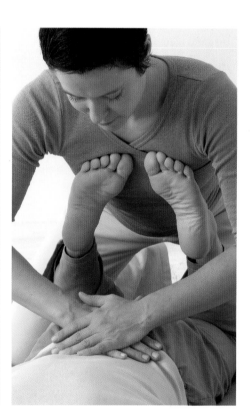

What is Thai Massage?

Traditional Thai massage, also known in the West as Thai massage or Thai yoga massage, is a powerful form of energy rebalancing and physical massage. A fusion of Buddhist spiritual practice and Indian Ayurvedic bodywork, it combines hatha yoga techniques and the spiritual commitment of working with "loving kindness". Working intuitively and without judgement in this way supports our body's natural inclination to heal itself.

Thai massage has been practised widely across what is now known as Thailand for several hundred years, exchanged among family members as a healing art. Only relatively recently has it become known in the West, where people are now discovering its ability to rebalance body and mind on many different levels, harmonizing the physical, the energetic and the emotional bodies to give the recipient a truly holistic treatment.

This is intended as an introduction to the joy and art of traditional Thai massage. You will find practical guidance on everything from preparing to give a massage with yoga and meditation, through a step-by-step breakdown of specific techniques for a full-body massage, to taking care of yourself and your partner after a massage. This has been written as a guide to help get you started, but the essence, the quality and the art of the massage will come from you, from your dedication to practise with an open heart and with sensitivity towards your partner. Once you have become familiar with the physical exercises in each sequence you can begin to shift your focus, massaging less from your head and more from your heart, surrendering yourself, more and more, to simply being present in the moment.

DISCOVERING THAI MASSAGE

My introduction to Thai massage came many years ago, when I received a treatment from a friend. I was highly impressed by the completeness of the massage, and it touched me in a way that I had not previously experienced with other forms of bodywork.

My first opportunity to find out more about this fascinating form of massage came totally out of the blue, with a last-minute trip to Thailand. I went to study with Asokananda, a German man who was living in a small tribal community in the north of Thailand and teaching northern-style Thai massage. I had repeatedly come across Asokananda in several other contexts in my life, and was intrigued by these recurring personal connections and by my new discovery of the delights of Thai massage. So, when the opportunity to learn more presented itself, I took it without hesitation.

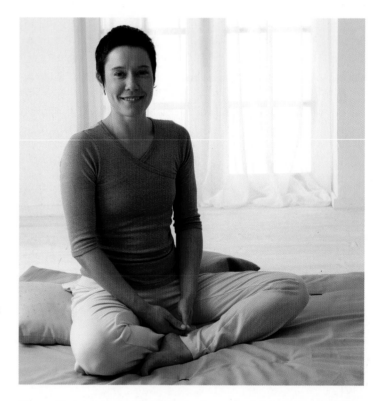

Above Thai massage has been a gift in my life and writing this guide has given me the opportunity to pass on this gift to others.

I already had an interest in bodywork through physical theatre, performance art and Western massage. But learning Thai massage started me on a deeper journey with myself, introducing me to meditation and a committed yoga practice, and setting me on a path of self-enquiry. My initial two-week trip extended into many months of study, exploring the world of Thai massage. Over the years I served a kind of apprenticeship, living in a Lahu hill tribe village and in Chiang Mai for several months at a time.

I feel personally that Thai massage connects me with my body. Its physical and dynamic nature opens my eyes to hidden parts of myself. Through both the giving and the receiving I learn about my own and other people's bodies. Its underlying spiritual principle of working with loving kindness also affords me the opportunity of accepting myself more fully and with greater compassion. The hands-on approach of Thai massage allows it to be absorbed bodily rather than mentally, encouraging a sense of feeling and "listening" through the hands, and it offers a wonderful breadth of techniques to suit all body types and abilities.

I feel blessed to have been able to incorporate the richness of Thai massage into my life, integrating its elements not only into my massage practice as a therapist and teacher but also into aspects of my everyday life.

HOW TO USE THIS SECTION

The first chapter in this section, *The Beginnings*, provides useful background and history, while the following chapter, *Preparing Body and Mind*, leads you through a variety of mental and physical practices that will lay the foundations for giving a good Thai massage. The third chapter, *A Complete Body Routine*, is the largest chapter. It takes you step by step through how to give a full-body massage, illustrating a

Below The teacher-student relationship is a crucial one. Take your time trying out different teachers, and trust that your intuition will lead you to the right teacher when you are ready.

balance of Thai massage techniques for you to practise and share with your friends or family. The routine is broken down into sequences for each part of the body, showing how to open up your partner's (the recipient's) body gradually, resulting in a well-balanced treatment. It is worth mentioning here that the techniques and the sequence shown in this chapter represent only one way of working within this incredibly broad and varied tradition. The next chapter, *After a Massage*, gives useful and effective grounding and relaxation techniques – what you do afterwards is just as vital as good preparation if you are going to look after yourself properly.

The section on Thai massage in this book is not intended as a substitute for hands-on teaching. If you are serious about wanting to learn, I hope it will inspire you to explore further under the guidance of an experienced teacher. If you are already a student of Thai massage, I hope it provides a stimulating addition to your practice. There are many excellent teachers and it is not necessary to go to Thailand to learn traditional Thai massage. What is important is that your teacher's approach should resonate with you. Try out different teachers by attending workshops and receiving massage.

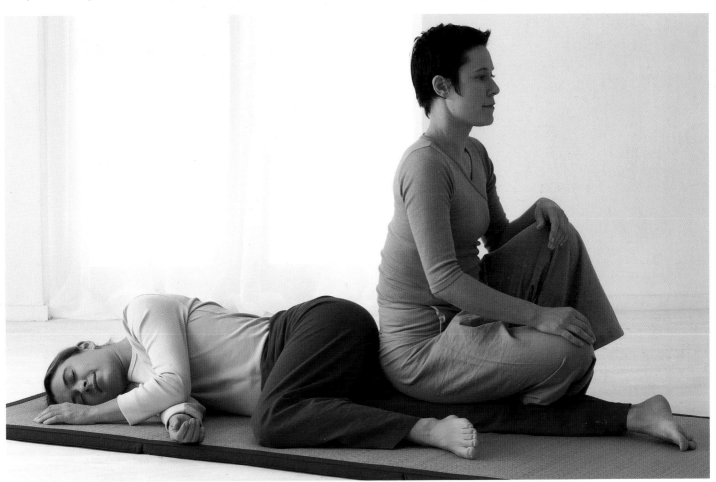

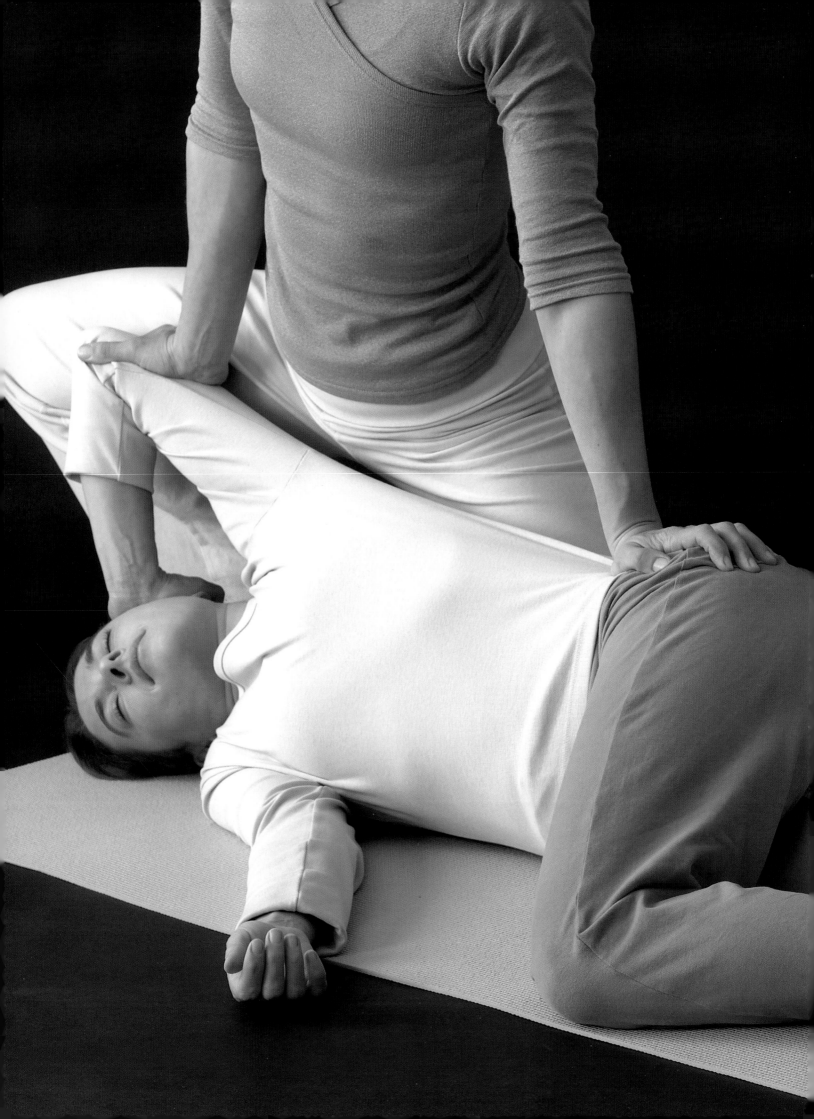

The Beginnings

Traditional Thai Massage, Thai Yoga Massage or Thai Massage are all different labels to describe a highly physical, hands-on branch of traditional Thai medicine. Other branches include the use of herbs or steam baths.

Learning a little about the origins of and history behind this form of bodywork, and about some of the underlying theories and practices, will start the process of understanding this extraordinarily simple, yet profoundly effective, healing art form.

The History of Thai Massage

Traditional Thai massage has its roots in India, in the Indian yoga tradition and in Buddhism. The practices that grew into Thai massage travelled to what we now call Thailand from India over 2,000 years ago. They were brought by Indian Buddhist monks and Ayurvedic practitioners who had been invited to northern Thailand by the Mon rulers of that region. Thai massage has been a part of traditional Thai medicine ever since.

In massage schools and practices right across modern-day Thailand, it is a man called Jivaka Kumar Bhaccha who is revered and honoured as the father of traditional Thai medicine. His name appears in ancient Buddhist scriptures as he was a physician to the Buddha himself, and to the spiritual community, around 2,500 years ago. Consequently, Jivaka Kumar Bhaccha became closely associated with what is now known as traditional Thai massage. In Thailand today, practitioners still offer up a prayer to him in thanks before they give each massage.

Detailed knowledge about the ways in which the practice of Thai massage developed over the centuries is limited, as most of the historical texts dealing with its theoretical background

were destroyed by a Burmese invasion of the old capital, Ayuthia, in 1767. However, some remnants of these texts did survive – and they form the basis for carvings that can be seen today on the walls of the Phra Chetuphon Temple (known as Wat Pho) in Bangkok.

PAST AND PRESENT PRACTICES

In most parts of Thailand, the practice and developing knowledge of Thai medicine and Thai massage was and still is passed directly from teacher to student, leading to a

Below These Buddha statues, from around the 1200s, are found at the ancient city of Satchanalai, in northern Thailand.

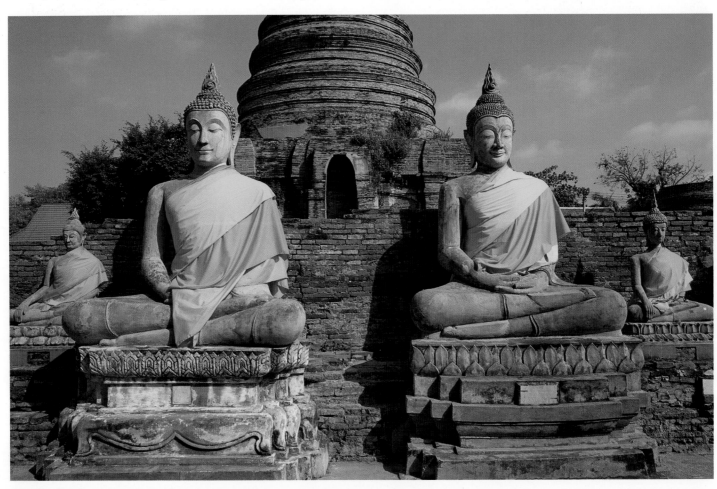

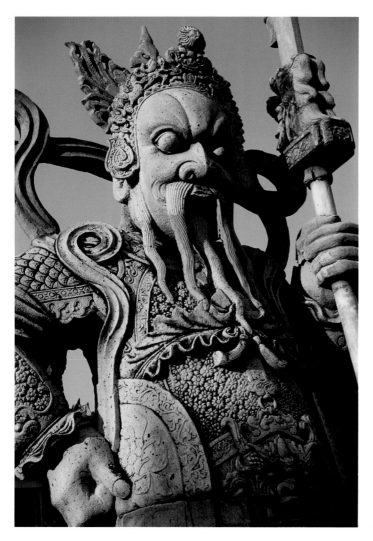

Northern-style Thai massage

There are two quite distinct styles of traditional massage that are practised in Thailand today: northern style and southern style. Both approaches adhere to similar principles, but their emphasis is slightly different. The methods described throughout this section broadly follow the tradition of northern-style Thai massage. This developed among the farming communities that lived in the hills of northern Thailand, and so the massage methods physically reflect their way of life by placing a particular emphasis on leg work and on dynamic stretches.

Left This 16th-century stone figure is a guardian statue at the temple of Wat Pho in Bangkok. Inside this temple lie carvings that tell us something of the early history of this healing art.

Below Today, traditional Thai massage is offered all over the country. Receiving this kind of massage in Thailand is a profoundly invigorating experience. The practitioners' relaxed manner and matter-of-fact approach to bodywork comes across very strongly.

wonderfully broad and eclectic approach to this ancient art. Traditionally, Thai massage was practised within temple compounds – not by monks, but by ordinary people who happily offered their healing arts to the community.

In modern-day Thailand, temples continue to function as the centre of the community, as a place where people come together and enjoy all kinds of social gatherings. Among Thai people, massage is still seen as a form of hands-on healing and therapeutic touch that is an everyday part of a normal and healthy life.

HEALTHY RESURGENCE

For many years, as Thailand began to open up to increased tourism, the only understanding that many Westerners had of "Thai massage" was in the context of the tourism and sex industries. However, over the last 15–20 years this rather sordid image has been shed and traditional Thai massage has enjoyed a serious resurgence within the country's mainstream culture. This revival was helped by Westerners, who were intrigued by Thai massage's unique combination of spiritual practice and physical therapy. As is the case with therapies in any country, there are still poorly trained masseurs who aim their services at the tourist trade, but if you avoid these you can now enjoy an excellent standard of traditional massage throughout Thailand.

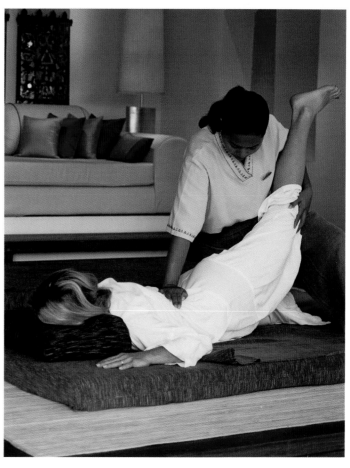

The Practice of Thai Massage

According to the Eastern philosophy underlying Thai massage, the body is made up of an interconnecting web of energy lines through which *prana*, or life energy, flows. This is the force that supports and maintains all the vital functions of the body. It permeates all life and sustains all living things. It is in the air that we breathe and the food that we eat. When this energy flows freely we enjoy good mental, physical and spiritual health.

If the energy lines become blocked and the flow of prana is interrupted, it causes disruption and imbalance throughout the system. So in Thai massage, practitioners stimulate the energy lines by using pressure and passive stretches to maintain a free flow of energy through the whole body.

THE ENERGY SYSTEM

Like yoga, Thai massage is based on the concept of a human being consisting of more than just their physical body. According to the Indian yoga tradition, we are made up of five different bodies, or *koshas*. These are the physical body (*anamaya kosha*), the prana or energy body (*pranamaya*

kosha), the memory body (*manamaya kosha*), the subconscious body (*vijnanamaya kosha*) and the all-encompassing cosmic body (*anandamaya kosha*), within which all the koshas are interconnected. This concept can be useful to embrace as a metaphor with which to appreciate the many layers of physical, mental and emotional experience within us.

It is the pranamaya kosha, the energy body, that we work with primarily in Thai massage and yoga. In the pranamaya kosha, yoga philosophy perceives many thousands of *nadis*, or energy lines. Thai massage has selected ten of these lines, called *sen*, which are all worked on during a treatment to rebalance the energy flow within the whole body.

THE NADIS AND CHAKRAS OF YOGA

Thai massage has strong links with yoga, not least in the yogic energy lines called nadis and the yogic energy centres known as chakras.

The links between the sen and the nadis are evident in the names of the three main nadis: *sushumna nadi* in yoga corresponds directly with *sen sumana*, and *ida nadi* and *pingala nadi* with *sen ittha* and *pingkhala*. Sushumna nadi runs through the spine; the other two run from each nostril down either side of the spine.

Chakras are energy centres located along the spine and up to the brow. Eastern treatments such as yoga and Thai massage aim to activate these, or their equivalents, in various ways.

—— Pingala nadi stands for the sun's awakening power

—— Sushumna nadi is the most important of the nadis

—— Ida nadi stands for the relaxing energy of the moon

● The crown chakra (*sahasrara*) is related to spiritual understanding

● The brow chakra (*ajna*), also known as the third eye, is related to intuition

● The throat chakra (*vishuddha*) is related to communication

● The heart chakra (*anahata*) is the centre of compassion and all-embracing love

● The solar plexus chakra (*manipura*) is the energetic centre for all bodily activities

● The sacral chakra (*swadisthana*) is the centre of unconsciousness and of sexual desire

● The base chakra (*muladhara*) relates to our fundamental survival needs

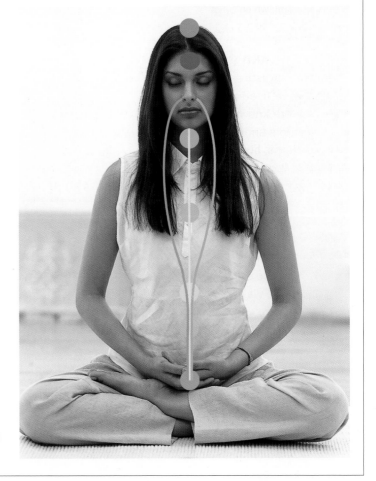

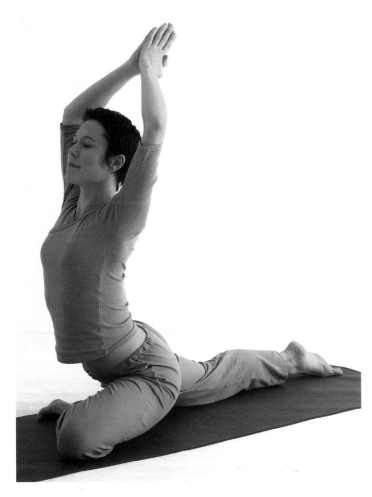

Above Both yoga (seen here) and Thai massage stimulate and open the spinal column, which is not only home to the nervous system that supplies the whole body but is also its energetic centre.

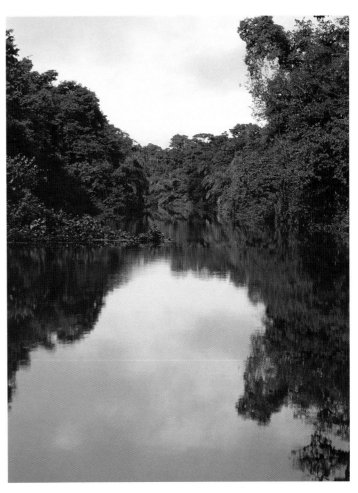

Above The body's energy flows just like water. If its pathways are kept clear, the energy can run freely, and this helps to maintain optimum physical and mental health.

THAI MASSAGE AND YOGA

Other healing practices, such as Chinese medicine and Japanese shiatsu, also view the body as a map of energy lines, which are known as meridians. There are many crossover points and areas of common ground among the Eastern systems, but Thai massage is more closely linked to the Indian yoga tradition. We can see quite strongly the links between yoga and Thai massage as it is practised today. It is often referred to as Thai yoga massage, highlighting the use of applied and passive hatha yoga stretches that give the massage its dynamic flow.

People often ask why Thai massage involves such a physically dynamic workout if it is a form of energy rebalancing. One way of looking at this is to understand that we manifest energy physically in the form of bones, muscle, skin and so on. So, the physical body can be seen as a point of access through which we are able to contact the more subtle aspects of the self. When we open the body with passive yoga stretches we feel it physically but, as in a yoga practice, the intention is ultimately to stimulate the energy flow within the body. This principle is important to remember – it is a reminder that Thai massage is not based upon the anatomical system that is understood in the West, but has its own logic and methodology.

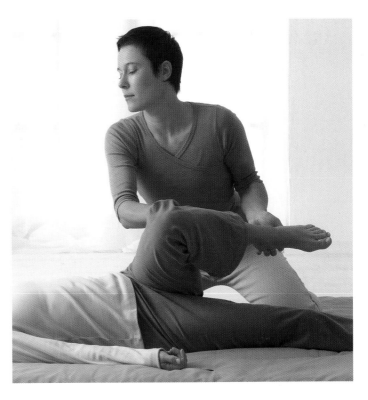

Above Energy is easily trapped in the joints; the constant, repeated movements of the body in Thai massage help to release deeply held tension in under-worked joints such as the hips.

The Sen

The practice of traditional Thai massage works on the sen, or energy lines, to keep the body in healthy balance. The sen, like the nadis of the yoga tradition, form a kind of map of the body that illustrates the subtle concept of the movement of energy within us. The sen lines sit neither inside nor on the body; they cannot be seen but only felt – as a subtle difference in the quality of the body.

When you are working the energy lines on your partner you may at times sense a kind of denseness, a feeling of something different from your own hands, a tingling or heat, a fullness or an emptiness. These kinds of sensation are extremely difficult to put into words, but you will know when you feel them. In order to give a good massage you don't have to understand such feelings; you should simply be open to experiencing them with your hands, and allow yourself to be guided by them.

The ten sen are always worked as an interconnecting unit. They do have their own individual strengths but as a general rule you would not select one line to work separately. Instead, you work all the energy lines throughout the body to create a feeling of balance. In the beginning it is not necessary to remember the functioning and exact therapeutic role of each line in order to give sensitive and relaxing massage. It can be useful to familiarize yourself with maps of the sen, but don't become so preoccupied with them that you forget to enjoy the scenery.

THE SEN AND THEIR FUNCTIONS

The diagrams featured on the following few pages indicate where the sen flow through the body. Though all ten lines are normally worked during Thai massage, each has a different therapeutic value and more experienced practitioners may place an emphasis on particular lines to achieve certain results.

Sen sumana

This line runs through the centre of the body. It supports the source of life – the breathing mechanism – affecting conditions such as asthma, bronchitis, coughs and colds.

Sen ittha and sen pingkhala

These are two aspects of the same line – the main treatment lines for problems with the internal organs. Sen ittha runs through the left side of the body; sen pingkhala runs through the right side. They are used therapeutically for abdominal pains, intestinal and digestive problems and diseases, diseases of the urinary tract and back pain.

Sen kalathari

This line criss-crosses the whole body, and its potency comes from this crossover effect. As it runs from left to right and from right to left, it joins the feminine and masculine elements within the body.

Sen kalathari supports or encourages emotional release, depending on how deeply and repeatedly it is worked. Stress is often related to the emotions, so it is good for tension headaches, sciatica and high blood pressure.

Sen sahatsarangsi and sen thawari

These two lines are simply different aspects of the same line. Sen sahatsarangsi runs down the left-hand side of the body and sen thawari down the right-hand side of the body. Working both these lines is especially effective for the treatment of knee pain.

Sen lawusang and sen ulangka

These are also two different aspects of the same line. Sen lawusang runs down the left side of the head and chest, and sen ulangka down the right side. Their main therapeutic use is for deafness and ear infections.

Sen nanthakrawat and sen khitchana

Both of these lines are part of sen sumana. Sen nanthakrawat splits into two: one aspect runs from the navel down through the urethra, while the other aspect runs from the navel down to the anus. Sen khitchana runs from the navel down through the vagina or penis.

In practical terms, both of these lines are accessed by working the abdomen from the navel down to the pubic bone. Their main areas of treatment are urinary problems, menstruation problems, infertility and impotence.

Right This artwork shows, in detail, the paths of the sen across the front of the body. Study this and the artworks over the next couple of pages to build up a picture of how these energy lines travel around the body, and where they interconnect and diverge. Notice also the places where certain pressure points lie on particular sen lines.

THE FRONT OF THE BODY

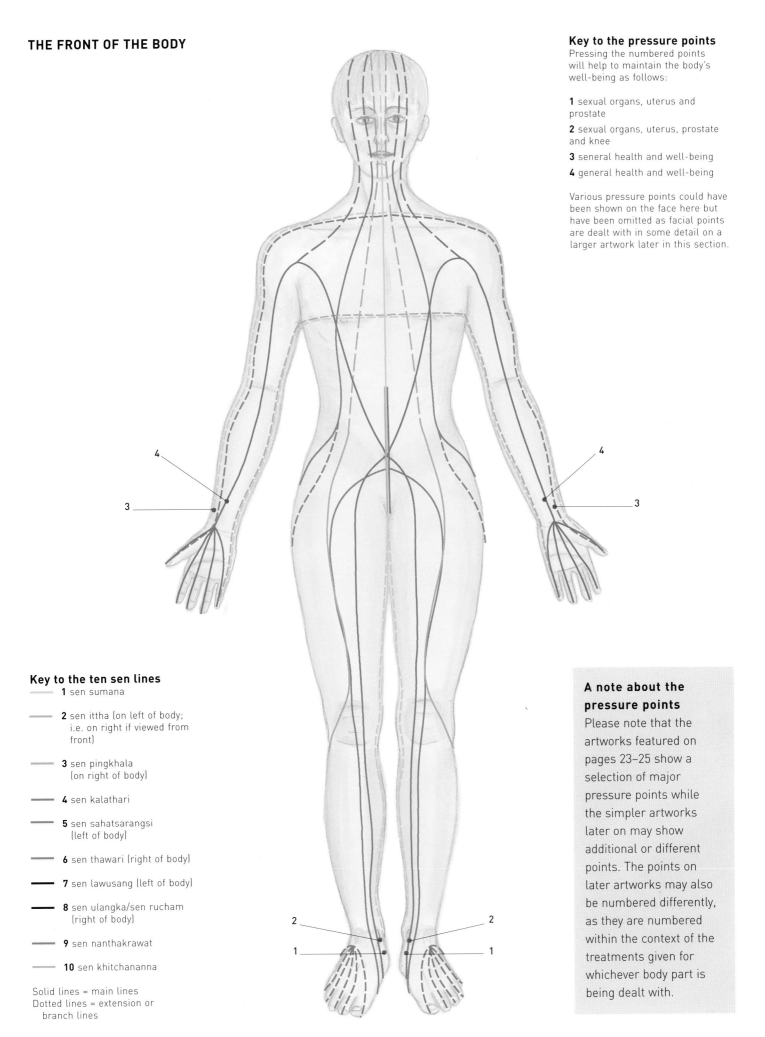

Pressing the numbered points will help to maintain the body's well-being as follows:

1 sexual organs, uterus and prostate

2 sexual organs, uterus, prostate and knee

3 seneral health and well-being

4 general health and well-being

Various pressure points could have been shown on the face here but have been omitted as facial points are dealt with in some detail on a larger artwork later in this section.

Key to the ten sen lines

1 sen sumana

2 sen ittha (on left of body; i.e. on right if viewed from front)

3 sen pingkhala (on right of body)

4 sen kalathari

5 sen sahatsarangsi (left of body)

6 sen thawari (right of body)

7 sen lawusang (left of body)

8 sen ulangka/sen rucham (right of body)

9 sen nanthakrawat

10 sen khitchananna

Solid lines = main lines
Dotted lines = extension or branch lines

A note about the pressure points

Please note that the artworks featured on pages 23–25 show a selection of major pressure points while the simpler artworks later on may show additional or different points. The points on later artworks may also be numbered differently, as they are numbered within the context of the treatments given for whichever body part is being dealt with.

THE BACK OF THE BODY

Right This artwork shows the paths of the sen across the back of the body.

For explanatory colour key, see previous artwork

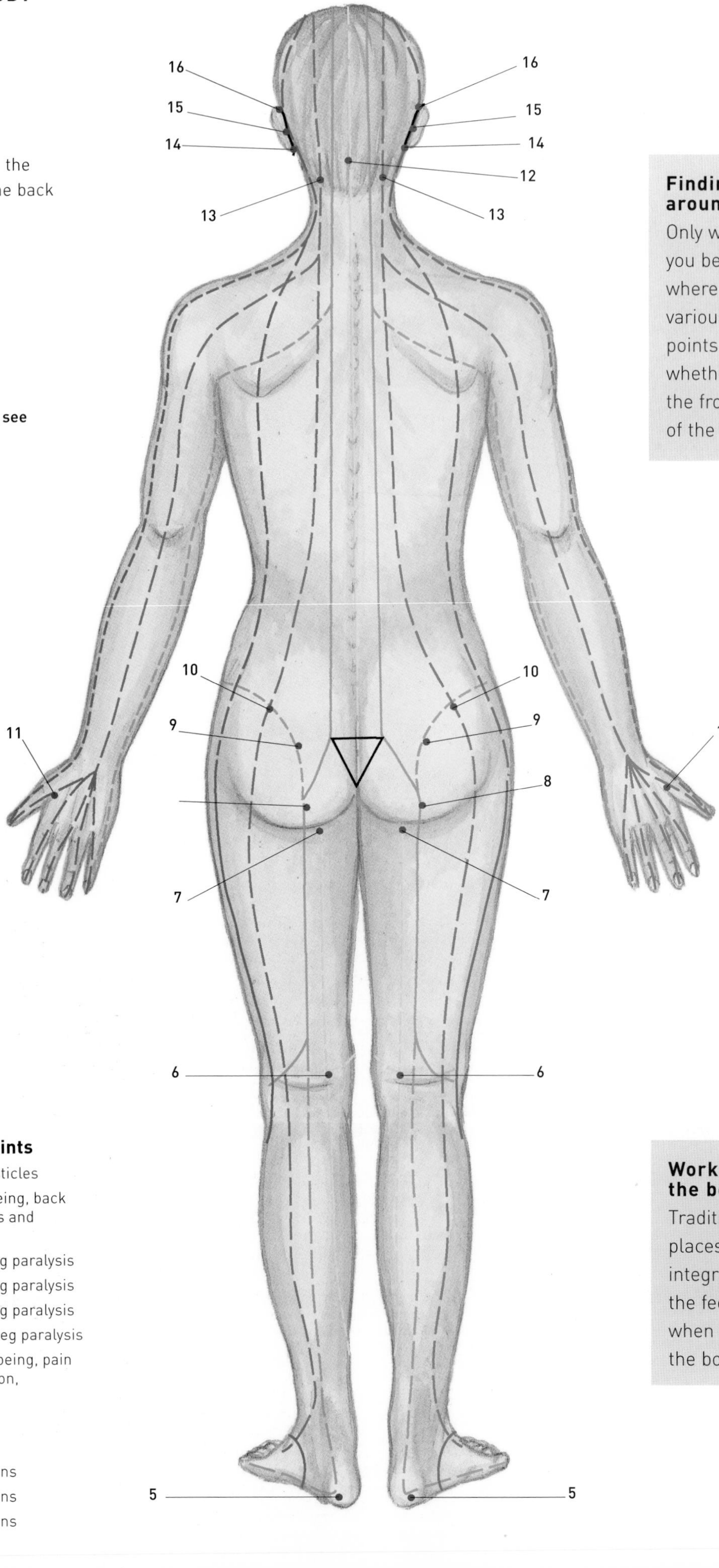

Finding your way around the body

Only with practice can you become familiar with where to locate the various sen and pressure points depending on whether you are working the front, back or side of the body.

Working the back of the body

Traditional Thai massage places emphasis on the integration of the legs, the feet and the back when working the back of the body.

Key to the pressure points

5 sexual organs, ovaries, testicles

6 general health and well-being, back pain, knee pain, leg paralysis and bloated stomach

7 lower back, sciatica and leg paralysis

8 lower back, sciatica and leg paralysis

9 lower back, sciatica and leg paralysis

10 lower back, sciatica and leg paralysis

11 general health and well-being, pain in general, lungs, constipation, tonsillitis, coughs and colds

12 headache and dizziness

13 headache

14 deafness and ear infections

15 deafness and ear infections

16 deafness and ear infections

THE SIDE OF THE BODY

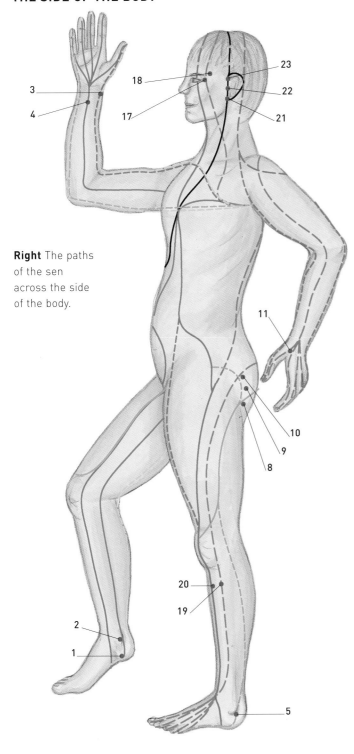

Right The paths of the sen across the side of the body.

THE TOP OF THE HEAD

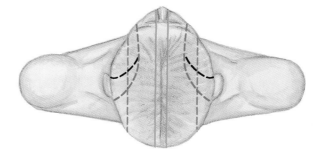

Above The paths of the sen across the top of the head.

THE SOLES OF THE FEET

Key to the pressure points
24 insomnia, foot pain, heart and mental disturbance
25 shock, sunstroke and hypertension

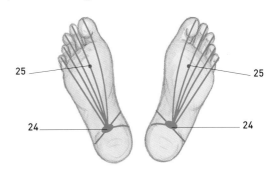

Above The paths of the sen across the soles of the feet.

Key to the pressure points
1 sexual organs, uterus and prostate

2 sexual organs, uterus, prostate and knee

3 general health and well-being

4 general health and well-being

5 sexual organs, ovaries and testicles

8–10 lower back, sciatica and leg paralysis

11 general health and well-being, pain in general, lungs, constipation, tonsillitis, coughs and colds

17 migraine

18 headache

19 general health and well-being, numbness, lower back and leg pain

20 general health and well-being, knee pain and bloated stomach

21–23 deafness and ear infections

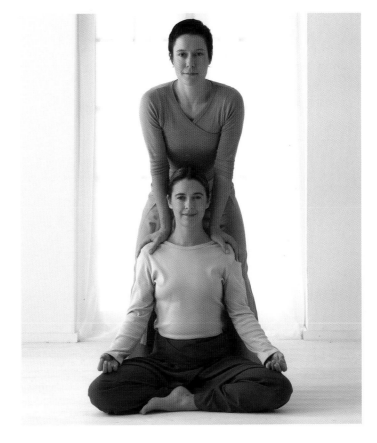

Above It is possible to work the energy lines in Thai massage from a variety of very different positions.

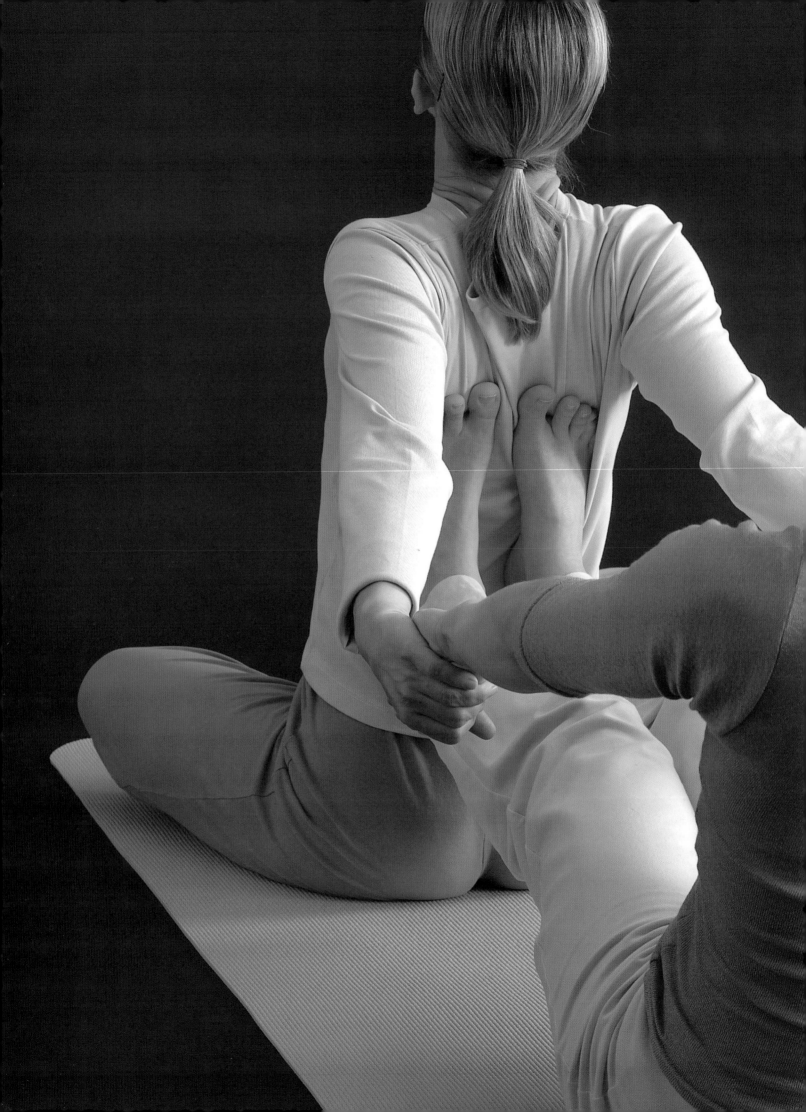

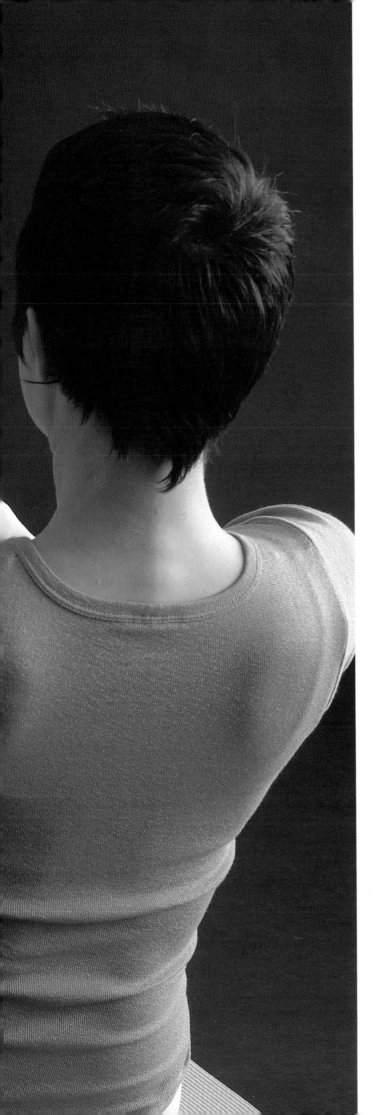

Preparing Body and Mind

In Thai massage the way you work is as important as what you do. As the giver, you need to ensure that the lines of energy are flowing freely in your own body so that you can be an example to your partner, the receiver. It is therefore vital to prepare yourself before giving a massage.

Exercise will make your body supple and flexible so that you can move smoothly through the routine, and a regular meditation practice will help quieten your thoughts, allowing you to approach the massage session in a state of mindfulness and with an open heart. The spiritual roots of Thai massage can be acknowledged by creating a sacred space in which to work.

Preparing Your Body

Thai massage is a physical experience for both the giver and the receiver. It is therefore important to open and prepare your body thoroughly so that you feel physically at ease when giving a massage. Once you begin to feel more comfortable in your own body, the massage you give will be a much more relaxing and enjoyable experience for both you and your partner. The simple but effective exercises shown below have been specially devised to open up the joints of the feet, hands and spine – all vital areas for the giver.

The Feet

Since Thai massage is given on the floor, you need to develop flexibility in your feet in order to feel comfortable in your working postures. Try to do these exercises daily.

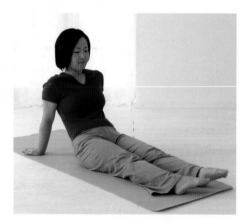

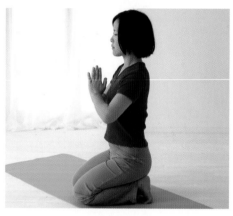

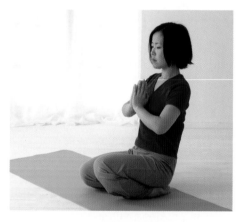

1 Circling the feet This opens and strengthens the ankle and hip joints. Sit as shown. With your feet at least hip-width apart, circle both feet slowly clockwise, and then anticlockwise.

2 Waking up the insteps Kneel down with the knees and feet together. Inhale and kneel up, tucking your toes under. Exhale and sink slowly back on to your heels. Repeat at least three times.

3 Knee lifts This opens the front of the ankles. Kneel down as shown. Lift one knee gently and return it to the floor. Work alternate knees, three times each. If you find this easy, lift both together.

The Hands

You will mostly be using your hands to apply pressure to the energy lines. Use these exercises to release any tension in your hands before or after giving a massage.

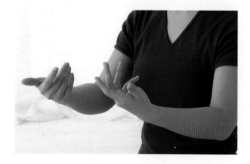

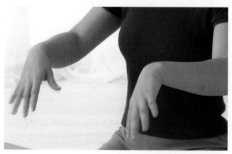

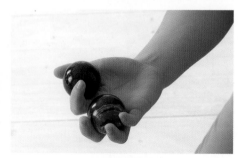

1 Wrist circles Check that your shoulders are relaxed and move your hands through full circles, both clockwise and anticlockwise, to loosen and strengthen the wrists.

2 Shaking the wrists This is a very effective and quick way to release excess tension and energy in the joints of the fingers and the wrists.

3 Strengthening the fingers Help to strengthen the hands and make your finger joints more flexible by rolling a pair of hard balls (ping pong balls are an option) around in your hands.

The Spine

When giving massage, aim to work with a sense of ease and freedom throughout your spine. This keeps you grounded in your own body and aware of your posture. These exercises help to free up the spine, from the pelvis all the way up to the base of the skull.

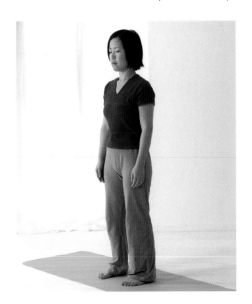

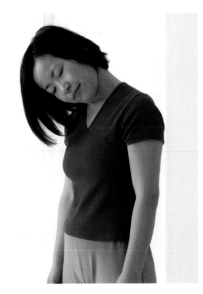

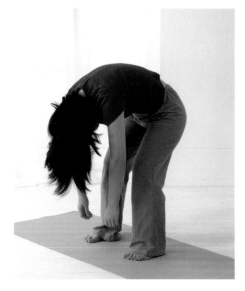

1 Standing Place your feet parallel and hip-width apart. Make sure that your weight is spread evenly throughout each foot – shift the weight until you feel yourself come to rest in the centre. Keep your knees straight but not locked. Let your tailbone drop towards the floor, and the back of your neck become very long. Stand like this for a short while, letting your breath flow freely and easily in and out of your nostrils.

2 Loosening the neck Drop your right ear towards your right shoulder, and let the weight of your head roll forward, keeping your shoulders relaxed back. Continue this soft, slow, rolling movement until the left ear is sinking towards the left shoulder. Repeat this semicircling three times. Do not roll your head back in a complete circle, as this would compromise the delicate spinal vertebrae.

3 Forward fold This provides a release between the spinal vertebrae. Stand with your feet hip-width apart, or slightly wider, with your knees a little bent to give the hips more freedom of movement. Let your forehead drop and feel each vertebra open, from the base of the neck down to the base of the spine. Fold from your hips, not your back. Exhale as you release forward, breathe smoothly and deeply as you fold fully. Roll slowly back to standing.

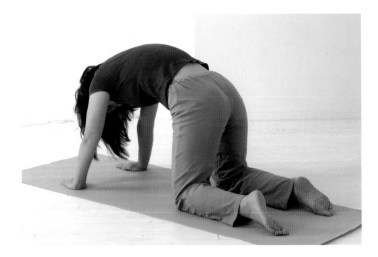

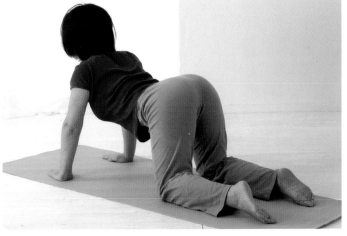

4 Cat tilt The cat and dog tilts bring greater flexibility to the entire spine. As you start to inhale, feel as if you are being drawn up between the shoulder blades, rounding your upper back. Tuck your tailbone under and let your chin move down towards your chest. Look between your legs. Feel your ribcage broaden.

5 Dog tilt As you begin to exhale, feel the whole of your spinal column lengthen. Lengthen your tailbone away from the crown of your head and open through the front of your body, looking up gently. Repeat this wavelike movement slowly and smoothly once or twice, letting your breath guide you.

Tuning into Yourself

The more aware you are of yourself and of exactly how you feel, the more aware you can become of how your partner feels, which in turn will allow you to give a much more sensitive and intuitive massage. Tuning into yourself not only makes you a better masseur, it also helps to keep you grounded in your own body while you are giving a massage. The following exercises show different ways of becoming aware of the more subtle feelings within your body. Try them all and see which ones suit you best. Allow yourself plenty of time to become fully aware of all the feelings and sensations that are arising in your body.

Self-massage

Massaging yourself is a wonderful way to re-energize the body. Notice how your body feels in different areas. Work gently or deeply depending on what feels good for you, but make contact only with the soft fleshy areas of the body; avoid tapping over bone.

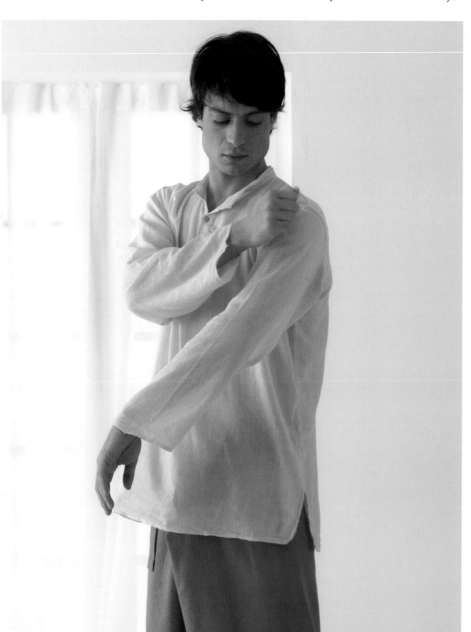

Left Beginning at the inside of your ankles, tap with your fists up the inside of your legs and gently clockwise round the abdomen. Continue up your breastbone and across your chest, and then work down the inside of your arm to the fingertips and up the outside of the arm to the top of the shoulder. Change arms. When you come to the face and head, use your fingertips. To work down your back, bend your knees and bend forward so that you can reach high up between your shoulder blades, using the backs of your hands. Tap either side of your spine. Straighten up and then work down the buttocks and outsides of the legs to finish at your feet.

Hand position
Make a loose fist to contact the body, remembering to keep your wrist soft. The self-massage should be stimulating but not painful.

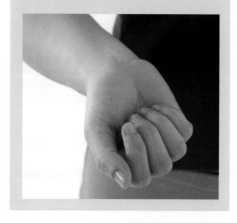

Listening to Your Body

Take time to be still and listen to the sensations in your body – it is surprising how much it will reveal to you. Notice where you feel any aches or pains, which parts feel relaxed and which feel "held", and where you let go and hold on to tension.

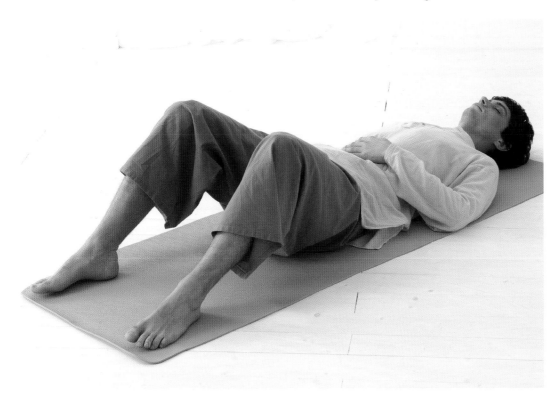

Left Lie comfortably on your back with your knees bent and your feet flat on the floor. Place one hand on your abdomen and feel it rise and fall as your breath flows in and out. Try to breathe through your nostrils. Allow the breath to be as it is – don't be tempted to force or change it in any way. Follow the flow of the breath with your attention, letting the weight of your body relax into the floor.

Prana Egg

This visualization exercise aims to build a protective shield of prana around your body, creating stronger energetic boundaries for yourself before you give a massage. It is especially valuable for beginners, who often take on too much of other people's energy.

Right Lie as shown in the yogic savasana pose (also called corpse or relaxation pose), totally at rest. Close your eyes, observe the rhythm of your breathing and, with your mind's eye, focus on a point a few centimetres below the soles of your feet. As you inhale, imagine drawing your breath up the right side of your body in a half egg shape until you reach a point a few centimetres above the crown of your head. As you exhale, draw the breath down the left side of your body, completing the egg shape at your feet. Continue this cycle of breath at least 12 times, so you become encased in a protective shield of prana. Reinforce it by visualizing a golden light or thread that moves with the breath.

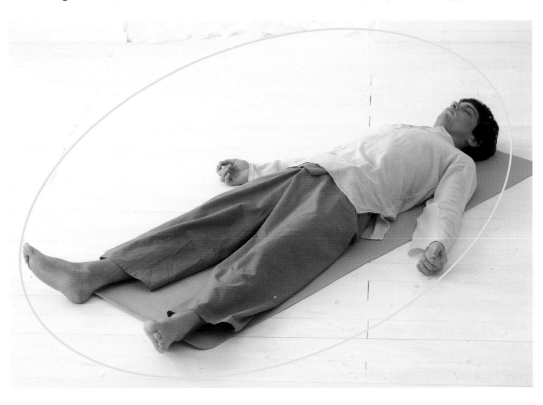

Preparing Your Mind

A good Thai massage is more than just a series of physical stretches and manipulations. Practising your massage in a meditative frame of mind enhances its potential for deeper healing. It is the influence of Buddhist spiritual practice that gives Thai massage its unique spiritual depth. By familiarizing yourself with some of these practices you can start to embody specific mental states so that they become a natural part of your massage work. The practices described below, of observation meditation, *metta* meditation and chanting, help to settle the activity of the mind and open the heart. It is these qualities of stillness and open-heartedness that we can aspire to bring to our practice of Thai massage. There are many different approaches to meditation. It doesn't matter which you choose as each individual needs to find a way that suits them.

Meditation of Mindfulness

This exercise introduces you to the practice of vipassana, or observation meditation.
This practice can be expanded to include an open observation of all sensations in the body
– hearing, smell, thought or touch. But begin here simply, by just observing your breath.

Right Sit comfortably and notice how your breath feels as it passes in and out through your nostrils, then notice how your abdomen feels as it rises and falls with the inhalation and exhalation. If your attention wanders, gently remind it to come back to your breathing. You can begin by sitting for five minutes and then gradually extend your practice for up to an hour.

Below Spiritual practice is an inherent part of daily life in Thailand.

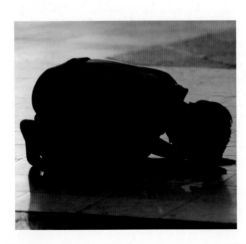

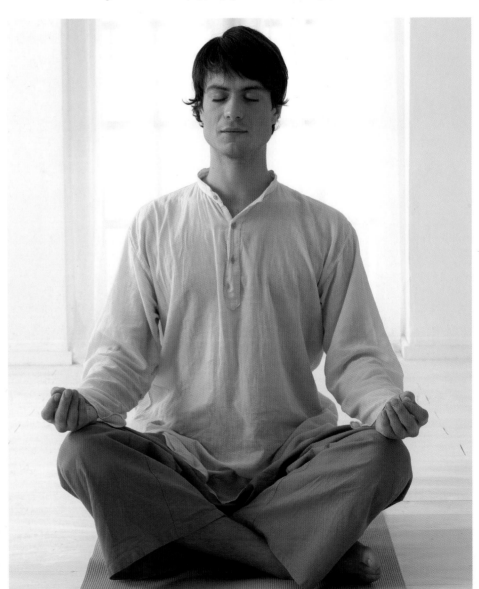

Metta Meditation

Metta is the word, from the ancient Indian Pali language, that means "loving kindness". Cultivating a compassionate and non-judgemental attitude is the foundation of Buddhist spiritual practice and is an important aspect of the spiritual practice of Thai massage.

When we choose to do this meditation of loving kindness it is important that we begin with ourselves. For only by fully accepting who we are, without any judgement, can we begin to extend this feeling out towards others. You can use the simple mantra below as a starting point.

May all beings be happy
May all beings be at peace
May all beings be well

Find a quiet, comfortable place to sit and allow yourself 5–15 minutes. Begin by focusing on yourself; on what you like and what you don't like or find difficult about yourself. You can repeat the mantra above with yourself in mind, focusing on the sensations around your heart centre. Imagine yourself in the role of your closest friend. If they were standing in front of you now, what would they wish for you? What would they say to you in order that you might feel more loving towards yourself? Receive this gift from your friend with an open heart. Once familiar with this practice, we can develop goodwill not just to relatives, friends and colleagues, but to everything around us and eventually the whole of creation.

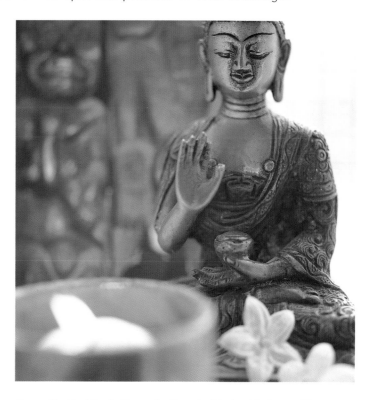

Above The Buddha is the embodiment of loving kindness. The development of loving kindness always begins with ourselves.

Om Mani Padme Hum

Widely used in Tibetan Buddhist practice today, this mantra originated in India and the Sanskrit language. Expressing this mantra evokes the qualities of the Buddha of Compassion.

Om is the sound vibration that is all existence.
Mani is the jewel, a diamond that uses the clarity and precision of wisdom to cut through ignorance.
Padme is the lotus, the symbol of beauty, purity and compassion, that rises and blooms out of the muddy depths of the clouded waters of ignorance.
Hum is the open heart that unifies all with kindness and love.

This lovely mantra or prayer can be very roughly translated as:
"May the jewel of the lotus flower send out a light of love and compassion to unite all existence as one."

It is a beautiful mantra to sing either out loud or in your head just before or even during a massage treatment. It opens up the heart centre and helps to focus your attention on working from your heart more than from your head.

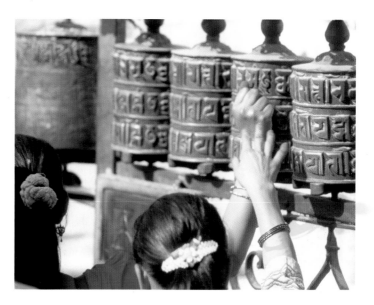

Above Prayer wheels inscribed with the *Om Mani Padme Hum* mantra are commonly used in Tibet and Nepal to ensure that the energy of the mantra is expressed continually throughout the day.

Nurturing Touch

For many people, nurturing touch is, sadly, very far from being an integral part of their everyday lives. Learning to give and to receive massage can be a wonderful way to reintroduce this important aspect of communication and to bring its benefits into your life. In order to give a good massage, you really do need to know what it feels like to receive a good massage. Receiving is always just as important as giving.

Through your sense of touch you feel your body and come to understand it better. Movement is also a way of getting to know the body, and people explore and express the feeling in their bodies in many different ways, such as through dance, yoga, swimming or sport.

Thai massage is movement and nurturing touch combined: as giver and receiver, you and your partner are in constant motion, dancing together. The dynamic quality of the passive yoga stretches makes them beneficial to the stiffest of bodies and helps to wake up those parts that may have been asleep for years.

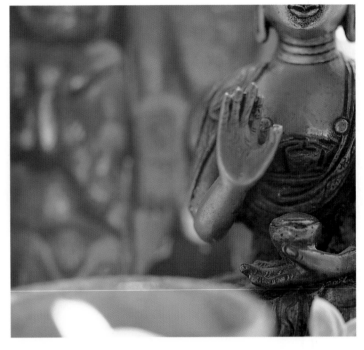

LEARNING THROUGH GIVING AND RECEIVING

Part of the learning process is to know what it feels like to surrender to the flow of the treatment. If you only ever give massage, and never receive it, you can become very unbalanced. A good practitioner is able to receive as well as they can give. It may sound obvious but it is surprising how many massage therapists don't take the time to receive massage and so never fully realize what helps them to relax. If you are a keen student it is recommended that you receive as much massage as you can from different people so that you can familiarize yourself with the feelings of release and letting go that come from a good massage. Your experience will, in turn, help you to facilitate greater relaxation for your massage partner.

Remember that Thai massage should be something that the giver and receiver share, like a conversation between two people. If you learn how to listen more acutely with your hands, it follows that you will develop far greater sensitivity and a more naturally intuitive approach to your massage.

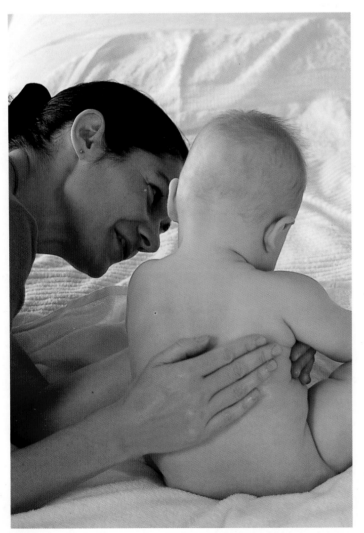

Above The feet are a good place to start giving nurturing touch – most people enjoy a relaxing foot massage.

Left Touch is a natural way for a mother to talk to her child. It is the first form of communication that we learn as babies.

Sticky Hands

This exercise is a playful way to develop your sense of touch. One person leads the other by suggesting a movement with their hand. Try to tune into where your partner wants to go and to move with them, keeping your eyes closed and working by touch alone.

1 (right) Stand facing each other. Place the palm of one hand very gently against your partner's. Your touch should be light but firm, your elbows bent and your shoulders totally relaxed. Close your eyes and feel the connection between the surfaces of your palms. Make sure you are standing with your feet apart and your knees slightly soft, in a stable stance, so that you can be ready to move comfortably and easily in any direction.

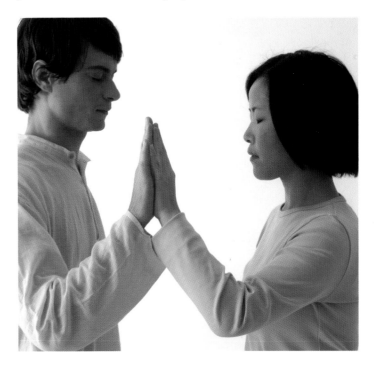

2 (below) Decide which of you is going to take the lead first. Now start to move around, keeping your palms together as you move in order to maintain that close connection with each other. Your movements can be either small or expansive, but you should always try to keep them as smooth as possible.

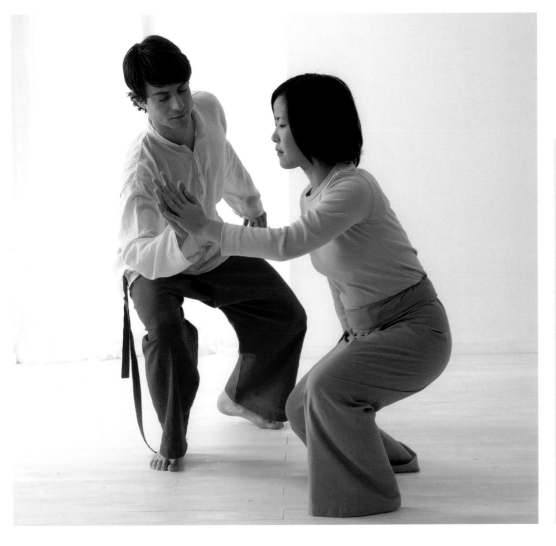

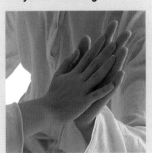

Ways of moving

Always keep your palms together, but softly – do not force it. Also, remember that when you are moving around in this exercise you are not trying to outwit your partner but rather seeing how much you can move together in synchronicity.

Preparing the Space

Setting up the room for Thai massage can be like a ritual, defining the space as somewhere special where you put aside everyday distractions. This preparation encourages a shift in your mindset by creating a place where thoughts quieten, the body slows down and deeper healing can take place.

Apart from the practical necessity of providing a space where your partner will be able to relax, it is important to create the right atmosphere in the room where you are giving the massage. Set up the space exactly as you would like it to be if you were receiving the massage yourself. Make sure that it is quiet and warm, switch off the phone and choose a time when you can ensure that there will be no interruptions.

Right A bed roll, a thick exercise mat, a foam mattress, or even a folded duvet or thick blanket are good alternatives to a proper futon, but any working surface must be padded, firm and non-slip.

Below The ideal equipment includes a futon, cushions and bolsters, foam blocks and a blanket, but you can easily improvise.

Burning a candle is recommended while you give massage. Not only does it provide a lovely soft light for working, but as fire is purifying you can use it as a means of clearing the energy in the room. The burning of incense or oils also has a cleansing and purifying effect on the space and creates a very welcoming and pleasant ambience, as long as the scent is not overpowering.

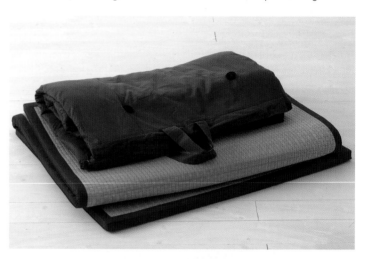

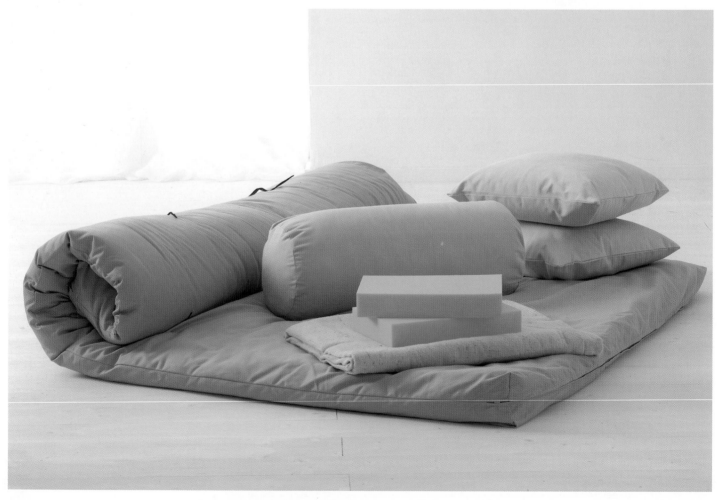

WHAT YOU NEED

Before you start your massage, ensure that you have everything that you will need close at hand. You may already have some of the following items, but if you don't you can always adapt similar everyday items that you own to use for your massage practice.

- **Futon or firm mat** This should preferably be wide enough so that you can kneel on it comfortably at either side of your partner.
- **Cushions or pillows** A couple of firm cushions will provide support for your partner's body.
- **Bolster** This will give additional support under the knees or the fronts of the ankles. Alternatively, you can use a rolled-up blanket.
- **Blanket cover** You may need to cover your partner at some point during the massage – their body temperature will drop as they become more relaxed.

- **Yoga blocks** A couple of foam blocks can be very helpful. They can be used as support either for your own posture or for your partner's, especially in the various seated positions.

WHAT TO WEAR

As Thai massage is a physical form of bodywork, you need to make sure that you are able to move very freely and easily, unrestricted by your clothing, while you are giving the massage treatment. You don't need any special clothing, but avoid anything with zips or buckles that could catch on your partner.

Your partner, the receiver, should also wear something unrestricting. Ideal garments are a t-shirt with sleeves and trousers rather than shorts. This is because covering up makes the acupressure part of the massage more comfortable to receive.

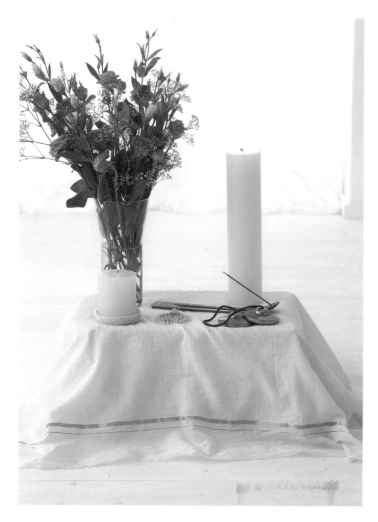

Above Making a shrine in the room where you give massage creates a sacred space. It is a personal place where you can honour elements that you feel are important to you within your practice.

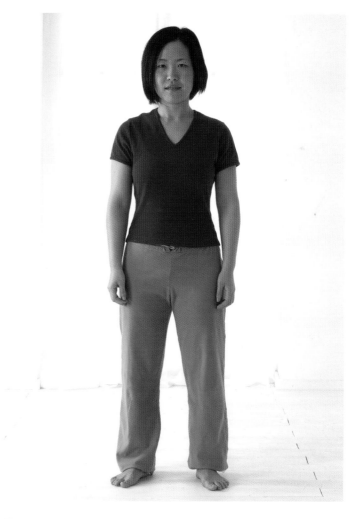

Above Wear something that is loose and comfortable for giving massage. Garments such as a simple t-shirt and stretchy tracksuit bottoms are perfectly adequate.

How to Use Your Body

Thai massage is a unique way of getting to know your body – whether you are giving or receiving. The beauty of this form of massage is that you are not restricted to the use of your hands alone. Thai massage uses the whole body, in soft, flowing movements, to create a kind of dance between giver and receiver.

Since Thai massage is a dynamic form of bodywork, it is important to focus on how to use the body safely and comfortably. The more at ease you, the giver, feel in your own body, the more relaxing the massage will be for the receiver. The following practical suggestions on posture will help to keep your body comfortable, so that the rhythmic, wavelike movements of the massage can flow freely and easily. Obviously, all the different exercises require different body positions, but it is useful to remember some general principles.

TERMS USED IN THIS SECTION

Throughout this guide you will find specific terms that refer to ways of working in Thai massage.

- **Inside hand** As you face your partner, this is the hand that is closer to the midline of their body.
- **Outside hand** Facing your partner, this is the hand that is furthest from the midline of their body.
- **The fix** This describes the position of the part of your body that is securing a pose – this may be your hand, your foot, or any other part of your body.
- **Being square on to the body** When palming, thumbing or working an acupressure point, this means keeping your body at 90 degrees to your partner's. It makes efficient use of your body weight while protecting your own posture.
- **Keeping your body open to your partner's** A useful way of checking your body posture in any of the exercises is to make sure that your heart is open to your partner's heart, that your belly is open to their belly. These open positions support the principle of working with loving kindness.
- **Working with the breath** Exhale as you work into a stretch and inhale as you release away from it. As you work with the more dynamic stretches, try to coordinate your breathing rhythm with your partner's.

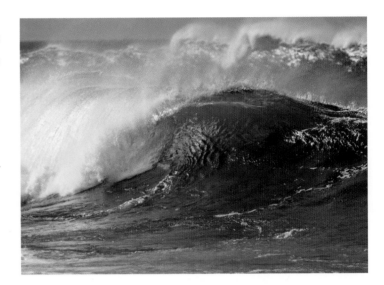

Above Like a wave ebbing and flowing, the rhythmic movement of leaning and releasing with the breath maintains a smooth and continuous flow throughout the massage, helping to unlock deeply held tensions within the body.

Getting it right

☒ Never press directly on to bone.

☑ Use your body weight, not your strength, and keep your back supported by a stable base. Bring your body weight up and over the area you are working, so that you can lean into your partner's body without any strain on your own.

☑ Get close to your partner. In order to use your body weight correctly you cannot give Thai massage at arm's length.

☑ Change your posture as often as you need to in order to stay comfortable. Be attentive to your own needs, too.

☑ Keep your movements economical: don't move your own or your partner's body unnecessarily. This helps you to see more clearly how exercises follow on from each other.

☑ Although you should work up and down the sen, the overall picture is of moving energy from the feet up towards the head.

☑ As a general rule, work in a measured and flowing way, with no sudden movements. Repeat each exercise about three times. Begin slowly and gently and work a little deeper with each repetition.

Caution

Some advanced positions appear in this section, to show the variety of poses that is possible, but you should only attempt them under the guidance of a professional teacher.

Wide-kneeling

Here, your base is wide and your centre of gravity is low. This is an extremely stable position that many people, especially beginners, find easy to use.

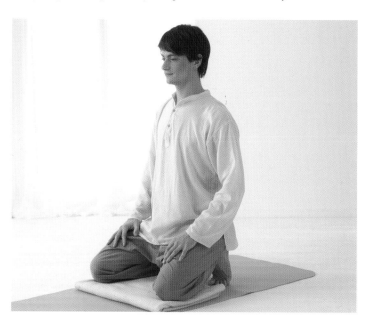

Above Keep your feet together and your knees apart. Remember to drop down through the tailbone, so you don't overextend into your lower back. You can alter your height very easily simply by tucking your toes under or sitting back on your heels.

Half-kneeling

This keeps your centre of gravity over the area you are working. The wide, stable base lets you overstep your partner without twisting your pelvis or back.

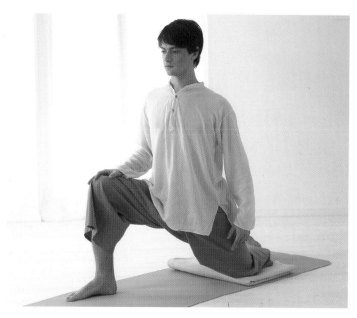

Above In this posture, focus on dropping down through the tip of your tailbone rather than lunging into the bent hip. Be prepared to change sides as often as you need to until, with increased practice, your hips open out more and your legs strengthen.

Palming

This technique applies general pressure to the sen and prepares the body for deeper energy work.

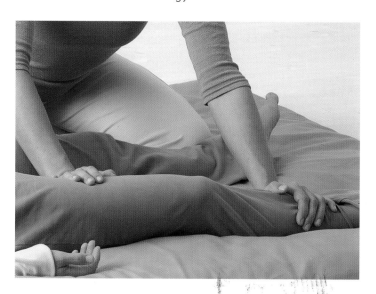

Above Use the padded part of the heel of your hand to apply most of the pressure and let your fingers relax around the body. Keep your arms straight, without locking the elbows. Relax your shoulders away from your ears. "Pour" your body weight down your arms so that the movement is slow and controlled. Gently rock your body weight from side to side, sinking into one palm then the other.

Thumbing

This technique is used for deeper energy work and for more focused pressure on the sen.

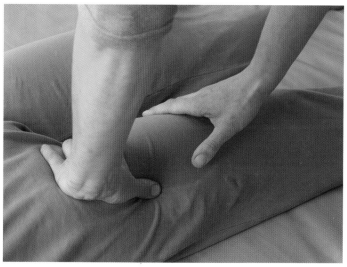

Above Use the soft, squashy part of your thumb rather than the point. To protect the thumb joint, spread the fingers wide for support and align the thumb with your wrist and elbow. Keep your arms straight but not locked and lean your body weight into one thumb and then the other, in a slow, rocking motion. Beginners may find that their thumbs ache, but practice should soon strengthen them.

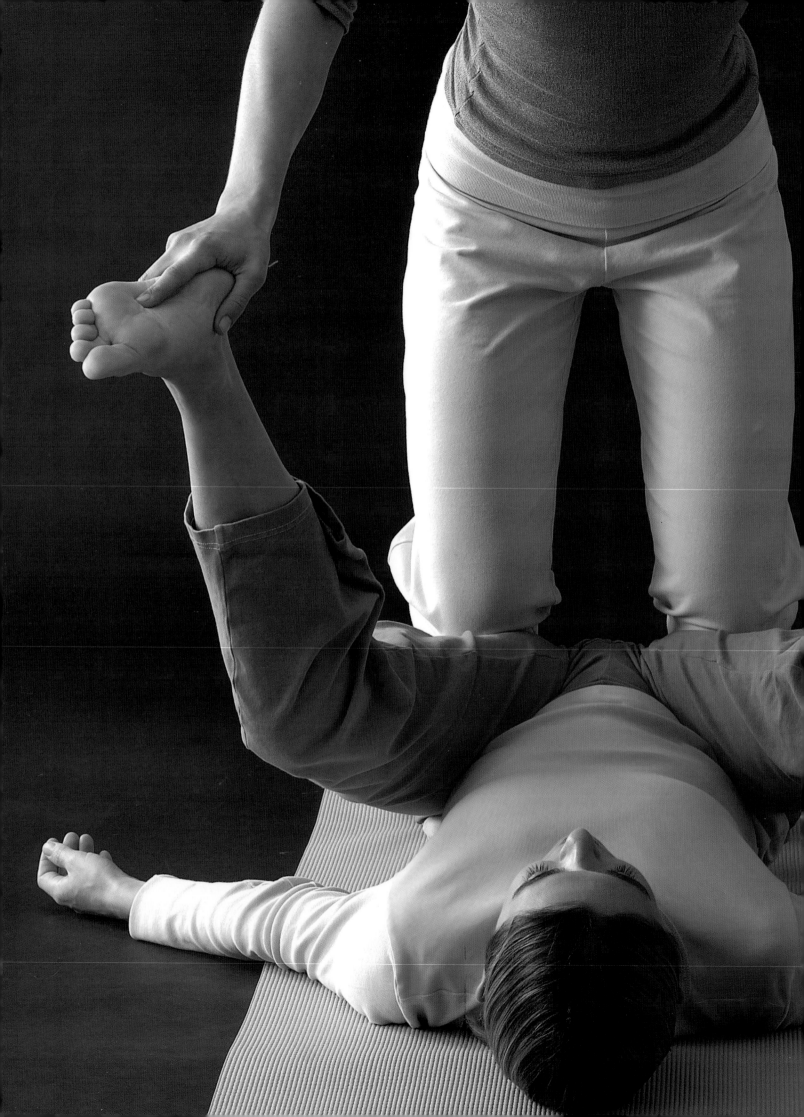

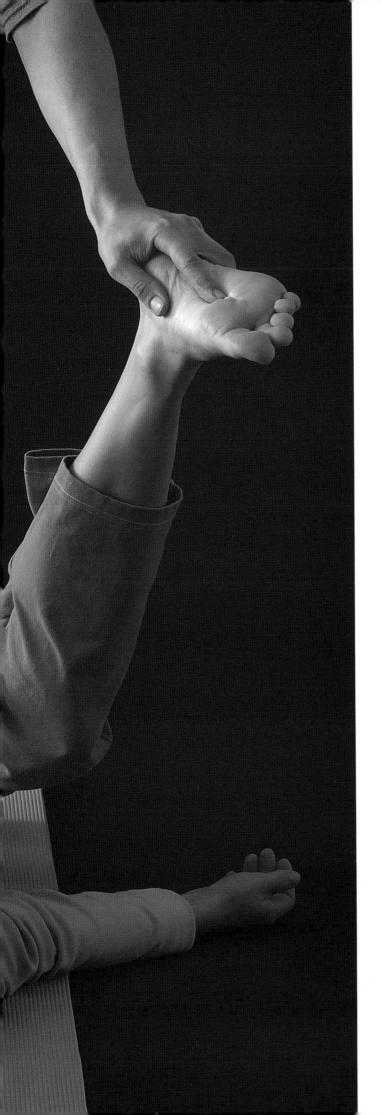

A Complete Body Routine

Traditionally, a full-body northern-style Thai massage lasts around two hours, flowing seamlessly from one part of the body to the next, moving energy from the feet towards the crown of the head. Nothing can replace this complete balancing of energy and the deep state of relaxation that follows. However, don't feel you always have to give a complete two-hour massage. A little goes a long way. Nor must you do all the exercises on every person – be guided by your partner's body type.

This chapter gives sequences for every part of the body and each ends with a visual summary – usually a selection of poses rather than a repeat of every one, to give an idea of the routine's overall flow. The sen on the artworks in this chapter are not multicolour-coded as at the start of the book, in order to focus on the main points being made. The chapter ends with routines for pregnancy and later life and for specific complaints.

Before You Start

This chapter will guide you through a complete full-body Thai massage. It focuses on one part of the body at a time, and it is suggested that you begin by practising each section separately. Take time to feel really comfortable and familiar with the work on each part of the body before trying to link all the sections together.

The sequence for each part of the body shows you how to open up the body gradually, moving from gentle exercises through to more dynamic stretches. The order of a Thai massage is not fixed: masseurs develop their own distinctive style and an experienced practitioner's treatments will vary from person to person. For a beginner, though, it is advisable to stick within the guidelines of this comprehensive structure, in order to give a complete and well-balanced massage.

COMMUNICATING WITH YOUR PARTNER

For a giver, the way to learn is to get feedback from your partner, so it is very important that you feel able to communicate freely during the massage. Although a significant aspect of Thai massage is the development of your intuitive skills and learning how to feel more sensitively with your hands, you are not a mind reader and you cannot expect to know how your partner is feeling. It is especially important when you are starting out as a masseur for you to ask your partner how the pressure and strength of the stretches feel for them.

As the giver, find out how much feedback is useful for you. Experiment and reach your own level – one that is helpful but that will not interfere with the experience of giving or receiving, and which allows space for silence and stillness within the massage. Take time at the end of each session to share what you enjoyed or didn't enjoy, so that you can learn from the experience.

ASSESSING YOUR PARTNER'S NEEDS

Thai massage is a powerful form of bodywork. It is a dynamic massage and involves passive stretching and mobilizing of the joints. You should be aware that not all the techniques in this section are suitable for everyone. So, before you start, it is essential to ask the right questions to find out about the state of your partner's health and how they are feeling. This will help you to decide on an appropriate and safe selection of exercises.

Massage is one of the oldest of the healing arts. If someone is in pain or suffering from illness or injury, its nurturing touch is a wonderfully supportive way of helping the body to heal itself. However, in the beginning, try to find a partner who is not suffering from any specific ailment, as

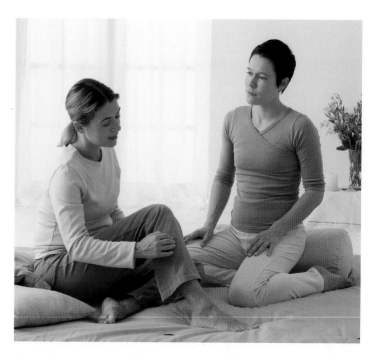

Above It's very important to ask the right questions to find out about your partner's health.

it is easier and safer to explore the techniques on a healthy body. Remember, too, that you as the giver need to look after yourself throughout the treatment. There is no point in taking care of your partner's body if you take no care of your own.

QUESTIONS TO ASK

The issue of contraindications is complex, and best assessed by a qualified practitioner with the skills and experience to judge what is and is not suitable for an individual. These general questions can help guide you but if you feel in any doubt about an exercise, don't do it. Specific dos and don'ts will be mentioned in each section.

- **Does your partner have any injuries?** You need to be particularly aware of spinal injuries and joint problems. Moving a damaged joint in the wrong way can be very dangerous. Avoid mobilizing any area of the body that is injured, inflamed or painful. Avoid pressing on bruises, cuts or recently healed wounds.

- **Is your partner muscle-bound?** Do they suffer from chronic tension? If your partner has very bound or tense muscles, don't press too hard or stretch too deeply as this will be counter-productive for them. It is more beneficial to do repeated energy line work and to introduce some easy stretches, so that you give your partner a feeling of release and ease.

- **Is your partner ill?** If their immune system is already working to combat illness, massage can sometimes be too much for the body to cope with.

- **Is your partner sensitive to pain?** Thai massage can be strong but should never be painful. Sometimes areas of the body that are unused to massage can feel highly sensitive to strong pressure. It can be very beneficial to work these areas provided you work within your partner's limits and encourage them to use their out-breath to help dissipate the strong sensations. If your partner is unable to do this, ease off the pressure and work more gently. The rule is that any feelings of "pain" should ease immediately after taking the pressure off the body.

- **Is your partner pregnant?** Many women find massage a wonderful means of relaxation throughout their pregnancy, but the routine shown in this section is not suitable for pregnancy. A full-body Thai massage for a pregnant woman must be given by a qualified professional. There is, however, a section at the end of this chapter highlighting some simple techniques that can be very beneficial and relaxing during pregnancy.

- **Does your partner have any specific medical conditions?** If your partner is suffering from any condition – and particularly if they need to take medication – they should consult their medical practitioner for advice before receiving massage.

The First Steps

You are now ready to start a Thai massage treatment. Give yourself plenty of time to enjoy these opening stages. You will soon discover that they are as important as the massage itself.

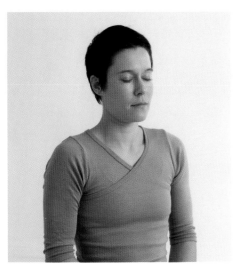

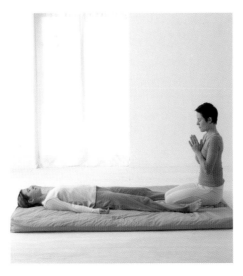

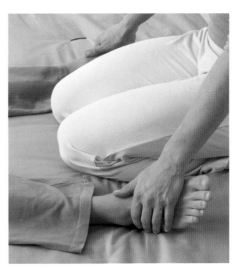

1 Quietening your mind Enjoy a moment of stillness with yourself. Listen closely to the coming and going of your breath. Allow your centre of gravity to settle. Relax. Notice how you are feeling in your body. Let yourself rest in this moment. Tuning into how you feel before you make contact with your partner can really help you to stay centred and grounded throughout the massage. It also gives space for your partner to settle into stillness.

2 The opening prayer Traditionally, each Thai massage begins with a prayer to the founder of Thai medicine, Jivaka Kumar Bhaccha. This moment of prayer acknowledges the deep spiritual roots of Thai massage and helps you to open to what is beyond rational thought. It can also be used as a moment to invite a deeper healing potential into your work.

3 Making the first touch The quality of the first touch is important as it sets the tone of the whole massage. Your hands should be warm and dry and your touch should be firm but gentle, helping your partner to feel safe and relaxed.

The Feet

Our feet are our roots, our point of contact with the earth. They carry and support us in all our movements, so they play an enormous part in maintaining a healthy posture. Just like the foundations of a building, our feet provide a solid foundation for the body. Working on them is very grounding, helping to bring your partner out of their head and into their body. The majority of people enjoy having their feet massaged, so it is an excellent place to start for those who may be apprehensive about receiving a full-body massage treatment.

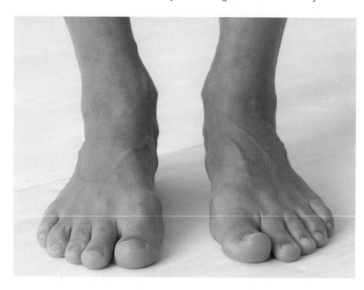

Above The feet are a vital part of our body, constantly carrying every movement and, quite literally, grounding us.

Getting it right

☒ Avoid pressing directly on cuts and bruises.

☑ Proceed with extreme caution if your partner has suffered any broken toes.

☒ If a joint is inflamed or painful because of arthritis, don't massage.

☑ Having some talc to hand for sticky hands and feet can make the foot massage more comfortable.

☑ Approach with a confident, firm touch, as some people can be ticklish or sensitive in the feet.

REFLEXOLOGY CHART

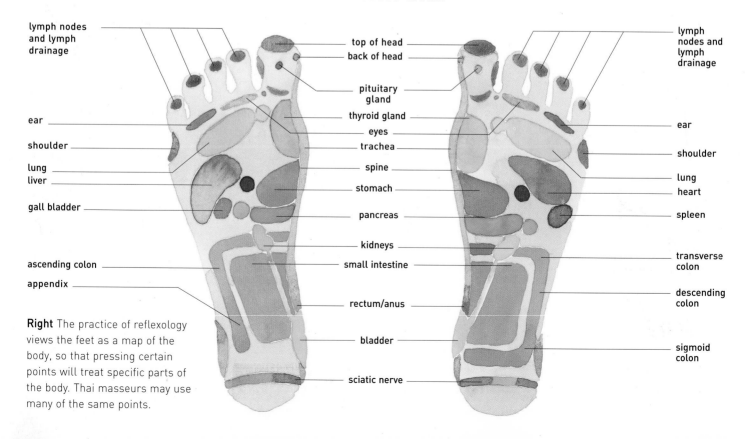

lymph nodes and lymph drainage

ear

shoulder

lung
liver

gall bladder

ascending colon

appendix

top of head
back of head

pituitary gland

thyroid gland
eyes

trachea

spine

stomach

pancreas

kidneys

small intestine

rectum/anus

bladder

sciatic nerve

lymph nodes and lymph drainage

ear

shoulder

lung

heart

spleen

transverse colon

descending colon

sigmoid colon

Right The practice of reflexology views the feet as a map of the body, so that pressing certain points will treat specific parts of the body. Thai masseurs may use many of the same points.

Preparing the Feet

These first four steps warm up the feet in preparation for deeper, more focused work. They also open up the ankles, which starts to open the hips gently. In this sequence work both feet simultaneously. Start near the ankle joint and work out towards the toes.

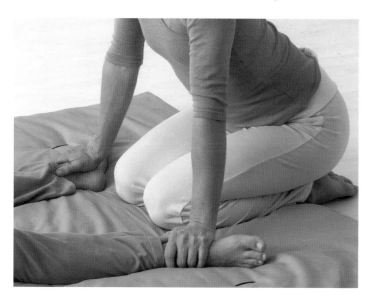

1 Warming up the instep Using the padded part of each hand, palm the whole instep up and down in a rhythmic rocking motion, leaning into and releasing out of the pressure. Begin near the heel and stop before you get to the ball of the big toe joint. Repeat several times until you feel the feet relax.

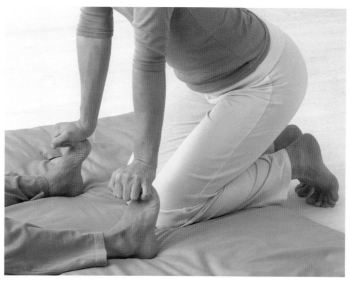

2 Opening the soles This stretch wakes up the foot. Place the heel of each hand, fingers pointing upwards, against the ball of your partner's foot, creating a point of resistance. Bend your elbows into your body and push against the sole of each foot so you see the whole leg move up into the hip socket. Maintain this resistance and slide your palms up until your fingers wrap over the toes. Now lean in and release. Repeat three times without changing your hand position. Use your body weight; your partner will tell you if it feels too much.

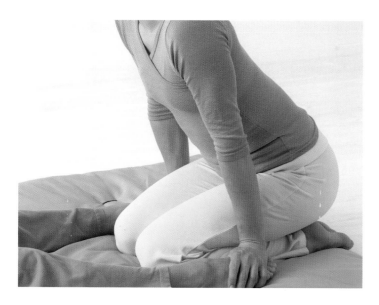

3 Lengthening the front of the feet This exercise will help to open up the front of the ankles while stimulating the energy lines that run through the top of the feet. Place your palms on top of your partner's feet, near the ankle joints. Lean down and slightly away, lengthening the front of each foot towards the ground. Now release and repeat, moving your hands down towards your partner's toes.

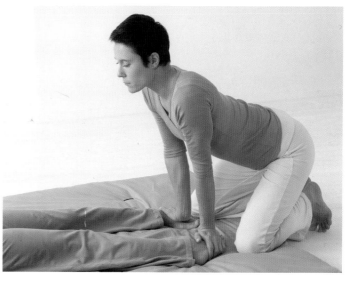

4 Opening the ankles and hips This is a wonderful position to open the hips while increasing mobility through the ankle joint. Cup your hands under the heels. Lift and lengthen the legs, turning the heels out and the feet in as you do so. Reposition your hands to fix on the tops of the feet, lean in with your body weight and lengthen the toes towards each other. See how the hips are affected.

Thumbing the Lines of the Feet

When thumbing the foot lines, check the pressure you are using with your partner – it is especially useful to establish the right depth of pressure at the very beginning of a massage, as it helps to put your partner at ease, allowing them to relax more fully.

THE FOOT LINES

The diagram seen here illustrates how we can work the energy lines and points on the feet in two ways. One way is in a fan formation, starting at the point seen in the diagram (and also in the photograph in the box below) and working out to the end of each toe. The other way is to work in straight lines, starting just above the heel and continuing in a line up to the tips of the toes. Working the fan is more effective for deeper relaxation as it repeatedly works the acupressure point for insomnia. Working in straight lines is more appropriate for a general relaxing massage.

Right Two approaches to working the foot lines (and points along their length) for a general relaxing treatment.

WAYS OF WORKING THE FOOT LINES

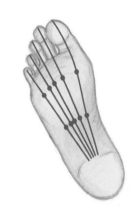
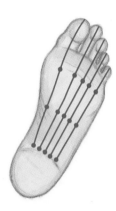

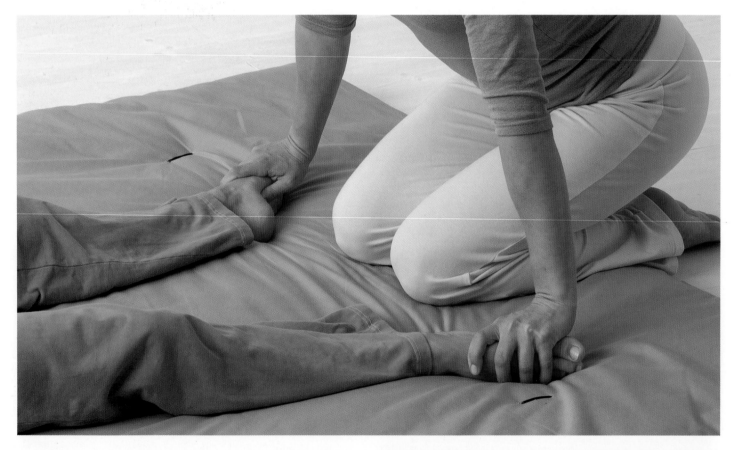

Above Work the lines on both feet simultaneously. Place your thumb on the line, lean in and release. Move the thumb gradually up the sole of each foot. Use the fingers to give counter-pressure, to stop the foot sliding away from you. Remember to work only on soft tissue: when you reach the bone of the ball of the foot, rub with firm circular movements.

How to thumb

Thumbing is not rubbing. With your thumb in position, lean in and out, using your body weight in a slow rocking motion. This picture shows the start-point for the fan technique.

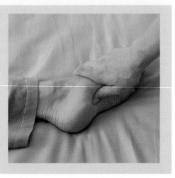

Working Single Feet

Up until now you have been working both of your partner's feet simultaneously. For the rest of the foot sequence, you will be working one foot at a time and will then repeat the whole sequence on the other foot.

Which side first?

In Eastern energy practices the body is seen as two halves of a whole: left and right, feminine and masculine, yin and yang. Traditionally you start by balancing the dominant side of your partner, and this applies throughout the whole body, not just to the feet. For a man the dominant side is usually masculine, or yang, so you would begin on the right side. For a woman, it is the feminine, yin or left side that is normally dominant. But people don't always fit into neat categories and there are many men with a dominant feminine side and women with a dominant masculine side. So make the choice according to what you sense to be true for your partner.

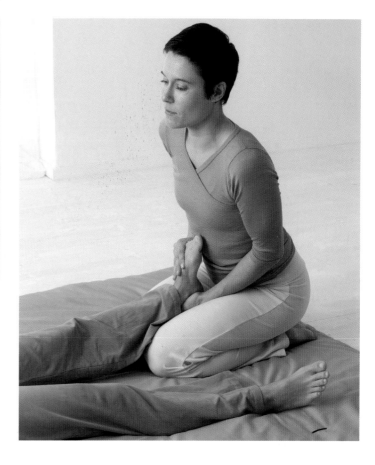

1 Ankle circles This motion opens up the ankle joint and also begins to warm up the hip joint. Align yourself with your partner's foot. Hold their heel in your lap and clasp the top of the foot with your other hand. Keeping the heel still, rotate your own body, taking the upper part of the foot with you. You will see the whole leg move if your partner is relaxed enough. Circle clockwise and anticlockwise, repeating three times.

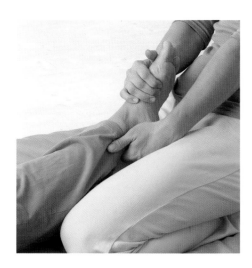

2 Twisting the foot Keeping the foot in your lap, wrap your hand all the way round the front of it, clasping your fingers around the instep. Using the heel of your hand as a lever, tuck your elbow in and lean gently away to twist the foot outwards, then release. Repeat this whole movement three times.

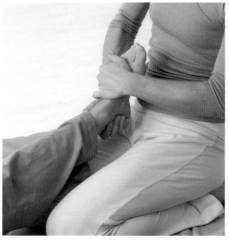

3 Now swap hands and repeat the movement, but this time twisting the foot gently inwards, to open the foot in the opposite direction. Repeat three times.

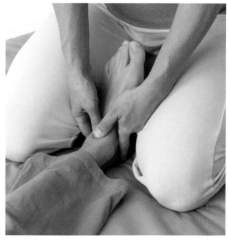

4 Knee pain point This acupressure point is excellent for relieving headaches and knee pains caused by overworking.

Place the foot on the floor and locate the dip on the top of the foot near the ankle joint (find it more easily by flexing the foot slightly). Place thumb on thumb over this dip and lean your body weight in. Check the pressure with your partner. Work in and out three or four times.

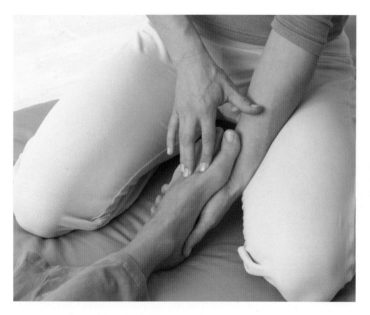

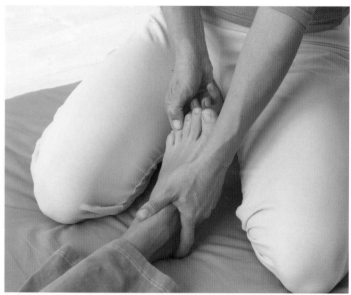

5 Working the top of the foot Keep the foot resting on the floor. Use one hand to support the sole and with the other work in between the tendons. You can use the flats of your fingers or your thumbs for a deeper pressure. This is an excellent way to work many valuable pressure points and create space throughout the front of the foot.

6 Squeezing the toes This produces a very satisfying feeling and lends a sense of completeness to the foot massage. Before you start, check for broken toes or arthritic joints and proceed with caution. Most arthritic joints benefit from mobilization as long as they are not currently inflamed.

Hold the foot firmly with one hand. With the other hand, work from the centre of the foot, squeezing and rubbing around all the joints of each toe. Work right to the tip of the toe and give the end a gentle pinch.

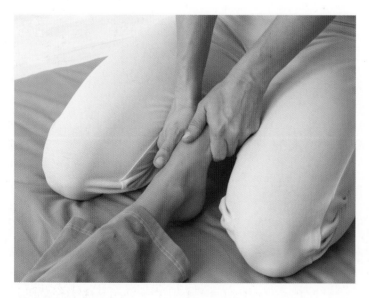

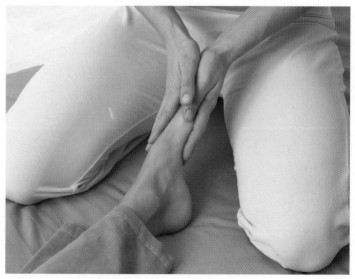

7 Kneading the foot This is wonderful way to relax the foot completely. The basic movement is a simple squeezing and releasing motion. Always start closest to the ankle joint and work out and away towards the toes. You can work both hands simultaneously or alternately. There is no fixed technique, so explore and enjoy.

8 Sweeping off the foot Finish the foot massage by smoothing the skin with a swift brushing movement. Hold the foot firmly yet gently between your hands and sweep from the ankle joint to the tips of the toes. Repeat two or three times.

Review: the Feet

Now repeat the sequence on the other foot – use the pictures below as a reminder of all the steps. Remember to use your bodyweight as much as possible rather than your strength, keeping your shoulders relaxed and your breath even.

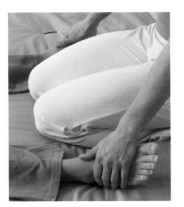

Making the first touch

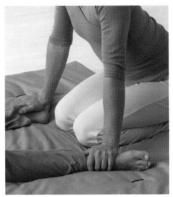

Warming up the instep

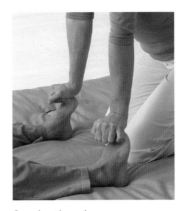

Opening the soles

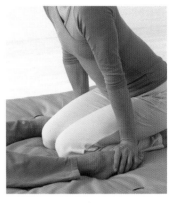

Lengthening the front

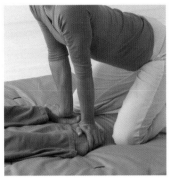

Opening the ankles and hips

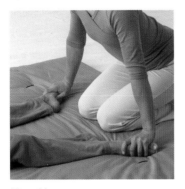

Thumbing

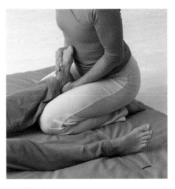

Ankle circles

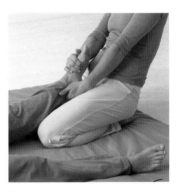

Twisting outwards

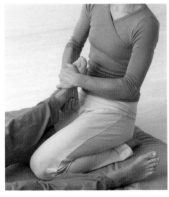

Twisting inwards

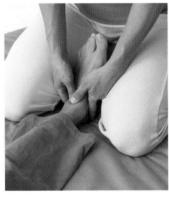

Knee pain point

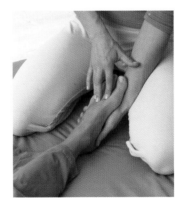

Working the top of the foot

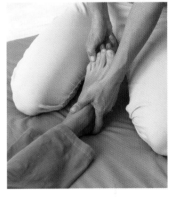

Squeezing the toes

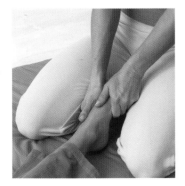

Kneading

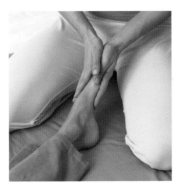

Sweeping off

Caution

People's feet take quite a pounding in everyday life and painful foot complaints of all kinds are very common, so always progress carefully prior to treatment. Examine your partner's feet thoroughly before you start and ask them about any problems. Can you see any cuts, bruises or swollen areas? Never press on these and avoid any joints affected by arthritis. Proceed with great care if any toes have been broken recently or in the past.

The Legs

Work on the energy lines of the legs stimulates the circulation of energy and blood. It eases tiredness and heaviness in the lower half of the body, giving renewed support for the legs and, in turn, for the rest of the body. It releases tension in the lower back and starts to open up the hips and pelvis for the deeper stretches. If worked slowly and rhythmically, the palming and thumbing of these lines can be deeply relaxing, laying the foundations for the rest of the massage.

Whichever side you chose to work first with the feet, start again on the same side for the legs. Always begin by working the inside of the leg: this will be on the leg that is furthest away from you. Palm all the lines on the inside leg first, then thumb all the lines and finish with another round of palming. When you have completed all the palming and thumbing here, repeat this pattern on the outside of the leg that is closest to you. Then, get up and move to the other side of your partner's body and repeat the sequence.

THE SEN OF THE LEGS

For demonstration purposes, the energy lines shown on the artwork (right) are numbered 1, 2 and 3 on the inside of the legs and 1 and 2 on the outside. There is a third line on the outside but it is more easily worked later, when your partner is lying on their side.

Inside leg

Line 1 runs from the anklebone along the underside of the shinbone to the knee. Above the knee, it begins at the lower edge of the kneecap and continues up the thigh to the groin. *Line 2* runs through the centre of the inside of the leg, from the depression below the anklebone into the soft, fleshy part of the calf and up to the knee. On the thigh it follows the more yielding groove of the muscle.
Line 3 begins at the back of the leg, on the Achilles tendon, and runs up the centre of the back of the calf, directly behind the knee. On the thigh, it continues just above the big tendon and runs up to the groin.

Outside leg

Line 1, from the masseur's point of view, starts at the knee pain point (see page 47) and continues – just outside the shinbone between the bone and the muscle – up to the knee. It then continues up the thigh from the outside edge of the kneecap; relax your hand to follow the line right up to the outside of the hip. *Line 2* is close to line 1. It starts just above the anklebone and runs up between the two bones of the shin, in the groove between the muscles. On the thigh, it starts a thumb's width lower than the first line and runs up to the head of the thighbone at the top of the leg.

WORKING THE LEG LINES

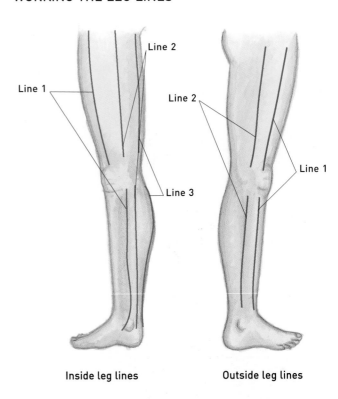

Inside leg lines   **Outside leg lines**

Above These two diagrams illustrate the path taken by the main sen energy lines in the legs – on the inner and outer leg.

Getting it right

☒ Do not press directly on to:
• bone
• any varicose vein (work only above the area under pressure)
• the knee (work gently either side of it)
• the groin area (this is painful and intrusive)

☑ Check the pressure and work sensitively. Each person has different levels of sensitivity and the pressure should be deep but never painful. If it feels strong, encourage your partner to focus on their breathing and to enjoy the new sensation of an energy workout for the legs.

☑ Remember to check for bruises and cuts; if the legs are covered you may not see them.

☑ Take care of your own posture. If you find yourself twisting to reach up and down the leg, move your body until you are square on to your partner's leg.

Palming and Thumbing the Legs

Steps 1–4 form a short distinct sequence that you can do first on one leg and then on the other. Different legs are seen being worked below, to show the poses from the clearest angles. Find a comfortable position and feel free to adjust it as you work.

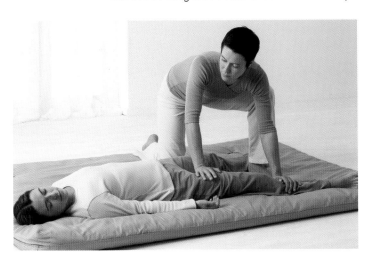

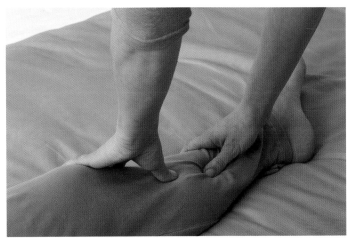

1 Palming the inside leg Begin with one hand near the ankle and one on the thigh just above the knee. Shift your body weight from side to side in a slow, rhythmic rocking motion, palming your hands up and down line 1. Repeat with lines 2 and 3.

2 Thumbing the inside leg As the pressure is deeper here, check that it is comfortable for your partner. Start with one thumb at the ankle joint and the other about a thumb's length away. Walk the thumbs up and down line 1. Repeat with lines 2 and 3.

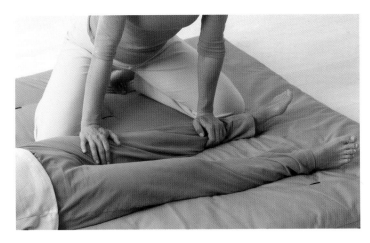

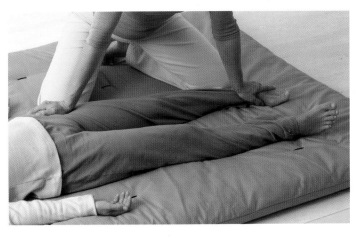

3 Palming and thumbing the outside leg Palm, and then thumb, lines 1 and 2 of the outside leg. (You may find that you want to change your body posture when you work the outside.)

4 Stretching the outside of the leg To complete the work on one side of the body, lengthen and stretch the outside of the leg before moving around to the other side of your partner's body to repeat the palming and thumbing from the other side. Fix one hand on the outside of the hip and the other on top of the foot. Now lean in and release. Repeat two or three times.

Getting into the flow

When palming, keep your breathing even, free and smooth. One way to develop a good rhythm is to sing to yourself. For example, the carol *Silent Night* has the rocking rhythm of a lullaby, mirroring the sinking and releasing that gives energy line work its relaxing quality.

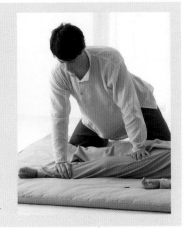

Technique tips

To palm, keep the lower hand on the calf, and the upper one on the thigh. Use the same smooth rocking motion for both palming and thumbing.

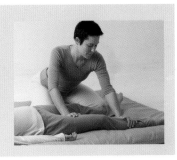

Single Leg Exercises

Like the feet, our legs work to ground and connect us to the earth. Northern-style Thai massage places a strong emphasis on working the legs. This sequence releases blocked energy and deeply held tension in the joints of the legs and the pelvis, bringing about deep feelings of release. Run through all the exercises on one leg and then repeat the sequence on the other leg.

As you work, keep your body movements economical and use your body weight to achieve the full depth of every stretch and line workout. If you have done the foot exercises prior to these single leg exercises, then start with the leg that is on the same side of the body. So, if you began your foot routine with the left foot, then work the left leg first.

Getting it right

☑ Check with your partner for any joint injuries, especially to the knee. Work with sensitivity and awareness and if in doubt leave it out.

☑ Keep communicating: as you are progressing to more dynamic stretches, it is important that your partner gives you plenty of feedback.

☑ Try to keep the movement flowing between each posture so that the sequence begins to feel like one continuous movement.

Relaxing the Leg

This sequence is beneficial for stiffness in the lower back, immobile hip joints and tightness in the legs. The energy line work on the thighs will not only relax that part of the legs, but will also rejuvenate tired knees.

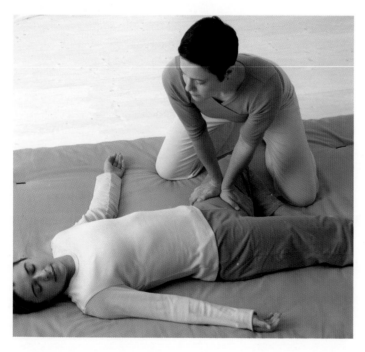

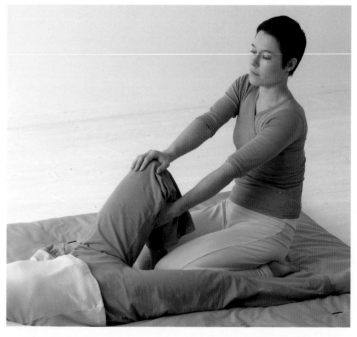

1 The tree Bend your partner's leg so that their knee falls out to the side. If the knee does not easily reach the ground, support it with a cushion. Align your body with your partner's knee. Place the heels of your hands in the centre of the thigh, close to the hip joint, and lean your body weight in and out. Adjust your hand position, working up and down the thigh. Avoid working too close to the knee joint.

2 Relax the calf Bring your partner's knee upright, placing their foot on the floor and securing it between your knees. Support the knee with one hand and clasp the other around the bulk of the calf muscle, scooping it away from the bone and leaning back at the same time. Change the fixing of your hands and work the calf from the other side. Make three or four scoops up and down the calf muscle.

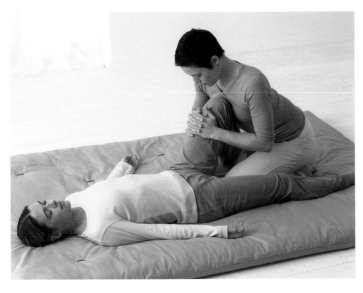

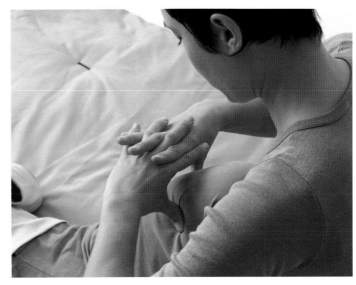

3 Butterfly squeeze: palming Keeping the knee upright, move closer so that your breastbone rests upon it. Clasp your hands together like butterfly wings and then place the heels of your hands on inside line 1 and outside line 1. Let your elbows drop and then gently squeeze your palms together. Work up and down the thigh two or three times.

4 Butterfly squeeze: thumbing This exerts deeper pressure on the lines of the thighs. Unclasp your fingers a little and place your thumbs along the inside and outside lines of the thigh. Using your elbows as levers, gently squeeze your thumbs, working up and down the leg as before.

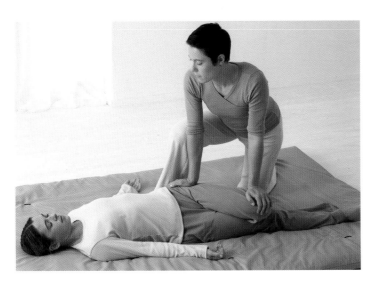

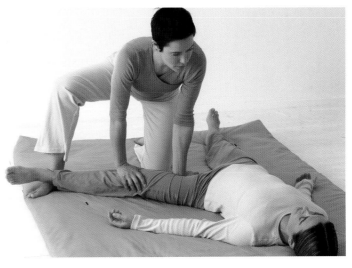

5 Cross hip stretch This exercise opens up the outside of the hip. Keep the foot where it is and let the knee drop across the outstretched leg. It is important to fix the knee in place with one hand, as any movement in this joint feels very uncomfortable. With your free hand, palm around your partner's hip and down the outside of the thigh. Start close to the hip joint and work towards the knee. Repeat three times.

6 Open leg stretch This opens the inner thigh and groin. Straighten your partner's leg and move their foot out to the side. Be aware of any strain behind the knee and don't take the leg to the edge of its stretch. To fix, cup your hand over your partner's knee. With the other hand, starting close to the hip, palm up and down the third inside line of the thigh. Do not press too close to the knee joint.

Step 5 tip
If the knee will not drop across easily for the cross hip stretch, place a cushion between the knee and lower leg to support it.

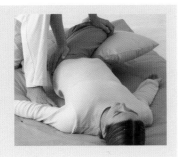

Step 6 tip
Support your partner's foot by placing their Achilles tendon against your knee pain point. This keeps their leg elevated slightly off the ground.

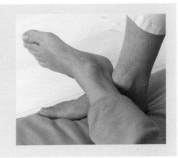

Opening the Hips and Groin

The following exercises are wonderful for all body types. They help to release energy held in the hips and groin and also start the process of stimulating the energy flow up into the lower back.

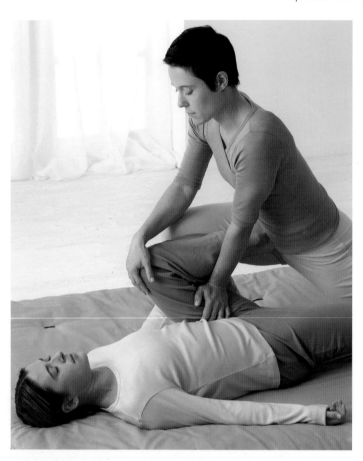

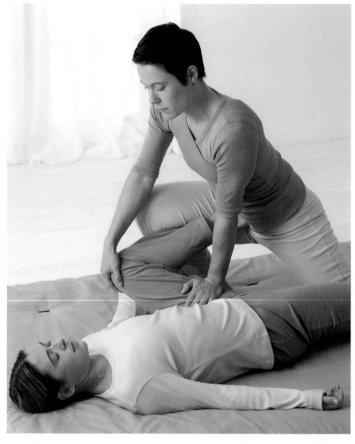

1 Hip opener I The joy of this stretch lies in the smooth repeated movement towards and away from the point of resistance. You will feel your partner's body gradually open up to the stretch and will be able to go a little further each time. If you feel that you are lunging too far, then simply move your body closer to your partner's head.

From the last position, support your partner's knee and heel with your hands and bring the instep of their foot up into the crease of your bent leg. Angle their knee so that it is pointing straight up towards their shoulder. Place your outside hand on the knee and, with your inside hand, palm the thigh as you sink into the stretch. Repeat a few times, working with your breath. Exhale as you gently lunge forward until you reach the point of resistance, then ease out. There is no effort required, since all the power comes from your centre of gravity.

2 Hip opener II This stretch is deeper than the previous one, and is often more satisfying for flexible people. Stay in the same position as for Hip opener 1, but move your supporting hand and leg away from your partner's body and let their hip drop out to the side. Work in the same way as before, exhaling into the stretch and inhaling as you release. Follow the natural direction of the leg up and out towards your partner's shoulder: you may find that it moves in an almost semicircular direction.

Caution
Avoid this stretch if your partner suffers from a hernia.

Getting a flavour of the dance

With the hip, groin and back-of-leg sequences shown on these and the following pages, you as the giver can really begin to appreciate and enjoy involving the whole of your body in your massage technique. The use of your body weight, along with the combination of working with your hands and feet together, will start to give you a flavour of a very special rhythm. It is this rhythm that leads many people to refer to Thai massage as a kind of "dance" – your movements become a rhythmic dance and you also engage in a dance with your partner.

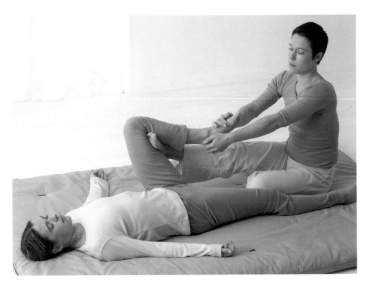

3 Kung fu foot This is a "transition" pose, leading you into the next step. Sit back but keep your partner's knee upright. Once you are sitting, take hold of their foot and place the outer edge of your foot (with toes pointing in and heel pointing out) at the back of their knee. Use your foot to guide their knee slowly out and down to the floor. You are now ready for the step 4 position.

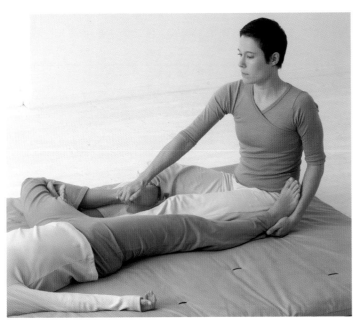

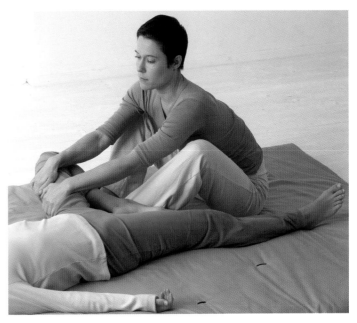

4 Paddle boat This is a wonderful exercise that releases deep into the groin and lower back. Use the instep, not the heel, of your inside foot to paddle up and down the thigh. Start near to the groin and work to the knee and back, being careful of the area around the knee. Begin with your knee bent and extend fully into the foot for a complete stretch. You can vary the strength of the stretch by moving closer or further away.

5 Foot sandwich This exercise relaxes the front of the thigh. Keep the knee where it is and sandwich your feet between the calf and the thigh. Shift your body closer to your partner so that you can reach between your knees to scoop around the back of the thigh. Work with alternate hands, leaning away slightly for a deeper pressure.

A close fit for step 4
Make sure that your partner's foot is tucked snugly behind your knee; hold their heel in place with one hand. With your other hand bring their outstretched leg close into your body and hold under that heel too. This snug fit gives the pose its stability.

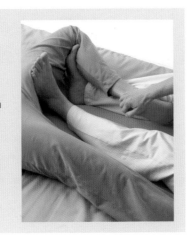

Making room in step 5
When tucking your feet in the bend of your partner's leg, you can try gently rolling your partner's calf muscle out of the way to make more room for your feet. If both of your feet still don't fit comfortably, then just take your outside foot away.

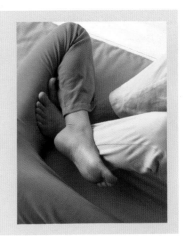

Opening the Back of the Leg

Staying with the same leg as for the previous exercises, we now finish the single-leg sequence. These steps stimulate energy flow up the back of the legs and into the lower back and hips. If your partner has tight hamstrings, work with sensitivity.

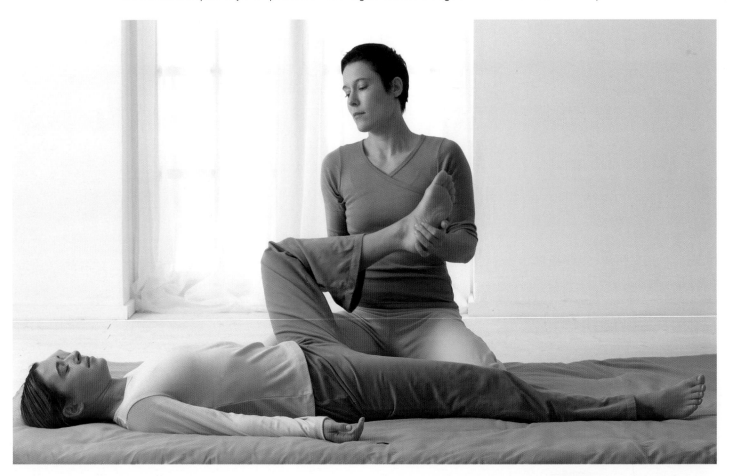

1 Leg circles This is a wonderful exercise for all body types. It encourages a deep feeling of letting go in the hip joint and can be used at any point in this sequence.

Before you start, make sure that your posture is comfortable and stable. Cup one hand under your partner's heel and your other hand under their knee. Keep their lower leg parallel with the floor. Now circle their knee, exploring the full range of movement as you do so. The movement can be big or small, fast or slow, whatever suits your partner. Circle the leg several times in both directions.

2 Hamstring yawn This exercise opens and energizes the leg from the hip to the heel. Keeping your body open to your partner's, stand with a wide stance. Bend your partner's knee across their body so that it is angled towards the opposite shoulder. Align yourself with the leg. Cup the heel with your inside hand, and with your outside hand palm the outside edge of the thigh. Encourage your partner to breathe with you. As you exhale, rock your weight on to your front foot, palming the thigh and pushing the heel in a smooth arc over the head. As you inhale, release the heel and thigh and rock back on to your back leg. Repeat three times.

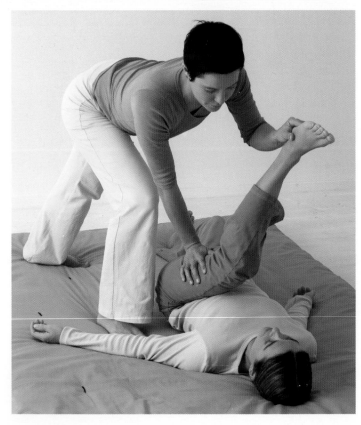

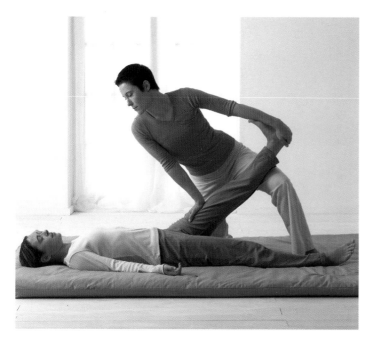

3 Pour the tea As its name suggests, this movement is a tilting motion; the weight is "poured" forward on to the thigh, opening up the back of the calf and heel.

From standing, drop down to half-kneeling, straightening your partner's leg and letting it rest on your thigh. Create a lever by cupping your fingers under the heel, making sure the toes are resting against your forearm. Rest your other hand on your partner's thigh, keeping away from the knee joint. Lean into the stretch as you exhale, and then release. Repeat three times, gradually working more deeply, but carefully sensing and controlling the strength of the stretch behind the knee.

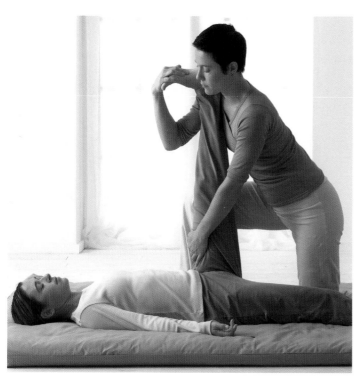

Variation to the Double Bass

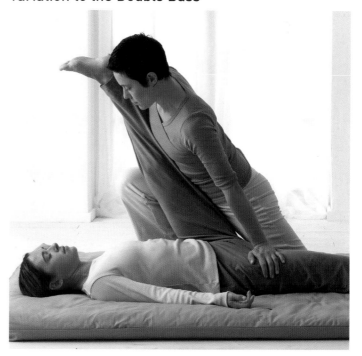

4 Double bass This stretches and stimulates the energy lines along the length of the leg. Not everyone can straighten their leg at 90 degrees, so if this feels a struggle for your partner, work at a more shallow angle where the leg can remain straight.

Drop down on to your other knee so that you are square on to your partner, with your body open to theirs. Take the leg up towards the vertical and let the foot rest on your outside shoulder. Fix one hand on the front of the thigh and the other on the ball of the foot. Use the top hand as a lever to gently open up the back of the leg. Encourage your partner to exhale as you lean down on to the ball of the foot. (This movement is quite small.) Once you have reached the point of resistance, release. Repeat several times, deepening the stretch as tension is released.

Above If your partner is a very flexible person, then you may want to try a version of the Double Bass that features a more dynamic stretch. Cup your partner's heel in your hand and tuck your arm close into your body. Fix your other hand on the thigh of the outstretched leg and sink your body weight forwards, taking the heel towards their head, to open more deeply through the groin.

Spinal Twist

Twists are invigorating as they help to stimulate the circulation and functioning of the internal organs. This twist releases tension throughout the mid spine, helping to create space in the ribcage and so encourage deeper breathing.

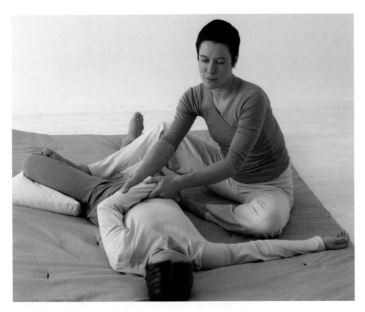

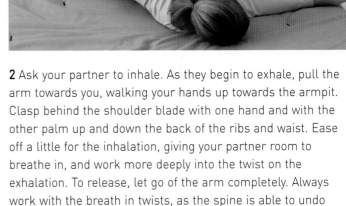

1 Put your partner's leg back into the tree pose (page 52). For most people a cushion under the knee is a good idea. Sit on the opposite side to the bent leg. You will need to move the arm closest to you out of the way. Fix the sole of your foot gently over the bent knee to give stability in the final stretch. Reach across the body and take hold of the other arm above the wrist.

Caution
People with spinal injuries or disc problems should avoid this movement.

2 Ask your partner to inhale. As they begin to exhale, pull the arm towards you, walking your hands up towards the armpit. Clasp behind the shoulder blade with one hand and with the other palm up and down the back of the ribs and waist. Ease off a little for the inhalation, giving your partner room to breathe in, and work more deeply into the twist on the exhalation. To release, let go of the arm completely. Always work with the breath in twists, as the spine is able to undo itself more freely on the exhalation. Repetition is not necessary – one twist is sufficient.

Technique improver

To begin with, the single leg sequence can seem quite overwhelming, as there are many different exercises all flowing into one another. To familiarize yourself with the sequence and the feeling of continual movement, it is a good idea to simulate it on your own body. The more that you are able to experience the techniques in your body, rather than just trying to remember them with your head, the sooner the exercises will make sense to you.

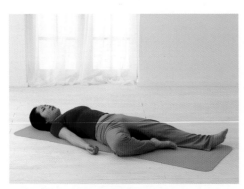

Tree pose

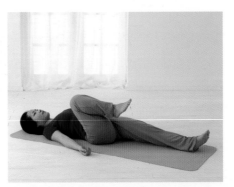

Hip opener

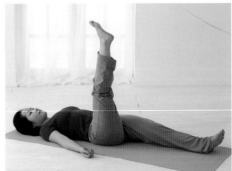

Double bass

Review: Single Leg Exercises

You are now ready to repeat the whole single leg sequence on the other leg. Use the pictures below as a reminder of the sequence. Take plenty of time to feel comfortable with the steps for each body section before moving on to the next one.

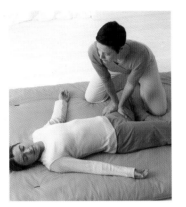

The tree

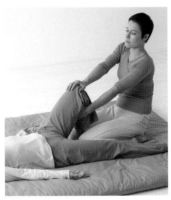

Relax the calf

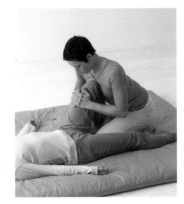

Butterfly squeeze: palming

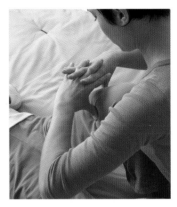

Butterfly squeeze: thumbing

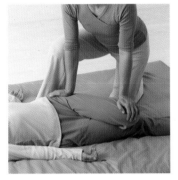

Cross hip stretch

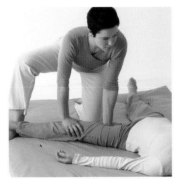

Wide leg stretch

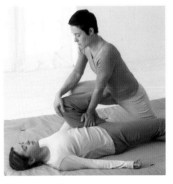

Hip opener I

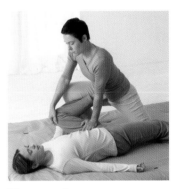

Hip opener II

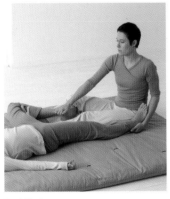

Paddle boat

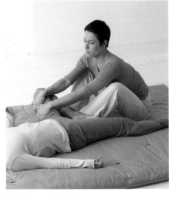

Foot sandwich

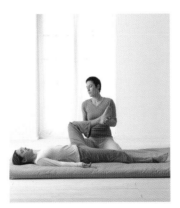

Leg circles

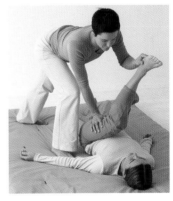

Hamstring yawn

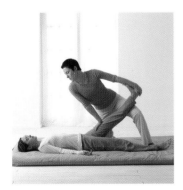

Pour the tea

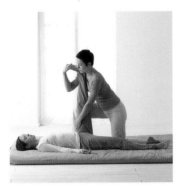

Double bass

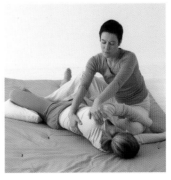

Spinal twist

Caution

Once again, check for cuts and bruises before starting and ask your partner about any joint problems. Their legs may be covered up and so areas to avoid may not be readily apparent.

Double Leg Exercises

This dynamic sequence works both legs simultaneously and focuses on opening the lower back and the hips. It introduces the body to inversions, back bends and forward bends, and is stimulating and invigorating for the whole system. The exercises are particularly helpful for those with low blood pressure or a sluggish digestive system.

There is enough variety in this sequence to find something to suit all kinds of body types, so do not feel that you have to try every exercise on every person. As some of these exercises involve deep stretches, it is important to establish good communication with your partner so that they can tell you when they have reached their limit.

Knees to Chest

A useful counter-stretch or relaxation pose, this is great for most body types. Your own posture is important here: place your feet apart as shown to create a stable base.

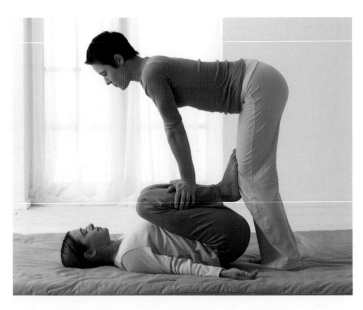

Above Place the soles of your partner's feet against your kneecaps, keeping your knees together and slightly bent. Place your hands on the outside of their shinbones and, as you sink your body weight into your knees, simultaneously lean your weight down into your palms. Ease in and out several times. If your partner is tight in the front of their hips or has over-developed thigh muscles, you may have to let the knees open slightly.

Crossed Leg Stretch

This works into the back and hips. Align your body with the direction in which you are working. The focus should be felt in the bent leg. Repeat the exercise on both legs before moving on.

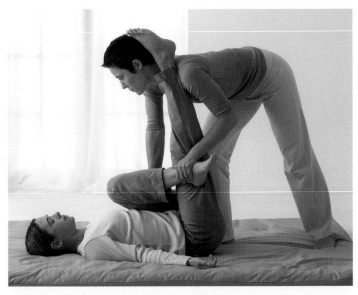

Above Ask your partner to bend one leg and straighten the other. Let the heel of the straight leg rest on your inside shoulder. Fix one hand on the ankle of the bent leg and the other on the thigh, just below the knee. Reposition yourselves so that the direction of the stretch is towards the opposite shoulder. With your feet wide, rock on to your front foot, palming up and down the outside of the thigh. Release and repeat three times.

Getting it right

☑ Watch your posture: work with a free spine, using the power in your legs, rather than your back.

☑ When practising the sequence, try to avoid putting your partner's legs down completely between the postures, which will make you tire very quickly.

☒ Don't use inversions for menstruating women, or those with high blood pressure, detached retinas or heart disease.

☑ As these poses are more dynamic, coordinate your breathing with your movements. Always move into a stretch on the exhalation and release on the inhalation.

The Plough

This stretch is an excellent one for toning and releasing tension in the
abdominal organs. It stimulates the sen sumana energy line
and the spinal column in general.

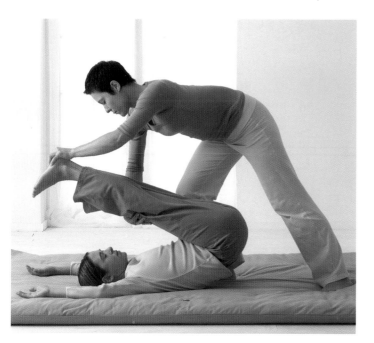

Left Hold both feet in your hands and reposition yourself so that
your back leg is directly behind your partner's sacrum. Watch your
posture: keep your feet wide for stability. Cup one hand behind
your partner's heels, keeping the feet together, and support the
fronts of the shins with the other hand to keep their body straight.

Exhaling, rock on to your front leg and take your partner's feet in
an arc above their head. Encourage your partner to exhale as you
move into the pose, as this will give a deeper feeling of release in
the spine. Their lower back will naturally come off the ground at this
point. Keep their hips in line with the rest of the body – don't let
them swing out to the side. As you inhale, release your partner's
hips back down to the ground. Work slowly in and out three times,
gradually increasing the depth of the stretch.

Easy and advanced variations to the plough

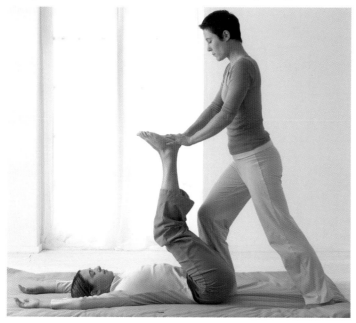

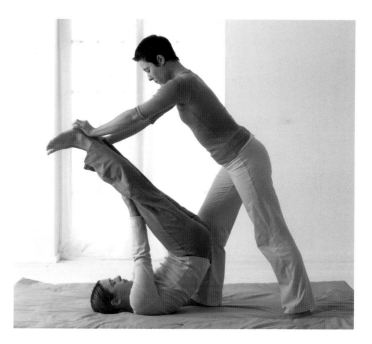

Above If your partner finds the regular plough pose too strong in the
back of the legs, or if you notice a shaking in the legs, ask them to
bend their knees a little to take the pressure off the hamstrings and
bring the focus of the stretch into the back.

Above The shoulder stand is an advanced pose that is an extension
of the assisted plough. It involves an additional release for the
shoulders and neck. This gives an indication of the kind of pose you
may be able to attempt once you know more about Thai massage.
It is better to work this pose with a fully qualified teacher and a
supple recipient.

Caution
Avoid the full plough stretch in cases of neck injury,
detached retina or heart disease, for people with high blood
pressure or for women during menstruation.

The Frog

This is a deep stretch to open the middle and lower back. It is not suitable for those with knee problems or injuries to the groin or spine. Make sure that you are working with the breath in this exercise.

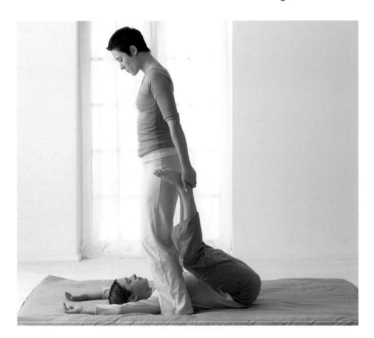

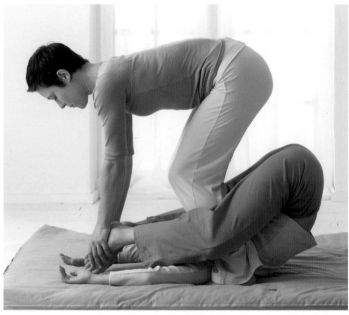

1 Hold one heel in each hand and encourage your partner to let the weight of their legs hang from your hands, with knees bent and hips relaxed. Ask them to place their arms above their head. Step in between their legs and stand as high up into their armpits as you can. Inhaling, lift their feet up and bring them round in front of your body so that the soles of the feet are together. It is normal for the hips to come off the ground.

2 Once the feet are together, settle them lower so that they are level with your pubic bone. Now, exhaling, push your partner's feet in a gentle arc over their head, extending your arms fully. Take the feet as far as they can go but do not force the body. When you reach your partner's point of resistance, release a little and repeat three times, without coming fully out of the posture each time.

The Butterfly

This time the direction of the stretch is straight down towards your partner's face. The pose focuses on opening the hips and groin. It is not appropriate for very stiff people or those with knee problems or injuries to the groin or spine.

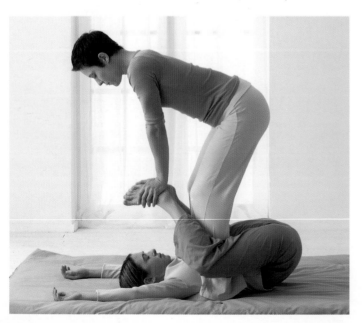

Left From the previous pose simply step away from the armpits until you are level with your partner's ribcage. Keep their feet together. You may feel some natural resistance, so check the pressure with your partner and then continue to sink your body weight down through your arms.

Undo the pose slowly. Move your partner's feet apart and, holding their heels, step back through their legs. Now rest for a moment, in the knees to chest pose featured previously.

Close-up on the fix
To fix this pose, place one of your hands over the other on the recipient's feet and lean your body weight down on to the feet.

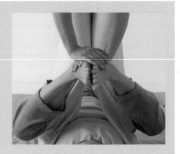

The Bridge

Do not be daunted by this pose. It benefits all body types (but avoid in cases of spinal injury). It opens the chest and the front of the hips, invites deeper breathing and stimulates the spine and sen sumana. It also boosts kidney function, helping to detoxify the body.

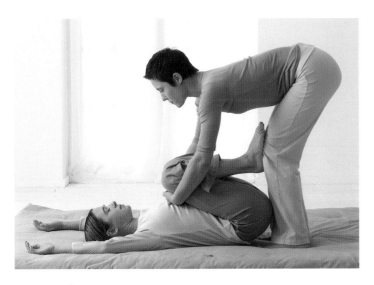

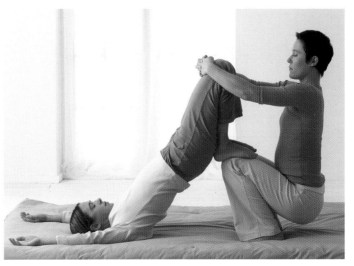

1 Position yourself as in the knees to chest pose and walk your feet as close as possible to your partner's buttocks. Make sure your knees are together and your feet are wide, creating a strong, pyramid-shaped base. Clasp your hands firmly around the fronts of their knees. This is your hold. Remember that you are using your body weight rather than your strength. Work with your breath to support your movements.

2 Sink your knees into your partner's feet and draw their knees up and over towards you as you squat down. Encourage your partner to go with the movement, without actually being active in it, by exhaling as they come up. Remember to squat rather than sit, otherwise you won't be able to stand up again. Enjoy the position. Check that your shoulders are relaxed and your chest is open. If you wobble, continue to hold the knees and don't let go. To release, ask your partner to drop their hips as you straighten up: this will give you the momentum to stand. Repeat three times.

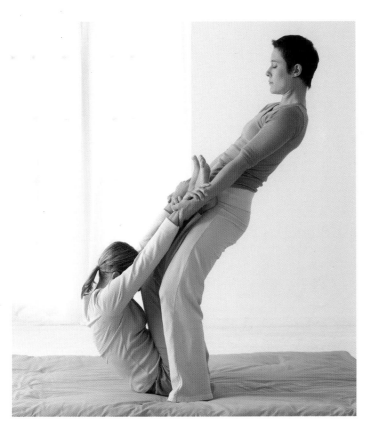

Forward Fold

This is a lovely counter-pose for all the deep stretches and back bends and is suitable for most body types. To protect your posture, use the power in your legs, rather than your back.

Left Rest your partner's legs up against your lower body. Depending on your height, their legs will stay together or will rest either side of your hips. Clasp each other's wrists. Bend your knees and, exhaling, straighten your legs and lean back, drawing your partner's upper body towards you. Their hips should stay on the floor. If they feel stiff in the backs of their legs, ask them to bend the knees slightly. Release their weight back down to the mat and repeat the pose three times.

Technique improver

This double leg sequence shows the direct relationship between the yoga tradition and the passive stretches used in Thai massage. Doing this will show you how your own body responds in these postures, which in turn will help you move your partner's body with more sensitivity and awareness. Try a variety of poses for yourself to feel how different shapes affect your body. Notice how moving with the breath can increase the feeling of release in your body.

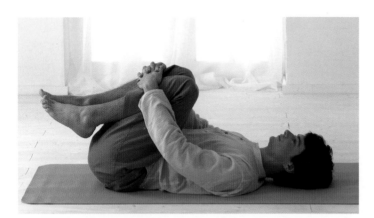

1 Knees to chest pose Lie flat on the floor with your knees bent. Bring your feet off the floor, allowing your knees to fall towards your chest. Try to keep the whole length of your spine in contact with the mat, using the weight of your arms and hands to draw your knees closer in towards you. Now relax your thighs completely and breathe. Take time to enjoy the feeling of your lower back and pelvis gradually broadening and sinking into the ground.

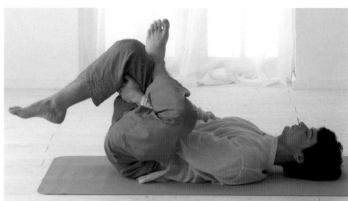

2 Crossed leg stretch From the previous position, place one foot down on the mat and let the other foot rest across your bent knee. Allow your knee to drop out to the side. Inhale and reach your hands up through the gap in your legs to clasp around the back of your bent knee. Now exhale and relax your upper body back down on to the floor. You should feel a stretch along the back of the crossed thigh and buttock. For a deeper stretch, use your elbow as a lever to encourage your knee to drop out further. Do not force anything. Hold the stretch for a few breaths, then release the leg and repeat on the other side.

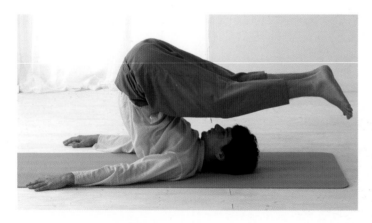

3 Halasana: the plough Start with your knees bent and your feet flat on the floor. Your arms should be alongside your body, palms down. Now bring your knees in towards your chest. Press your palms down into the floor and extend your legs up and over your head. If they start to shake, bend them a little. Once in position, let the weight rest on your shoulders, not on your neck. To release, unfurl the spine slowly back on to the floor. Don't attempt this pose if you have a spinal injury, disc problems or neck problems.

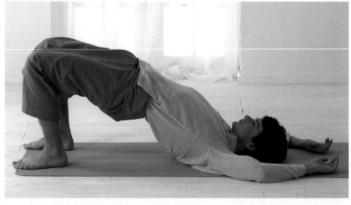

4 Setu bandhasana: the bridge Begin with your knees bent and feet flat on the floor, hip-width apart. Place your arms above your head, with your elbows slightly bent, feeling the whole of the back of each arm fully in contact with the floor.

Work in harmony with your breath, using it to give the pelvis the momentum to lift slightly off the floor. Exhaling, sink the soles of your feet into the ground and feel your knees move slightly away from you. On the next exhalation, use the power in your legs to elevate your pelvis a little higher off the ground. Be careful not to push or pull too much in the buttocks or front of the hips. Keep your feet, knees and hips in alignment.

To release, slowly sink your weight back down to the ground and rest before repeating the exercise two or three times.

Advanced pose – the assisted bridge

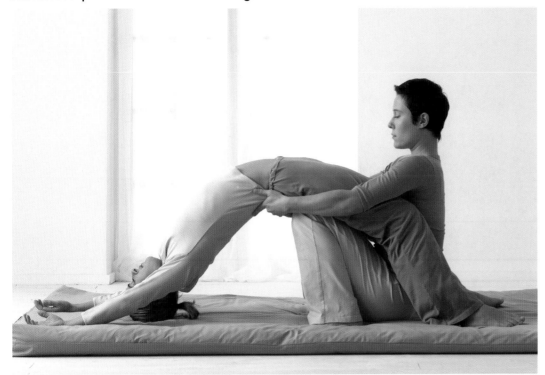

Left The assisted bridge pose is an advanced exercise that illustrates how Thai massage correlates directly with yoga asanas. This pose provides a deep opening for the front of the hips and a sense of expansiveness through the chest and upper back. Given passively, as part of a Thai massage, it gives the receiver a wonderful sense of freedom throughout their body. Remember, you will only be able to attempt poses like this once you are well-versed, and following the guidance of an experienced teacher.

Review: Double Leg Exercises

Use the pictures below as a reminder of all the exercises featured in the double leg sequence. Remember that not all of the exercises are suitable for every kind of body type, so allow yourself to be selective, according to your partner's individual needs.

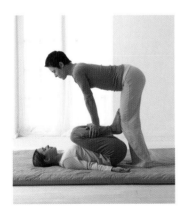

Knees to chest

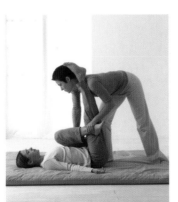

Crossed leg stretch

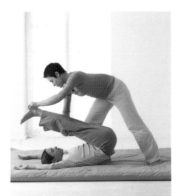

The plough

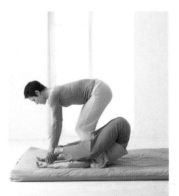

The frog

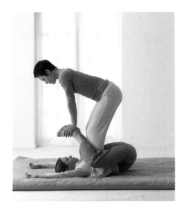

The butterfly

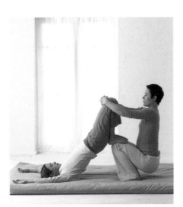

The bridge

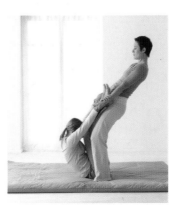

Forward fold

Caution

When giving double leg exercises, always be very careful to protect your back in order to avoid any strain. Remember that you should use the power in your legs, rather than your back, and keep your spine relaxed and free.

The Abdomen

As all ten sen pass through the abdomen, this is the energetic centre of the body. It is also the centre where we digest and process not only the food that we eat but also all of our experiences and emotions. The abdomen is extremely responsive to changes in our emotional state, so we can assess how relaxed we are by tuning into our belly, learning to sense if it feels soft and yielding or hard and resistant. The more we can release tension here, the more we can let go of tension throughout the whole of the body.

Working the abdomen stimulates a sluggish digestion and eases constipation. It encourages deeper breathing into the lower part of the lungs and helps to quieten and relax the entire body. It releases stiffness and tension in the lower back, ideal for back pain sufferers who find it too uncomfortable to lie on their front to receive a back massage. Repeated energy work to the abdomen can provide much-needed relief to the lower back.

Getting it right

☑ Work with the rhythm of your partner's breathing. If you have difficulty hearing or feeling it, ask them to breathe more deeply and audibly, but without forcing the breath.

☑ Many people are unused to having their abdomen massaged and may be sensitive. Approach with care and ask your partner to tell you what feels comfortable.

☒ Don't work this area of the body if there is any acute abdominal pain or if your partner has had any abdominal surgery in the last two years.

☒ Don't work on a full stomach: it is advisable to wait at least two hours after a meal.

Technique improver

Feeling the movement of the breath in your own body will help you to gain another level of sensitivity for giving abdominal massage. It is also a very effective way to relax your whole being, both physically and mentally. As you breathe in and out the belly expands and contracts.

When massaging the abdomen, you are simply following the natural rise and fall of the belly, helping to accentuate this movement for deeper relaxation. Repeat this exercise a few times until you feel familiar with how working with the breath can release tension in the belly.

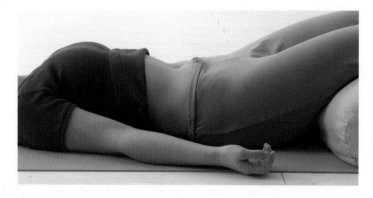

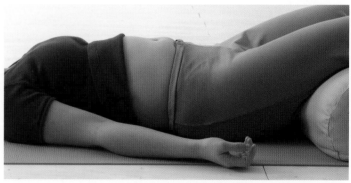

1 Lie on the floor with your knees bent; you may want them supported in some way. Close your eyes and listen quietly to the flow of your in- and out-breath. Rest one hand on your belly and notice how your hand moves up and down as you breathe in and out. Don't worry if you can't feel anything at first: tuning into the breath can take a little time.

Inhale normally and, as you exhale, draw your belly muscles in towards your spine, so that your abdomen is completely sucked in. Suck it as far in as it will go and empty your lungs completely.

2 Pause slightly at the end of the exhalation. When you need to inhale, do nothing except let go of your belly muscles. The belly will inflate of its own accord, like a balloon, and the in-breath will be sucked into the body, filling the lungs completely.

Repeat for at least five breaths, then relax. Let yourself breathe normally, noticing any differences in your body.

Relaxing the Abdomen

Make yourself really comfortable here, or your partner will pick up on the tension through your hands. Sounds from your partner's belly are to be welcomed, as they indicate movement of energy and a release of tension.

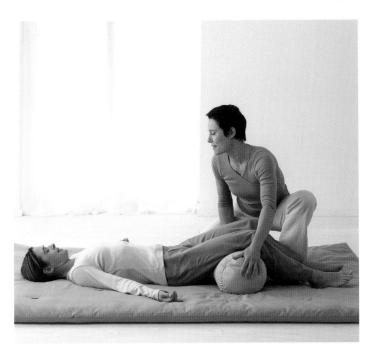

1 Getting comfortable The position of your partner is very important. As a rule, the knees should be bent up, to help the front of the body to relax more fully. This is especially important for women as it also protects the ovaries. Put a couple of pillows, a rolled-up blanket or a yoga bolster under the knees.

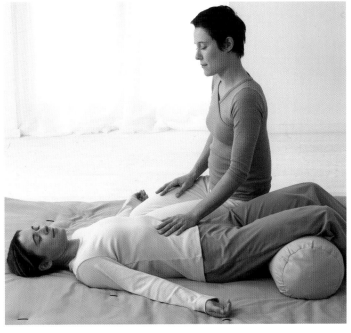

2 Tuning in Sit close in to the side of your partner. In this position you can listen to your partner's breath, noticing how fast or slow, deep or shallow it is. Allow your body to settle and become aware of your own breathing. Now place a relaxed hand on the belly. Let the weight of your hand rest without actively applying any extra pressure.

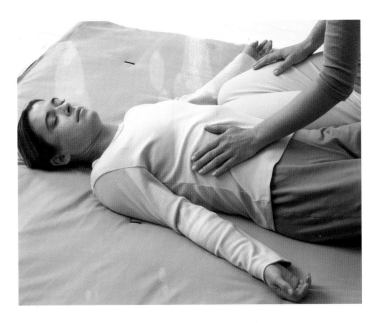

3 Relaxing circles This initial movement is superficial. Simply make circular clockwise motions across the surface of the abdomen. Work slowly and smoothly, with broad general strokes.

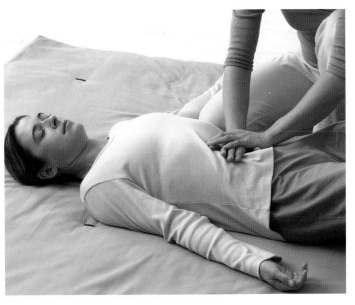

4 Making waves This movement is a little deeper. It's very relaxing and can be used at any point in the abdominal massage. Place hand over hand and work into the soft fleshy area between the ribcage and the hip. The heel of your hand and the flats of your fingers should move in an undulating wavelike motion across the belly.

Working the Abdomen

Traditional Thai massage work on the abdominal area involves working with energetic pressure points. The skill that you are aiming to develop here is to coordinate the pressure that you exert with your partner's breath. The idea is that you sink in as they exhale and then release as they inhale.

When working this part of the body, one good approach is to start with a round of palming, and then follow this with a round of deeper pressure, using the flats of your fingers. Finish off by palming the points again. If the belly is extremely sensitive or tense, your partner may not feel able to take the deeper pressure – if this is the case, then simply repeat the palming.

Right Do not suddenly start work on the abdomen (or on any other part of the body for that matter) without any preliminaries. Before starting your abdominal massage work, make the all-important initial contact by placing a relaxed hand on your partner's belly.

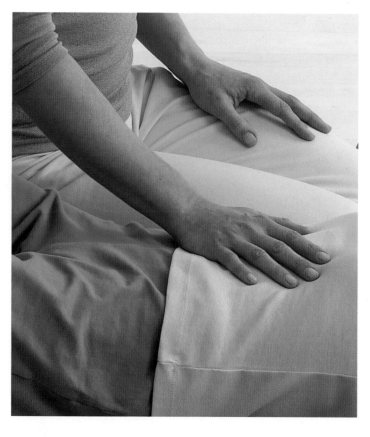

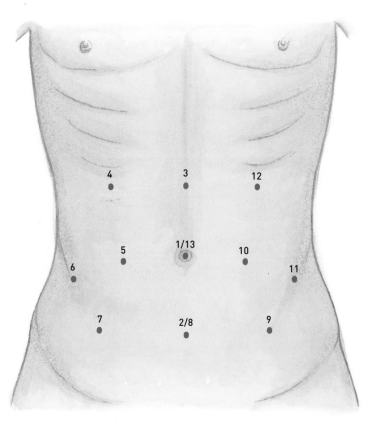

USING PRESSURE POINTS ON THE ABDOMEN

Key to the pressure points
1/13 navel and intestines
2/8, **5**, **7**, **9**, **10** intestines
3 stomach and solar plexus
4 liver
6 and 11 kidneys
12 spleen and stomach

Left This artwork shows the pressure points to be worked for an abdominal massage. For sluggish digestion or constipation, work clockwise, as this follows the natural direction of the digestive system and encouraging this movement will help to stimulate elimination. Use the flats of your fingers in a circular rubbing motion and work the points in this clockwise order: 1, 2, 7, 6, 5, 4, 3, 12, 10, 11, 9.

For a general relaxing stomach massage, begin at point 1, then go to point 3, and then follow the numbers round, but this time working anticlockwise.

Palming and Thumbing the Abdomen

Remember when pressing to use the flats of your fingers – don't dig in sharply with your fingertips. Communication with your partner is especially important here as this can be a very sensitive area of the body for many people.

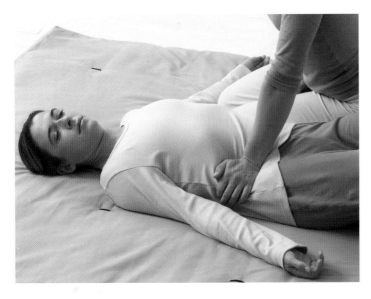

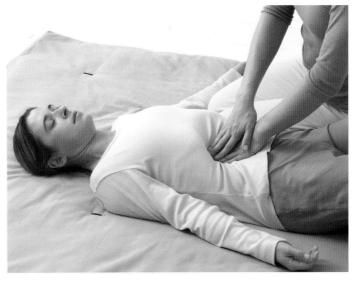

1 Palming Check that your arms are straight, but not locked, and your shoulders are relaxed. Sink your body weight down through the heel of your hand. If the belly yields, don't be afraid to sink all the way in; just check that the pressure suits your partner. If the abdomen is feeling very sensitive, work more lightly.

2 Finger pressing For a more focused pressure, use the flats of your fingers. For greater control and a deeper workout, place one hand on top of the other. Work in the same way as for the palming, sinking your body weight down through the flats of the fingers.

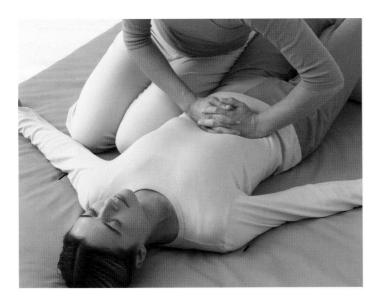

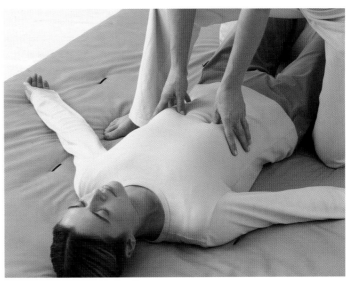

3 Wind release This is an optional exercise that is very effective for releasing trapped gases in the abdomen. Clasp your fingers together and take your elbows wide. The action is a scooping movement. Begin just below the ribs and work down with several scoops until you can feel the pubic bone against the sides of your fingers.

4 Thumb points For this exercise, overstep the body in a half-kneeling position. Focus on the six points that run either side of the belly button. Work points 4 and 12 simultaneously, then points 5 and 10, then points 7 and 9. On your partner's exhalation, sink your thumbs in slowly, pause for the inhalation and work slightly deeper on the next exhalation. You can work surprisingly deeply, so long as you maintain a slow, smooth rhythm in and out. Take time for at least three breaths in each position. Complete with some gentle belly circles.

The Chest

The routine shown here works with your partner's natural breathing rhythm, helping to open the lung cavity and encourage deeper breathing. It also directly stimulates sen sumana – the central energy line that runs up through the core of the body, incorporating the spinal column and all the chakras. This line not only affects the mechanical workings of the ribcage and lungs but also links directly with the energetic heart centre of the body. Be aware that although the techniques are simple, they can have a powerful effect on your partner.

Chest Routine

These exercises help to protect against coughs, colds and lung and throat infections, as well as stimulating the immune system as a whole.

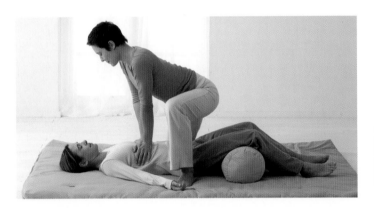

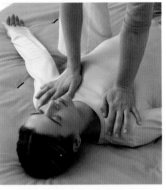

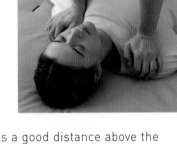

1 Palming the chest Overstep your partner's body and make sure that you can drop your weight down directly over the ribcage. Keep your arms straight and your shoulders relaxed. Place your hands on the ribs well below the nipples. Allow your partner's ribs to expand as they inhale; when they begin to exhale, sink into the ribcage, following the breath out as far as your partner will allow. Now repeat the exercise about two or three times.

2 (above left) Place your hands a good distance above the nipples. Palm in and out, following the breath. Take more care with women with larger breasts, as this area can feel quite sensitive.

3 Shoulder nest (above right) Find the "nest" (bowl-shaped dip) just inside each shoulder joint. Place the heel of the hand gently into this dip and sink in and out two to three times.

Getting it right

✗ Don't press directly on the area around the nipple.

✗ Never push or force the breath out, or hold beyond your partner's natural limit. The chest and ribcage area can hold a lot of tension, so approach it with sensitivity.

✓ Work slowly and smoothly: it is important to maintain an even rhythm as you move in and out of the postures.

✓ Make sure that you are comfortable, as a comfortable posture will enable you to listen with greater sensitivity to the responses of your partner's body.

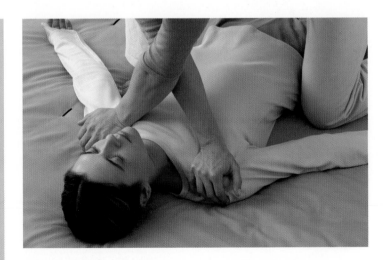

4 Crossing the shoulders Now cross your arms so that the opposite hand sits in the nest. As you sink your body weight in, sense a feeling of opening up the chest widthways.

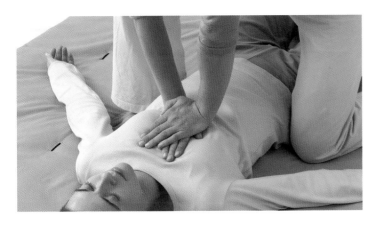

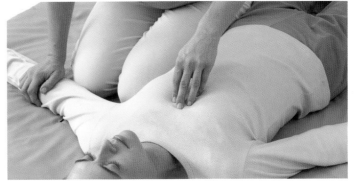

Variation to sternum press – sternum circles

5 Sternum press Place hand over hand across the centre of the sternum (breastbone). Make sure that your fingers are slightly out to the side so they don't press against the throat. Be equally careful not to press too low, as there is a fragile piece of cartilage at the base of the breastbone. Work with the breath. Repeat three times.

Above If step 5 feels too strong, use circles as an alternative. Position your first three fingers so the middle one presses on the sternum and the outer two work into the small pockets between the ribs, close to the bone. Make firm circles with the flats of your fingers, working from the base of the sternum up towards the throat.

Review: Abdomen and Chest

Use the pictures below as a reminder of the abdomen and chest exercises. Take time to feel comfortable with the steps for each body section before linking sequences for different sections together.

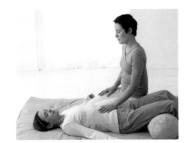

Tuning in

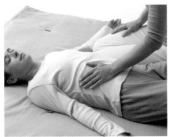

Relaxing circles

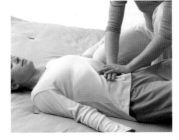

Making waves

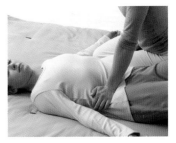

Palming the belly

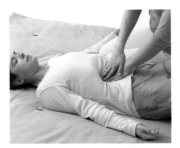

Pressing the belly

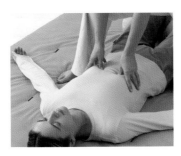

Thumb points

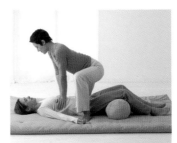

Palming the chest

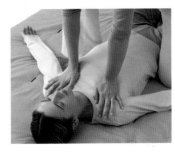

Palming the chest

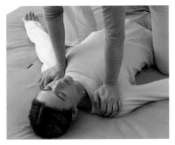

Shoulder nest

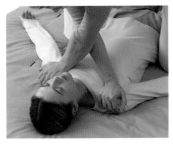

Crossing the shoulders

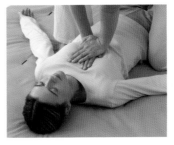

Sternum press

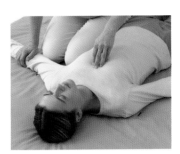

Sternum circles

The Arms

We use our arms to express what we want in life. We reach out and draw towards us what we love, or we hold back and push away things that are harmful to us.

Having stimulated the energy flow up through the abdomen and chest, you can now continue to unblock the flow along the arms, providing an enormous sense of release in the upper body.

After what can be emotional work on the abdomen and chest, working the arms (and the hands, which we will come to soon) can prove to be a fundamentally grounding experience for the receiver.

SEN KALATHARI

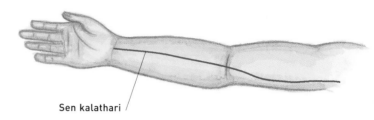

Sen kalathari

Above There are three sen that run through the arms. For beginners, it is best to focus on the central line, sen kalathari, which is shown here. Working this line has the most relaxing effect.

Working the Arm Lines

With this sequence of exercises, work the dominant arm and hand of your partner first, then move round to the other side of their body and repeat the whole sequence on their other arm.

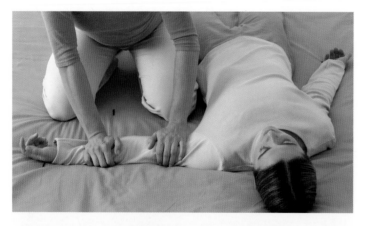

1 Palming the arm line Extend your partner's arm out to the side and palm up and down the inside of the arm, starting with one hand near the wrist and the other above the elbow. Palm in the same rhythmic fashion as with the leg lines, smoothly rocking the weight from one hand to the other. Check that your posture is relaxed and steady. Do one round of palming, then a round of thumbing. Palm the whole arm up and down to finish.

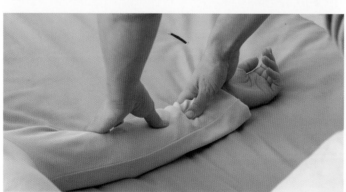

2 Thumbing the arm Thumb the lower and upper arm separately as they require slightly different techniques. Begin between the tendons just above the wrist and walk the thumbs alternately up to the elbow joint and back down again.

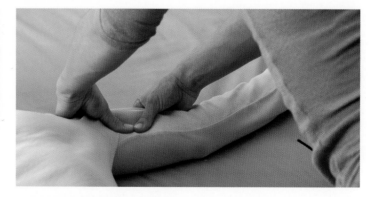

3 Thumbing the upper arm Use both thumbs simultaneously instead of the usual alternate pressure. Place the tips of your thumbs together and roll and squeeze the bicep muscle up, away from the bone. Use your fingers to give counter-pressure on the back of the arm. Start with your thumbs above the elbow and work up towards the armpit.

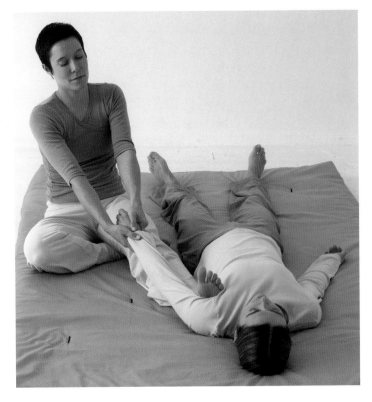

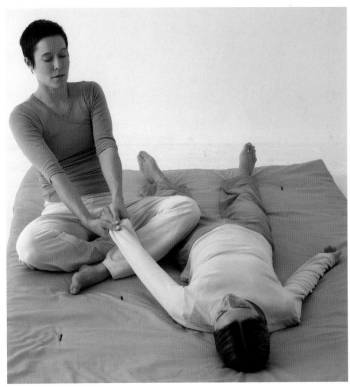

4 Arm stretch I Sit back, taking your partner's hand with you. Create space in their armpit in which you can fix with the sole of your foot. Hold the arm just above the wrist to protect the joint. Gently lean back into the stretch, then release. Repeat two or three times. This opens up the armpit and stretches the outside of the upper arm. Don't expect the body to move very much as it is a very contained stretch.

5 Arm stretch II This second stretch focuses on creating space between the shoulder and the ear, gently stretching the neck. Clasp firmly above your partner's wrist and lean away until you see their head roll slightly. Release the stretch slowly and let the head roll back. Repeat two or three times.

Technique improver

Of all the senses, our sense of sight is probably the most developed. When we are learning massage we often rely on what a pose looks like to judge whether or not we are getting it right. However, it is the quality of your touch that is important, so developing your sense of touch will add depth to your massage.

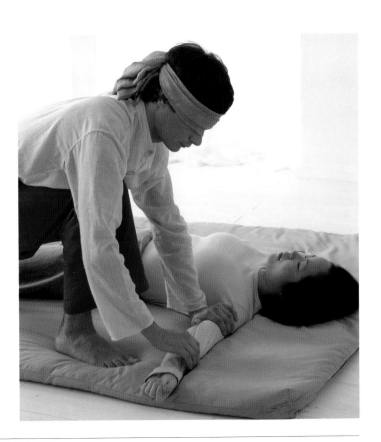

Right Covering your eyes, so that you temporarily remove your sense of sight, gives you an opportunity to explore working with touch alone. This is highly valuable, as it enables you to tune into the feeling in your hands. Palming the arm is a simple and safe place to start with the blindfold exercise, although of course you can eventually expand this practice to the whole of the massage.

The Hands

Our hands are incredibly dexterous, complex and strong structures that are constantly in motion and at work. Time spent focusing on the hands will enable you to work into all the joints and pressure points and will give a sense of completeness to the massage.

Small repetitive hand movements have become part of most people's daily lives, and can lead to repetitive strain injuries. Stimulating the acupressure points and creating space within the joints relaxes the hands and influences the flow of energy throughout the upper body. The sequence shown here is only a general guide – feel free to explore and play with what feels good for your partner.

Right This artwork shows specific acupressure points that can be worked on the hands in a Thai massage.

Getting it right

☒ Don't massage cut or bruised areas. Be careful of arthritic joints and don't massage when they are inflamed.

USING PRESSURE POINTS ON THE HANDS

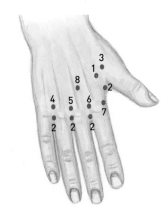
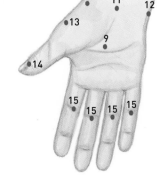

Key to the pressure points

BACK OF THE HAND:

1 hegu point, for all kinds of pain

2 and 3 headache and toothache

4 sciatica and hip pain

5 sore throat and toothache

6 tension in neck

7 shoulder pain

8 tension in neck, shoulder and arm, plus migraine and various stomach pains

PALM OF THE HAND:

9 heatstroke and nausea

10 asthma, plus pain in chest, back, shoulder and wrist

11 wrist pain and arm paralysis

12 insomnia

13 coughs, asthma, fevers, sore throat and tendon problems

14 sore throat, fevers, fainting and respiratory problems

15 whooping cough and arthritis of the fingers

Working the Points on the Hands

Like the feet, the hands have specific acupressure points to focus on. For a general relaxing massage use the outline below, then for specific conditions you can focus on working particular acupressure points.

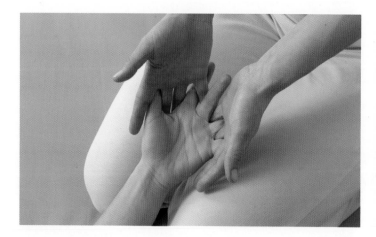

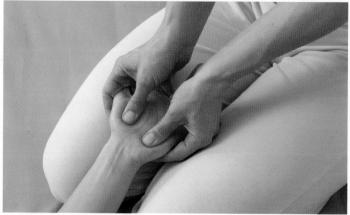

1 Palm opener Sit comfortably and let your partner's hand and wrist rest in your lap. Turn your hands palms up and slide your fingers between your partner's, leaving their middle finger free. Use the resistance of your fingers against the back of their hand to open their palm.

2 Stroking the palm Using your thumbs, firmly stroke from the wrist down to the centre of the palm. Use your fingers at the back of the hand as counter-pressure. Most people find this very relaxing, so work here for as long as your partner likes, exploring the whole palm with your thumbs.

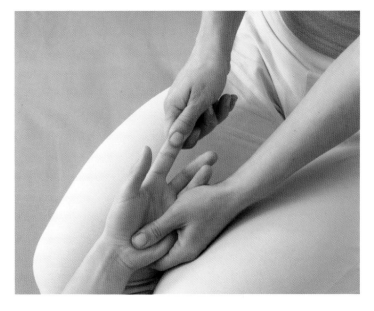

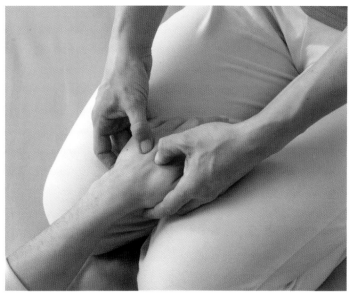

3 Finger squeeze This exercise creates space in the finger joints and relieves and enlivens stiff, tired fingers. Firmly hold the palm of your partner's hand in place and use your thumb and forefinger to rotate around all the joints of each finger, working from knuckle to tip and squeezing and lengthening each finger in turn.

4 Opening the back of the hand Turn the hand over and work as you did the top of the feet. You can stimulate the many points on the back of your partner's hand by working in between the tendons. Use your thumbs to massage firmly from the wrist up towards the knuckles, giving a gentle pinch to the webbing between the fingers.

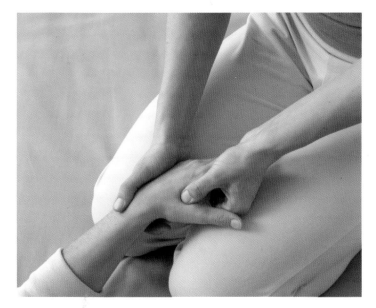

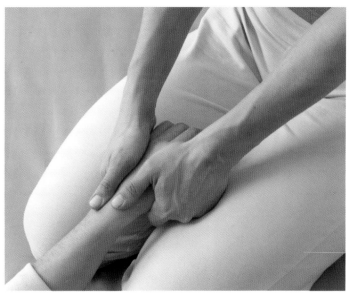

5 Hegu point To locate this point, turn your partner's hand slightly on its side. Go right up into the webbing of the hand and come away from the joint slightly. Angle towards the finger joint. Pinch firmly with thumb and forefinger for maximum effect – if it feels painful you've hit the spot. Encourage your partner to breathe. For a relaxing massage you can rub around the area, but for therapeutic use, work with very strong pressure and hold for as long as possible before releasing. The feeling should be one of a good pain, which eases as soon as you ease off the pressure. Now repeat several times.

6 Kneading hands This is a very relaxing movement so explore and enjoy it. You can work the hands in a slow pulsing, squeezing movement from the wrist towards the fingertips. Use your hands alternately or simultaneously.

Caution
The hegu point is used in Chinese medicine as a natural painkiller and powerful detoxifier. Often called the Great Eliminator, it is specifically good for headaches and toothache. Never use during pregnancy, due to its strong eliminating effect.

Opening the Wrists

The wrists are extremely sensitive, much-used joints that often suffer from compression and strain. These exercises bring a wonderful feeling of freedom and release to the wrists.

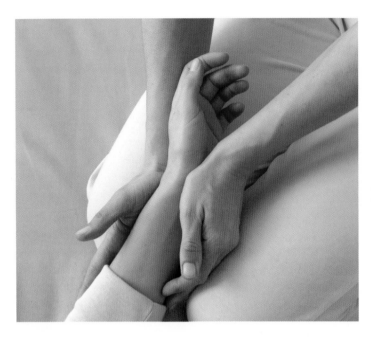

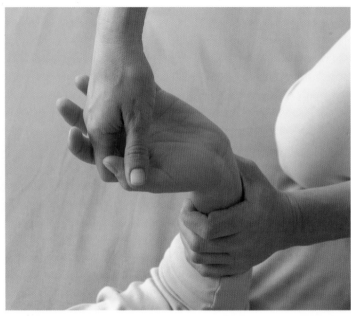

1 Wrist rub Hold your partner's wrist between the heels of your hands and let their hand relax completely. Rub your hands together, letting their fingers flop back and forth as you do so.

2 Opening the wrists The wrists are often restricted in their movement because the forearms are tight, so this exercise focuses on opening the wrists and the forearms simultaneously. With one hand on the forearm, press your partner's elbow down into the mat. Place the fingers of your other hand between their fingers and lengthen their fingers away, creating space throughout the front of the wrist.

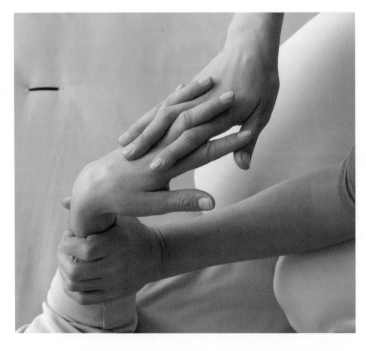

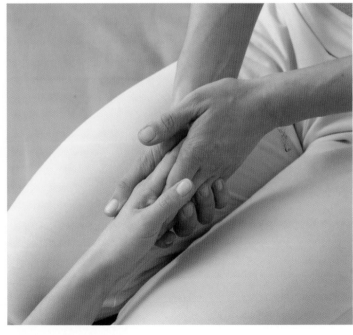

3 Maintaining a feeling of length through the palm, take the fingers over to the other side and stretch open the back of the wrist and the back of the forearm. Repeat gently back and forth three times.

4 Hold and sweep To finish the hand massage, hold your partner's hand between yours and sweep firmly from the wrist to the fingertips. Repeat several times.

Review: Arms and Hands

Now repeat the whole arm and hand sequence on the other side of the body, using the pictures below as a reminder. As before, make sure that you are confident about working this part of the body before moving on.

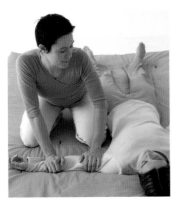

Palming the arm

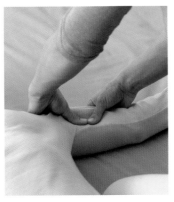

Thumbing the arm

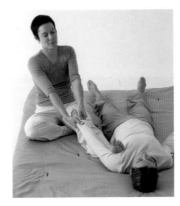

Arm stretch I

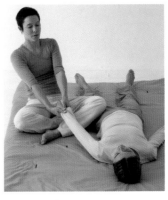

Arm stretch II

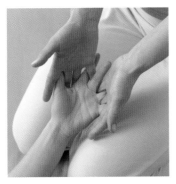

Palm opener

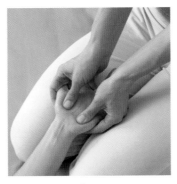

Stroking the palm

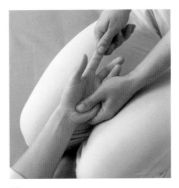

Finger squeeze

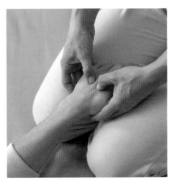

Opening the back of the hand

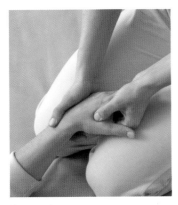

Hegu point

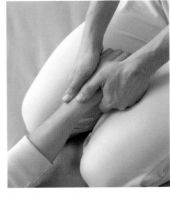

Kneading hands

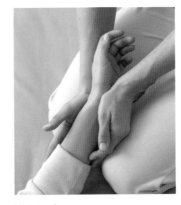

Wrist rub

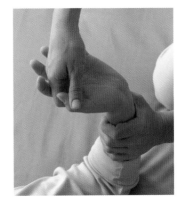

Opening the wrists

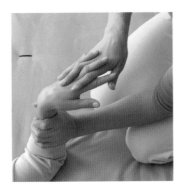

Opening the wrists

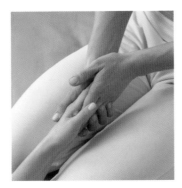

Hold and sweep

Working the hands

Don't skimp on the hand routine as this part of the body is so important. Also, always make sure that you work right to the very tips of the fingers.

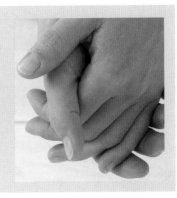

The Side of the Body

Working with your partner's body in the side position has many benefits. It is so versatile that you can in fact give a full-body Thai massage with your partner lying on their side. It is a very comfortable position for anyone who suffers from back problems, as you can use cushions against the belly and under the bent knee to provide full support for the body.

WORKING THE LEGS

In the side position you can complete the palming of the leg lines by working on the line that you couldn't reach when your partner was lying on their back – the third outside line. You could, of course, palm all of the leg lines in this side position, but for a beginner to Thai massage, most lines are easier to locate when your partner is lying on their back.

Working the third outside line of the leg is especially beneficial for people who are suffering from lower back pain, and there are also several powerful acupressure points around the hip joint itself. Worked therapeutically, these points are extremely effective at releasing tension held deep inside the hip joint and in the lower back area.

Practise your massage technique by working the leg in two halves to begin with – first the lower leg and then the upper. This will save you from changing your posture too much and from therefore breaking your rhythm.

THE THIRD OUTSIDE LEG LINE

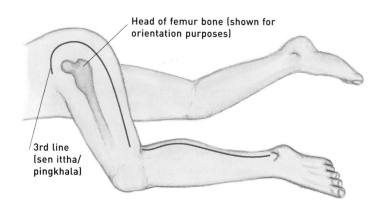

Head of femur bone (shown for orientation purposes)

3rd line (sen ittha/ pingkhala)

Above This artwork shows the position of the third outside line, which runs from below the ankle joint up to the hip joint.

Left This advanced Shiva pose, named after a well-known yoga asana (position), shows how we can involve the hands and feet to open up the body. Advanced poses must only be done once you have considerable experience, under the guidance of a fully qualified teacher.

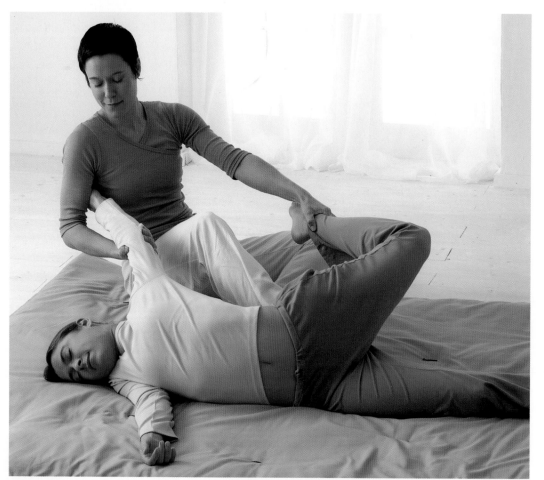

Getting it right

☑ Always check carefully for varicose veins, or ask your partner if they have any, before you begin your massage routine on this part of the body. Never work directly on varicose veins – just massage the area above them.

Working the Third Outside Line

Notice that you palm this line in a slightly different way to the other leg lines. Use the same slow, rhythmic rocking movement, but keep one hand on your partner's hip for support while your other hand palms up and down the leg, from the ankle to the hip.

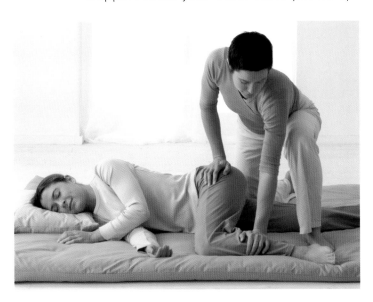

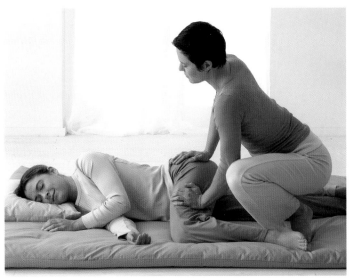

1 Palming the third outside line Begin by palming the lower leg. Your posture is important here: half-kneel and overstep your partner's outstretched leg as this will give you better scope to palm the whole line without having to move around too much. Start just below the anklebone, in the small dip above the Achilles tendon. Work up to the knee and then back down again.

2 To palm the thigh, simply lift your knee and swivel on the ball of your foot so that you are facing the top of the mat. Use your knee as a support for the arm that is doing the palming. In this way you can use the full power of your body weight more effectively. Start above the knee, in the hollow just above the large stringy tendon at the back of the knee. Palm up to the hip and back down again.

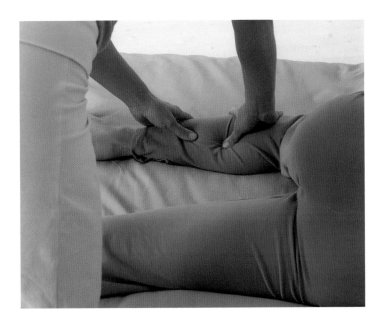

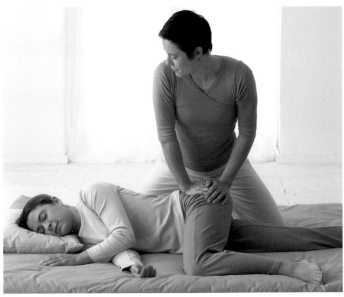

3 Thumbing the third outside line Again work the leg in two parts. Thumb from ankle to knee and back, and then from knee to hip and back. Thumb the line in the usual way, as for the rest of the leg lines. Work up and down and then complete the leg with a round of palming.

4 Hip points Change your posture to a wide kneel directly behind your partner's hip joint. Tuck your toes under so that your centre of gravity is up over their hip. Place hand over hand and, with the heel of your hand, circle firmly around the ball of the hip joint into the soft fleshy area. Palm firmly into areas where your partner feels that they need more attention. Bear in mind that for some people this area can be very sensitive.

The Shoulders and Neck

You will discover that the side position is a particularly effective one for helping to free up energy that has become blocked around the shoulders and the neck.

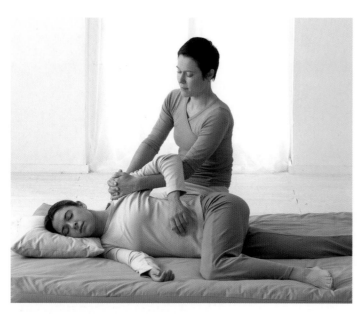

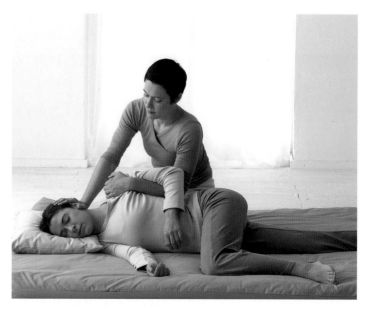

1 Shoulder circles This is an easy general movement that relaxes the neck and the whole of the shoulder joint. For very stiff people it helps to free up the chest area. Kneel behind your partner's shoulder blade and slide your body close up against their upper back. Circle your arm under theirs and clasp one hand around the front and one hand around the back of the shoulder. Make sure your partner's forearm is nice and floppy. Now slowly rotate the whole of the shoulder joint, drawing as big a circle as possible. Rotate several times in both directions.

2 Neck stretch Now that you have loosened the shoulder, this stretch will work deeper into the neck and up into the base of the skull. Keeping the front hand clasped around the top of your partner's shoulder, slide your other hand up the neck so that its heel rests against the occipital ridge at the base of the skull. Fix your hand here and lean away to create space between the shoulder and the ear. Check the pressure with your partner as it can be deceptively strong.

Shiva Pose

This mirrors the yoga pose, Natarajasana (Lord Shiva's pose). It gives a wonderful expansive feeling through the front of the body, opens up the front of the hip and belly and stimulates the sen in the front of the abdomen, as well as the spine and sen sumana.

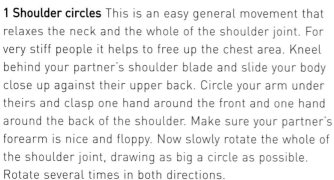

1 Kneeling behind your partner, reach forward and support their knee with your hand and their lower leg with your forearm. Keep your elbow wide, as if there is a circle emanating from your breastbone to your fingertips. This will help maintain the framework of the stretch. With your other hand, push yourself back to upright, using your partner's hip joint to support you.

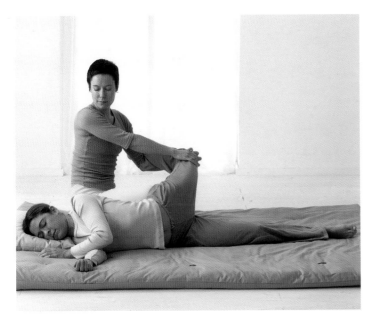

2 Raise your knee (keep the toes flat) and place into your partner's buttock. Clasp both hands around the front of their knee for support. To move into the stretch, sink your knee into the buttock and lean away with your upper body. Ease in and out of the stretch three times without undoing the pose totally. To end, keep a good support under their knee and circle the leg down to the floor.

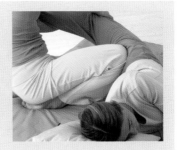

Step 2 positioning
Note the position of the masseur's knee and foot. This is a similar position to the knee lift featured in the physical preparatory exercises.

Variations to the Shiva pose

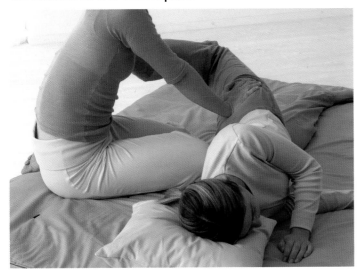

Above For a gentler stretch, use this alternative method. Kneel down and place your hand on your partner's buttock. Sink your hips down to one side of your feet. Keep your arm straight and lean into your hand, bringing the movement out through their thigh and knee. Continue the circle with their leg by leaning away with your other arm. Work to the point of resistance, then ease off. Repeat three times before releasing the whole posture.

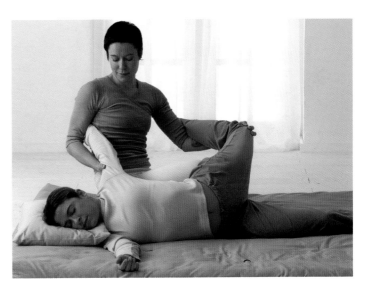

Above There are a large number of different variations of this pose within the Thai massage tradition. The one shown here adds a shoulder stretch, in order to open up the chest and the armpit.

Getting it right

✗ Don't do this exercise if your partner suffers from disc problems in their lower back or from lower back pain. Also, avoid it if your partner is much bigger and heavier than you.

✓ Make sure you are working with the breath, exhaling as you move deeper into the stretch.

✓ Ask whether the stretch is too strong – you can't see your partner's face to judge their reaction.

✓ You need to support your partner's body throughout so that they can stay very relaxed in the thigh and buttocks. Remind them to let the weight of their leg drop completely into your arm.

✓ Always keep your partner's knee in alignment with their hip joint. To maintain the correct angle, imagine that you are drawing a circle with their leg so that if the foot carried on round it would eventually reach the top of the head.

Technique improver

Practising Lord Shiva's pose improves your balance and is a useful way of getting a feel for the movement that your partner's body makes. However, avoid it if you suffer from a knee injury or lower back problems. The trick with this pose is to keep the hips level so your knee doesn't swing out to the side. If the knee does do this, it upsets the integrity of the posture and can put undue strain on this fragile joint: try to do it in front of a mirror so that you can see what your hips and knees are doing.

Right Stand with your feet hip-width apart and your weight evenly spread throughout each foot. Shift your weight gradually on to one foot. Bend your other foot up behind your buttock and catch it with your hand. Let the weight of the knee drop towards the floor so that the front of the thigh and hip begin to "undo".

Raise your opposite arm. Now press the front of your foot into the palm of your hand – this opens up the hip and thigh. Go only as far as feels comfortable. Breathe and feel a circle emanating from your belly through your thigh and knee and out through the tip of your toes. Keep this feeling of the circle in mind as you take your partner into the pose. Put the foot down and change to the other side.

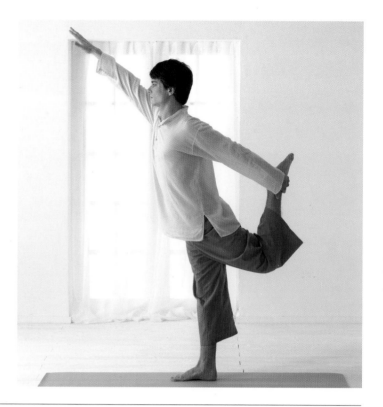

Open Spinal Twist in Side Position

When working in the side position, the recipient's body is totally at rest and so the effects of stretches can be maximized. Twists are a way of "undoing" the body and can provide a deep sense of release.

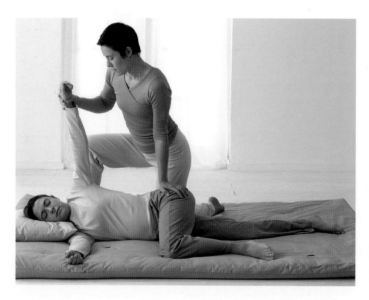

1 This good general spinal twist suits all body types, as you can work according to the level of your partner's flexibility. It releases tension through the entire back, opens the chest and ribs and stimulates internal organs. Half-kneel, level with your partner's torso. Fix one hand on their hip and ask them to inhale as you extend their arm upwards, creating space through the chest cavity. This preparation gives maximum length through the body, helping your partner release more fully into the final stretch.

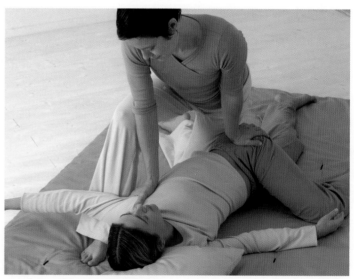

2 As your partner exhales, take their arm out to the side and let their head follow through. Keep one hand on their hip to fix the pose and, with your other hand placed above their armpit, gently stretch through their body. Don't worry if their arm doesn't touch the floor – it is better to start with the hip fixed and the arm slightly off the ground. Stay in this pose for three breaths, easing off as your partner inhales and deepening into the diagonal stretch as they exhale.

Advanced twist – the rag doll

Right Traditional Thai massage offers a wonderful variety of twists to invigorate, stimulate and release energy in the body – energy that often gets trapped in the body as deeply held tension. The rag doll position is an advanced, deep twist for flexible people. It gives a strong release in the lower part of the back and in the waist and is wonderful for stimulating the internal digestive organs.

As well as being very flexible, your partner has to feel completely relaxed before you attempt deep twists such as this. You yourself have to be very experienced. Getting into this pose is quite complex, so work under the guidance of an experienced teacher to achieve it in the safest way possible.

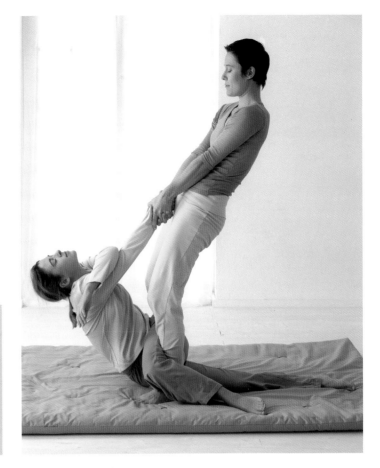

Getting it right

X Avoid twists with people who have spinal injuries or disc problems.

✓ Remember to work into the twist on an exhalation, working gently towards a deeper stretch.

Review: the Side of the Body

Now ask your partner to roll over and work through all the exercises on their other side, using the pictures below as a reminder. You may not want to repeat every exercise, depending on your partner's body type and needs.

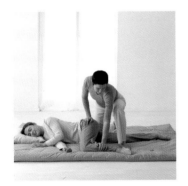

Palming third outside line

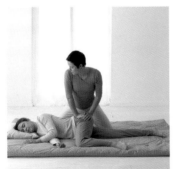

Hip points

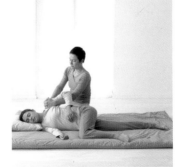

Shoulder circles

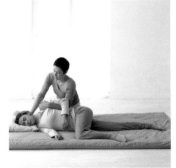

Neck stretch

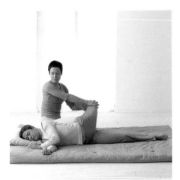

Shiva pose

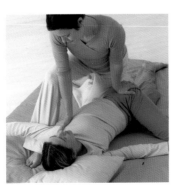

Open spinal twist

Caution

The stretches done with your partner in the side position involve working the back, neck and shoulders – all areas that are notorious problem spots and where even the fittest people can tend to hold tension. You must avoid dynamic stretches in these areas if your partner suffers from any injuries here – especially if they have a lower back condition. Also, watch out for varicose veins while working the outside line of the leg.

The Back of the Body

The back of the body is like a protective shell and is where we tend to habitually hold tension, often over many years. The massage sequence given over the following pages aims to soften this shell and re-integrate the energy previously held as tension, letting it flow freely through the body from the feet to the head.

The exercises directly influence the structure of the spine, which provides fundamental support for the whole skeleton. It works with deep layers of tension held around the spine, which can restrict the flow of energy and blood to the spinal nerves, with implications for the whole nervous system. Most people feel very relaxed lying on their belly, so this sequence provides a chance to consolidate the stronger work of the side position.

Below Thai-style palming done in this position is a very traditional way of working the back. Its beautiful contained shape shows how one body can support the other.

THAI MASSAGE AND BACK PAIN

Back pain is something that many of us suffer from to some degree during our lives. Many cases are not too serious and are the result of tight or aching muscles. However, back pain may be caused by injury, and one common spinal injury is a slipped or herniated disc. You may have experienced this for yourself or be massaging someone who has, so it can be useful to have a little understanding of what it involves.

The spine is a column of 26 vertebrae interspersed with discs, which are gel-like shock absorbers. The spine is healthy and flexible only if the discs remain healthy. Movement keeps the inside of each disc nourished with a good flow of blood, but if the spine is not used to moving in all directions, a disc can become weak. If it is then put under too much stress, it may become herniated: fluid leaks out of the disc membrane. When this happens at the back of the spinal column the

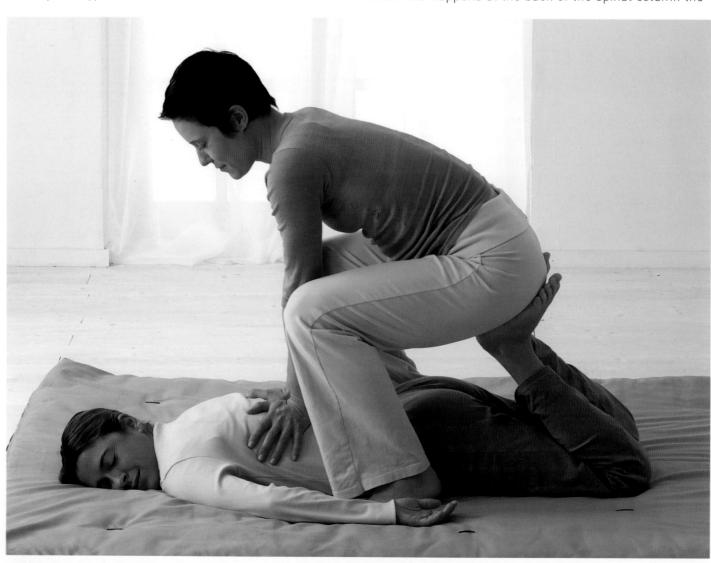

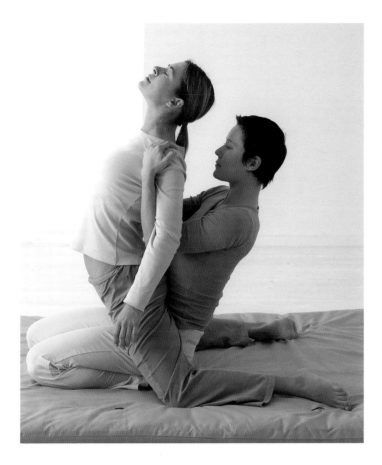

Getting it right

☒ Do not use stretches on those suffering from spinal injuries or disc problems. If you are in any doubt about the state of your partner's health following an injury or back problem, then you must consult an experienced physiotherapist or osteopath.

☒ Remember not to work directly on the bone itself.

☑ Work with the breath. It can be useful to remind your partner to focus on their breath. Work with a slow and smooth rhythm as you apply and release pressure. Sink with your body weight, don't push with your strength.

☑ Check the strength of the stretches and pressure with your partner as you will not be able to take cues from their facial expressions.

Left The King of Cobras is a beautiful pose, suited only to advanced practitioners and recipients, that shows the potential of a healthy back, allowing an opening all the way through the spinal column.

fluid presses on the spinal nerves, causing pain. It can also occur at the front of the spine. As there are no nerves here no pain is experienced, but the integrity of the body is still affected.

We need exercises that help prevent these weak areas from developing. We need to keep the joints in the spinal column well nourished with good blood flow and strong, healthy energy flow. This increased flow can come about only through movement, and Thai massage, with its emphasis on dynamic and passive movement, is very beneficial for maintaining a healthy spine.

SLIPPED DISCS
Avoid working on your partner's spine if they are suffering from, or have recently suffered from, a slipped (herniated) disc. The condition may take up to three months to heal, and during this time it is very important to avoid any movements that might aggravate the

situation. However, you can help to alleviate the discomfort and tension around the affected area by gently working the energy lines of the back. Work with your partner's permission and constant feedback.

MAKING YOUR PARTNER COMFORTABLE
Ensure that your partner is as comfortable as possible so that they are able to relax fully. Some people are unused to lying flat on their front with their arms down by their side, in which case you may need to provide a little extra support. A pillow or folded blanket under the chest or hips can help create more space through the upper spine so that the neck feels free. Support under the front of the ankles can alleviate any pressure or discomfort in the knees. If your partner suffers from a very weak or painful lower back then you may need to raise the feet slightly higher, again using some padding under the front of their feet.

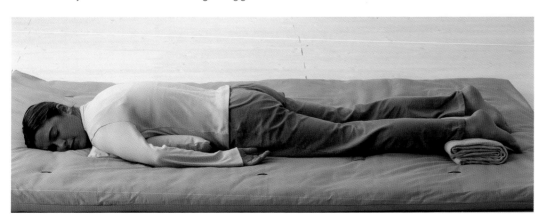

Left You may need to add extra support – with pillows or folded blankets for example – to ensure that your partner is totally comfortable and relaxed.

The Sequence for the Back of the Body

There are many different aspects to working the back of the body. As this is a long sequence, it is advised that you practise it section by section until you feel more confident about putting all of the aspects together. The initial section of the sequence focuses on additional work for the feet and ankles, before providing some gentle warm-up exercises for the legs and hips. The sequence then moves on to exercises that cover ways of working the energy lines of the back, as well as stretches that provide a deeper level of opening.

Integrating the Back of the Body

This exercise, like the ones that follow, acknowledges the all-important energetic and physiological connection between the feet, the legs and the back.

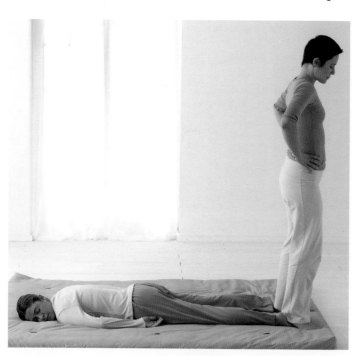

1 Walking on the feet This is very easy and very satisfying for your partner, but do not attempt it unless their heels fall comfortably out to the side with their ankles touching the mat. Facing away from your partner is easier – use a chair for support, if necessary. Stand with the front of your feet on the mat and place your heels on your partner's insteps. Shift your weight from side to side, as if you were walking on the spot. Check the pressure with your partner (most people love the sensation).

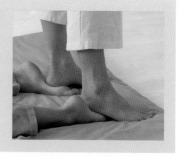

Step 1 foot position
Make sure that your heels are well away from the balls of your partner's feet – to avoid putting direct pressure on the joints.

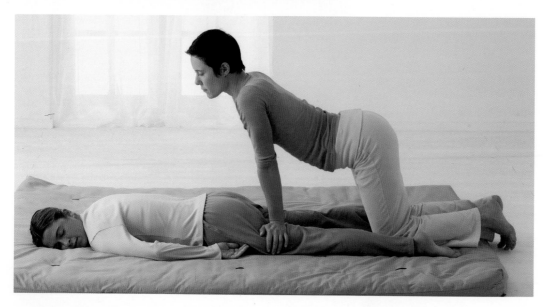

2 Palming the backs of the legs Palm both of the legs simultaneously. Work from the Achilles tendon directly up the legs until you feel the buttock bone. Ease off the pressure as you pass over the knees. This additional palming for the backs of the legs will help to relax both the hips and the lower back.

Feet to Sacrum

This exercise helps to open the lower back and works to lengthen through the front of the hips and into the thighs, as well as opening the ankle joints. Three variations are shown here for varying degrees of flexibility.

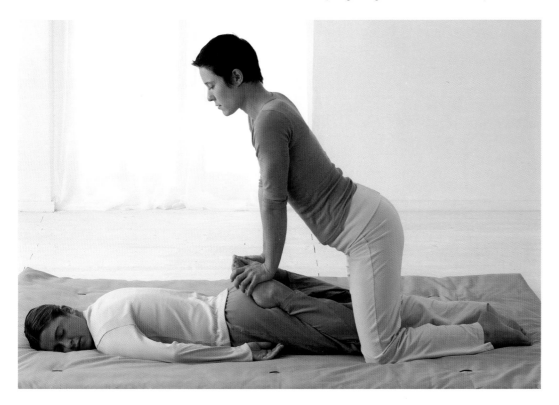

Pose 1 This is the main version, suitable for a wide range of people. Position yourself at your partner's feet. Take both their feet up towards their buttocks, and lengthen through the front of their toes. Keep your posture wide and your arms straight. Sink your body weight on to their feet so that their heels press in towards their buttocks.

Variation for less flexible people

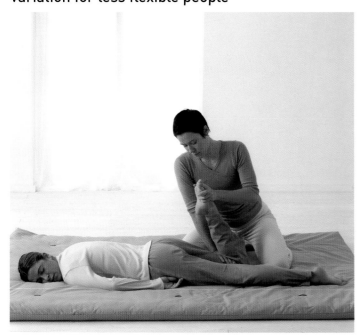

Pose 2 This version is for stiffer people who experience restriction through the fronts of the thighs or discomfort in the lower back. Kneel at the outside of the leg, facing sideways on to your partner. Place your upper hand behind the knee and take the front of the foot up and towards the buttock as far as it will go. Encourage your partner to remain relaxed and heavy in the front of the hips.

Variation for protecting the back

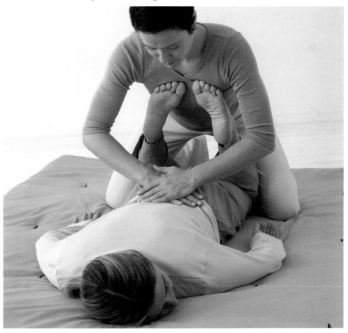

Pose 3 This pose lengthens the sacrum as you bring the feet in towards the buttocks, so it is ideal for those whose lower back needs protection and stability. Wide-kneel at your partner's feet. Lift up their feet to rest against your chest. Cup your hands over their sacrum, with your fingers pointing in and your elbows wide. As you lean forward with the feet, scoop the sacrum back towards you with your hands.

The Locust

In this pose, lengthen through the sacrum to create a deep opening into the front of the hip and thigh. The Locust can be a strong posture, so ensure that you work smoothly with the breath.

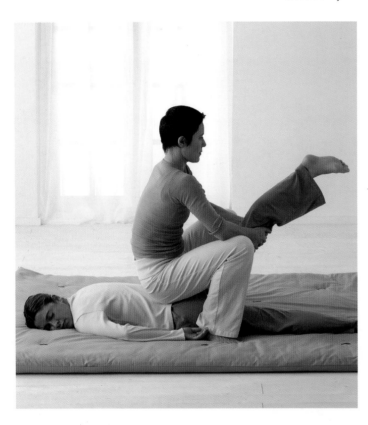

Left Squat lightly over your partner's hips, keeping most of your weight in your legs. Work one leg at a time. Cup your hands under their knee and firmly interlace your fingers, so that you have a good grip. Fix your tailbone against your partner's sacrum, then lift the knee off the ground and rest your elbows on your thighs. This is your lever and your fix in the pose.

To achieve the stretch, work on the exhalation. Make a scooping action with your hips to create length through the base of your partner's spine and lean back, lifting their knee up and away. Ease in and out two or three times, but without completely undoing the pose. Repeat the exercise with the other leg.

Getting it right

☒ Don't try this pose if your partner has a weakness in the lower back, or if they found feet to sacrum challenging. Do not attempt it if your partner is much bigger or heavier than you.

☑ As the pose can be quite strong, make sure you maintain a good level of communication with your partner.

Take a Break

This is a wonderfully relaxing pose for both you and your partner, as you can really enjoy using your body weight. The rolling action can be repeated for as long as feels good for your partner.

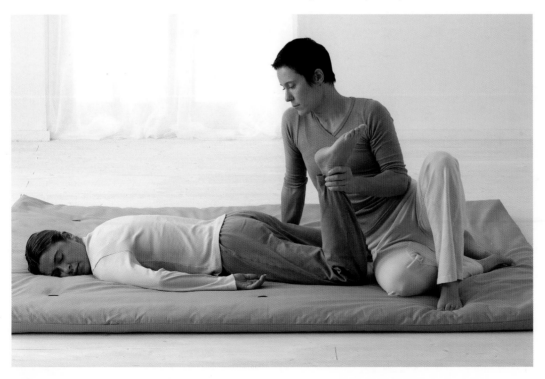

1 Get close to your partner. Bend their knee up and, with your lower hand, hold firmly around the ankle joint. Support yourself properly by placing your other hand on the floor.

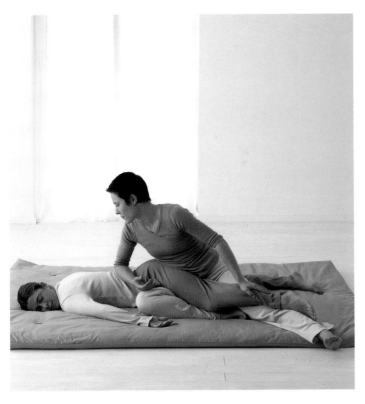

2 Catch hold under your partner's knee and lift their leg high so that you can slide your thigh all the way up under the front of their hip. Extend your lower leg to provide support for their calf. Fix your lower hand on their calf.

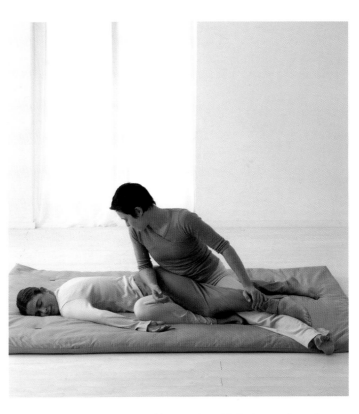

3 With your upper arm, roll over the thigh, buttock and lower back of your partner, using the fleshy part of your forearm. As you roll, keep your other hand securely on their lower leg, as shown.

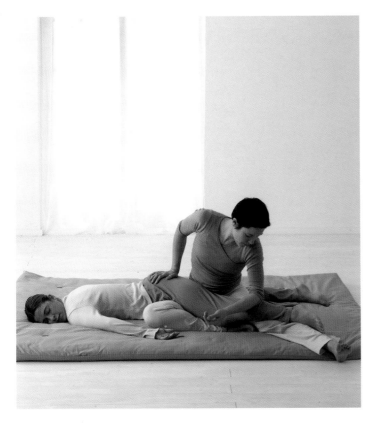

4 Now fix your upper hand on the hip and, using your lower forearm, roll away across the calf, working only on the fleshy part of the leg.

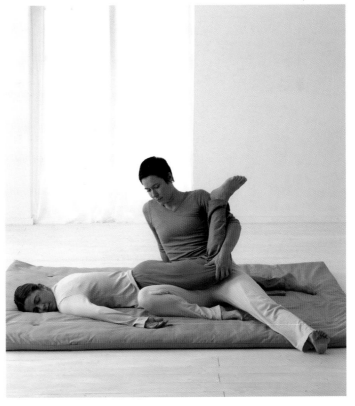

5 Your partner should be extremely relaxed by now, so ease your way out, causing the least disturbance possible. Support your partner's knee as you gently lift their thigh in order to slide your body out carefully. Repeat the exercise with the other leg.

Working the Energy Lines of the Back

Working the back lines is an important part of the massage as it affects the whole body. Sen sumana runs through the spinal column and is regarded as the location of the body's main chakras, or energy centres.

Two energy lines run up the back. Line 1 has two aspects: sen ittha, running up the left side of the body, and sen pingkhala, which runs up the right. To work line 1, begin just above the sacrum and apply pressure into the shallow dip either side of the spinal column. Line 2, sen kalathari, begins just above the hips, about a thumb's width out from line 1. You may notice a muscular ridge running either side of the spine. This is the pathway for line 2: work up and down this ridge.

YOUR POSTURE

To tune into your partner properly, you must establish a comfortable, stable working posture. Half-kneel astride your partner, with your hips in line with their back. Change legs as often as you need to. Depending on the length of your partner's back, you may need to adjust your pose several times in order to keep your centre of gravity directly over the area that you are working.

THE BACK LINES

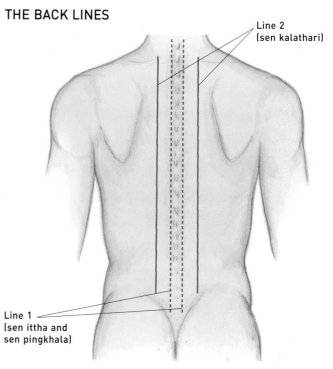

Above This picture shows the paths of the two sen, or energy lines, that are worked on the back.

Palming and Thumbing the Back Lines

Use exactly the same kind of slow and rhythmic rocking movement as for the leg and arm lines, but instead of working alternately, apply the pressure with both of your hands simultaneously.

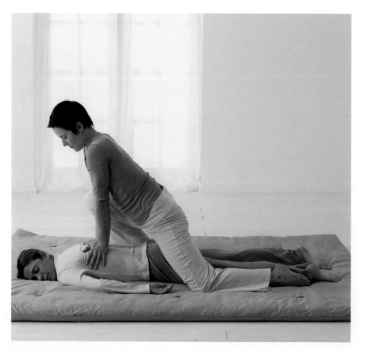

1 Palming the back lines A broad, general pressure on the sen deepens and slows the breath and prepares the body. To begin, place your hands lightly on your partner's back to get a feel for their breathing rhythm. As they inhale, let their ribcage expand under your hands and, as they exhale, sink (don't press or push) your body weight down through your arms and hands, helping to expel their exhalation. Reposition your hands and work with the breath up and down line 1. Repeat for line 2.

Line 1 hand position
Palm with the pressure coming down through the heel of your hand. Your fingers should be relaxed around the ribcage.

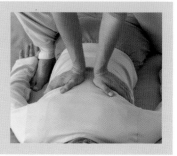

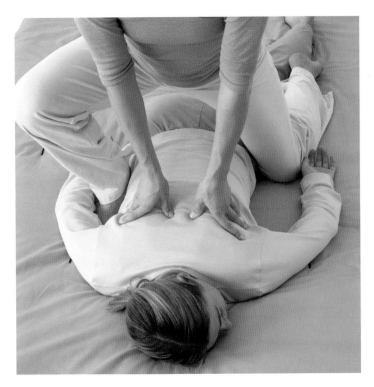

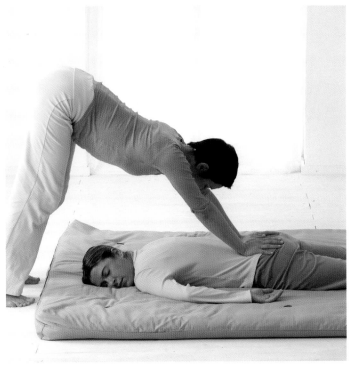

2 Thumbing the back lines Use your thumbs for a more focused deeper pressure on the sen. Start as for palming, but adjust your hand position so that you work with the flats of your thumbs. To support your thumbs, spread your fingers wide and align your thumbs with your wrists and shoulders. The position shown is for working line 1. Work with the breath, sinking your weight in and slowly releasing out. Thumb up and down lines 1 and 2, working from the base of the spine to between the shoulders. Finish with another round of palming.

3 Sacrum lengthener Get into a kneeling position above your partner's head and slide the heels of your hands down to their hipbones. This is your fix on the pose. As your partner exhales, lift up your hips. Enjoy a few breaths, feeling the opening of your own body as your partner enjoys the openness in theirs. This delicious stretch creates length all the way through the spine. It is particularly soothing for tired and tight lower backs.

Accessing the upper back

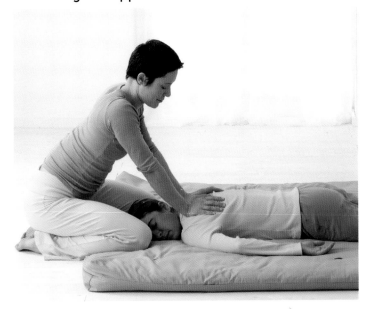

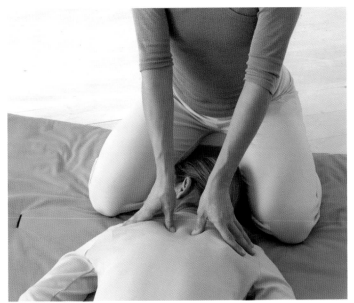

Above In order to work lines 1 and 2 effectively right up into the upper back, you will find that it is often easier and much more comfortable for you if you change your position. Wide-kneel above your partner's head and work your hands alternately, like a cat pawing in a relaxed way.

Above To thumb your partner's back lines much more easily, tuck your toes under, in order to raise your centre of gravity. Work with both of your thumbs either simultaneously or alternately – whatever feels best for you.

Dynamic Back Stretches

After you have warmed up the body thoroughly by working the two back lines and stimulating the flow of energy up and down your partner's spine, you can now move on to some more dynamic stretches to stimulate the back of the body. You'll see that the selection of stretching exercises that follow each involve some active lifting of your partner. When doing these stretches, remember to move into them sensitively and with awareness, using your body weight and breath to help you.

The Cobra

This energizing back bend stimulates the upper spine, chest and shoulders, while also encouraging deeper breathing. As the focus is on opening the upper back, the lower back should feel no discomfort.

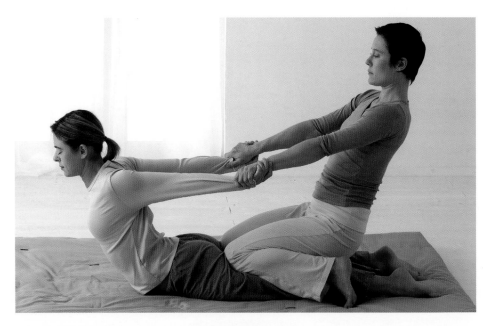

Left Make sure that your partner's toes are pointing inwards and their ankles outwards. Kneel gently on their thighs, keeping your feet outside their legs. Leave a space between your knees and your partner's buttocks so that they have enough room to come up fully into the pose. Ask them to place their forehead on the floor and to take hold around your wrists as you hold theirs.

Gently lean back, lifting their upper body off the ground. You can work on either the inhalation or the exhalation. The former gives a greater lift and opening through the front of the body; the latter gives more control and lengthens the spine more effectively. Explore which feels best for you and your partner. Work in and out of the posture three times, resting completely on the ground between stretches.

Variation to the pose

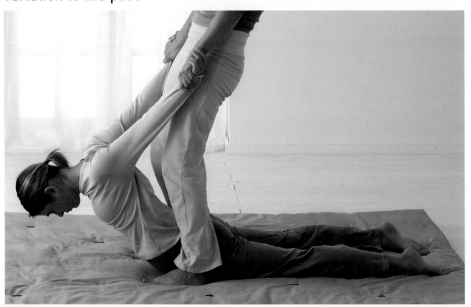

Left The shoulder lift This is a gentle alternative to the cobra for stiff or heavy people. Fix your feet very snugly against your partner's hips. Bend your knees, keeping your back straight. Hold on to each other's wrists. As you exhale, stand up using the power in your legs. Encourage your partner to let their arms and head relax. Repeat three times.

Cross-legged Forward Bend

This is a lovely counter-pose for the cobra position. Remember that you can alter the degree to which your partner's legs are crossed in order to stretch both of their hips to whatever level feels comfortable to them.

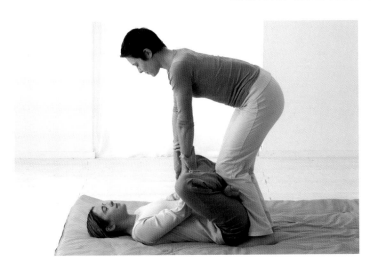

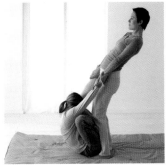

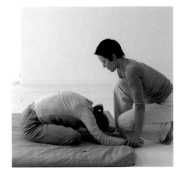

1 Ask your partner to roll on to their back and bring their knees up to their chest as if they were sitting cross-legged. Stand with your knees together and your feet wide, as close up against your partner's shins as possible. Make sure that their feet are crossed below your knees to fix the pose. Bend your knees and clasp around each other's wrists.

2 (above left) On the exhalation, straighten your legs and, leaning away, lift your partner's upper body off the mat. Keep your shoulders relaxed. Sink your knees inward slightly for a deeper stretch. Release your partner back down to the mat.

3 (above right) Repeat three times, but on the third stretch, step away with your feet and extend your partner's arms to rest on the mat in front of them. You can give them extra support here by placing a bolster or cushion underneath their upper body.

Percussion

The vibration of these percussive techniques penetrates deep inside the body. They are very invigorating for the energy system and have a grounding effect on the body. Keep your shoulders and wrists relaxed, and remember to avoid contact with the spine.

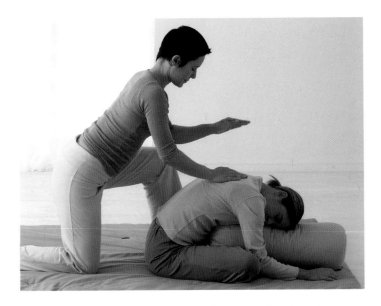

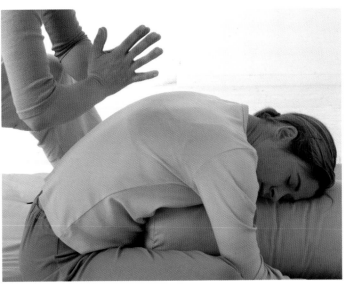

1 Cupping Make a shallow cup with each palm, keeping your thumbs tucked in and your wrists soft. Alternately cup up and down either side of the spine, experimenting to find a rhythm and speed that suits your partner.

2 Prayer hands "Glue" the heels of your hands together and imagine that the pads of your fingers are stuck lightly together. Keep your elbows wide and make a chopping action with your hands. Contact the body with the sides of your little fingers. You will know when you have it just right, as your fingers will make a very satisfying clacking sound.

Technique improver

Occasionally you may work with someone who is suffering from severe pain or acute sensitivity in their back and who is unable to receive any of the dynamic work or acupressure of traditional Thai massage. However, they may still benefit enormously from some hands-on therapy and there are alternative ways of working the energy lines of the back that are very soothing and effective – namely, using herbs and oils.

Traditional Thai medicine has several different aspects, of which physical massage is just one. Herbs are also used therapeutically, and in Thailand it is common to see herbal steam baths offered alongside Thai massage treatments. These baths are a wonderful way to complement the relaxing and detoxifying effects of a Thai massage.

Most of us do not have ready access to steam bath facilities. However, you can easily introduce herbal therapy in the form of compresses, for use during the massage. These compresses are very effective at helping to ease congestion and tension. Traditionally, each practitioner would make up a blend of herbs appropriate to an individual patient's condition, but a simple compress of something warming and stimulating such as ginger can be just as beneficial.

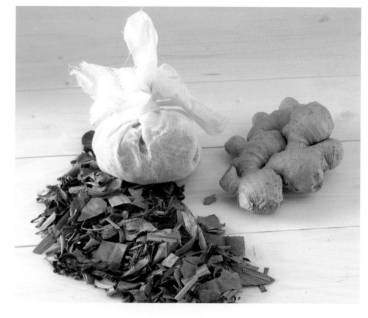

Above Preparing a ginger compress To make a simple compress, roughly chop plenty of fresh ginger into a pan and then add boiling water and let it simmer so that its warming properties are released. Wrap the ginger in a piece of muslin (cheesecloth) and then, checking that it is not too hot, apply the compress directly to the energy lines, using a padding movement, in the same smooth rhythmic way as when palming the lines.

Right Using oil Although not a standard part of traditional Thai practice, working with oil is a very soothing alternative to applying direct acupressure to the energy lines. No special oil is required: you can use grapeseed, sweet almond or even sunflower oil. Try to use organic oils if you can, so that no impurities are absorbed into the skin.

Make sure that your partner is warm enough. Use the same body posture as when thumbing the energy lines but instead of applying downward pressure, simply glide your thumbs up and down the path of the energy lines, checking the pressure with your partner.

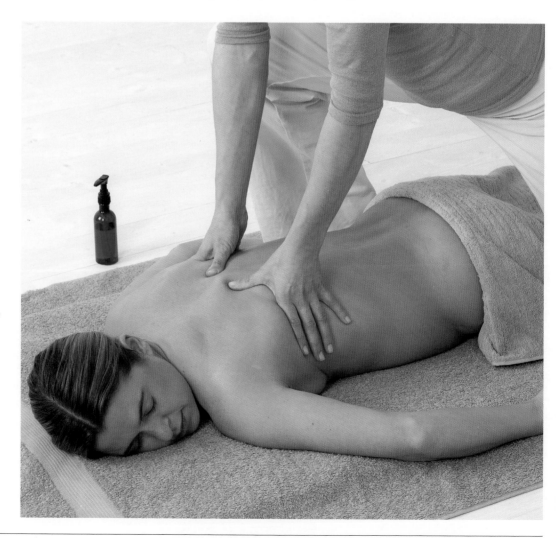

Review: the Back of the Body

Use the pictures below as a reminder of the main flow of the sequence. As before, take time to feel comfortable with massaging this part of the body before moving on to the next, and work to your partner's specific needs.

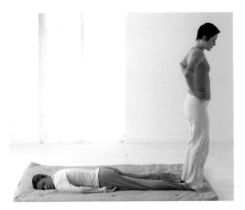

Walking on the feet

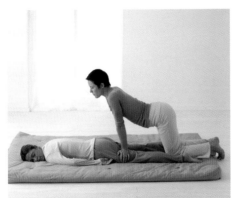

Palming the backs of the legs

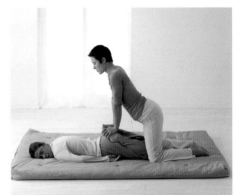

Feet to sacrum

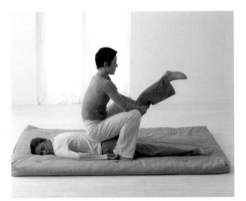

The locust

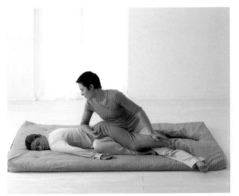

Take a break

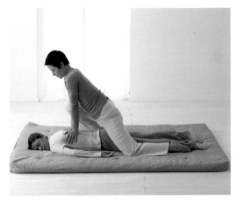

Working the back lines

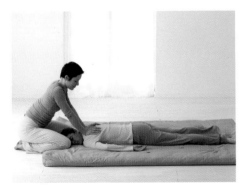

Palming and thumbing

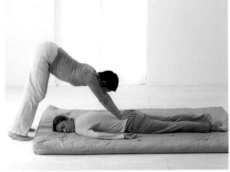

Sacrum lengthener

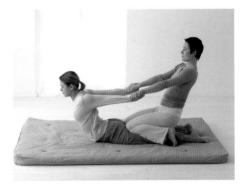

The cobra

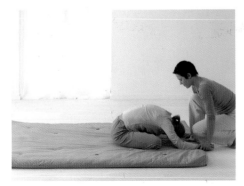

Cross-legged forward bend

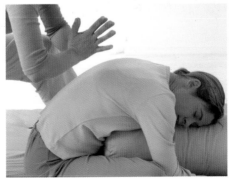

Percussion

Caution

Remember when carrying out percussive techniques that you should keep your hand contact soft and never strike your partner's spine directly.

Seated Sequence for the Upper Body

For the exercises that follow, featuring the head, neck and upper body, your partner will be in a seated position. This makes these exercises very versatile, as it means they can be done anywhere, unrestricted by lack of space or equipment. Most of the exercises could be given with your partner sitting on a stool or low chair.

Modern lifestyles can leave us feeling depleted, tired and weighed down, particularly in the upper chest, shoulders and neck. The stimulating sequence that follows eases the upper body and helps clear the mind. The work here focuses on releasing what is often long-term tension held in the upper body.

SITTING WITH EASE AND LIGHTNESS

To ensure that your partner gains maximum benefit from this sequence, take time to check that they are relaxed and supported in their sitting position, so that the whole of their spine, right up into their head and neck, feels light and free. Maintaining a healthy posture is beneficial not only for the physical body but also for the energetic body, which is central to Thai massage.

Below It can help to raise the hips slightly higher than the knees, using a folded blanket or block. If necessary, place extra support under the knees to prevent any strain in the joints.

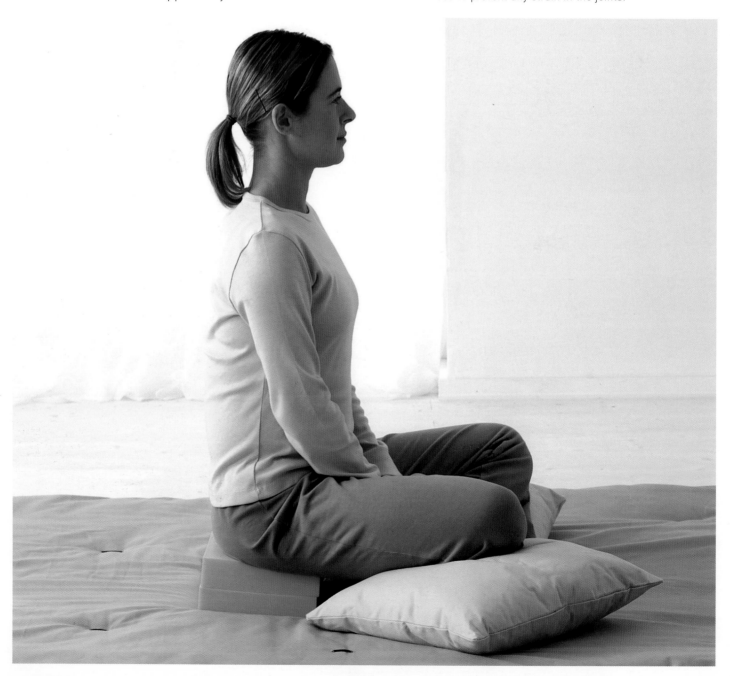

Warming up the Shoulders

Working this area helps to release habitual tension in the shoulders and neck and stimulate deeper breathing. It creates a feeling of space between the shoulders and ears, encouraging greater freedom of movement in the neck.

ENERGY POINTS IN THE SHOULDERS

The exercises shown below work along three important acupressure points located on the top of the shoulders. These are very effective for releasing tension in and around the base of the neck and upper back. They are described in the order given below for learning purposes only, but once you are familiar with their location it may feel more natural to start at the base of the neck and work outwards.

Getting it right

☑ Ask if your partner has suffered from any neck injuries, including whiplash, and if so proceed with due sensitivity and caution.

☑ Be aware of how much tension people can hold in their upper body. Some people find deep pressure very beneficial while others are extremely sensitive.

☑ Work with the breath. Encourage your partner to focus on their exhalation, so that they actively release the tension in the shoulders.

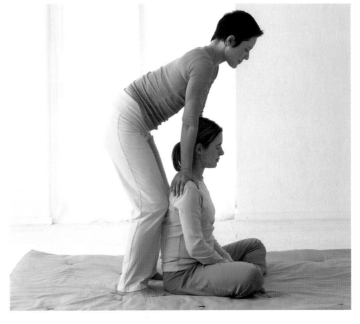

1 Palming the shoulders This general pressure loosens and warms up the shoulders. Come close in to your partner's body so they feel supported from behind. Make sure you are stable and your feet are relaxed. Turn your wrists forward, with your fingers pointing back towards you, and place your palms on the fleshy part of the shoulders, as shown. Use your body weight to sink into the shoulders. Slowly apply as much pressure as your partner enjoys.

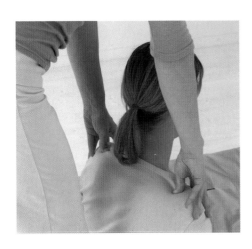

2 Thumbing the shoulder points Work into these points with the pads, rather than the tips, of your thumbs. Stabilize your hand position by spreading your fingers wide. Locate point A by sliding each thumb away from the neck and coming to rest in the small dip at the "V" where your partner's collarbone and shoulder blade meet.

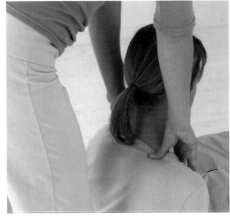

3 Where the shoulder meets the neck, drop back slightly off the top of the muscular ridge of the shoulder to find point C.

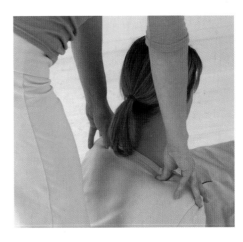

4 Midway between points A and C is point B. It often has a slightly different quality to it, and may naturally feel quite dense.

The Head and Neck

This part of the sequence concentrates on smaller, more sensitive movements for the neck and head. The energy flow can readily become blocked here and this can result in feeling "stuck in the head" and slightly disconnected from the sensations and inner cues of the body.

THE OCCIPUTAL RIDGE

The area at the base of the skull, where the spinal column feeds up into the head, is known as the occipital ridge and can be described as being like a physical junction between the body and the mind. Keeping a free flow of energy here maintains a healthy supply of blood to the brain and scalp. It also helps to preserve an integrated sense of the body, where the body and the mind are held in equal regard and where neither the sensations of the body nor the chattering of the mind dominate the other.

Right This artwork shows some of the acupressure points that you can work around the base of the skull. They can be located by letting the head drop back slightly until the thumb falls into a natural dip up against the bone.

USING PRESSURE POINTS IN THE NECK AREA

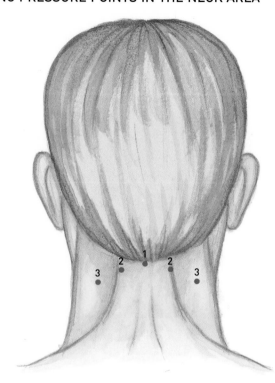

Working the Occiput

By working the acupressure points along the occiputal ridge and easing tension from the neck, you help to keep the energy flowing freely and the body and mind in balance.

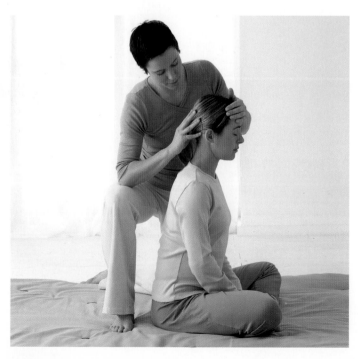

1 Half-kneel behind your partner – making sure that you are in a stable and comfortable position – and lightly support their forehead with your hand. Use the thumb of your other hand to work on the points. Keep your fingers spread wide for support against the back of the skull. Work with an inward and upward motion, using slow, firm pressure.

Remember that these points can be sensitive but you can work them more deeply if your partner consciously works with their breath as you apply the pressure. As with all the other exercises it is important for masseur and receiver to communicate well with each other throughout.

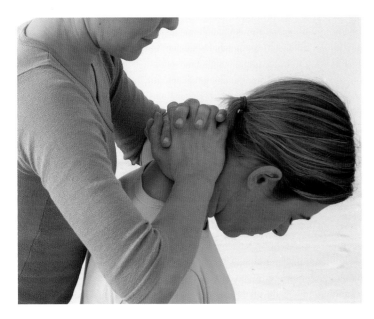

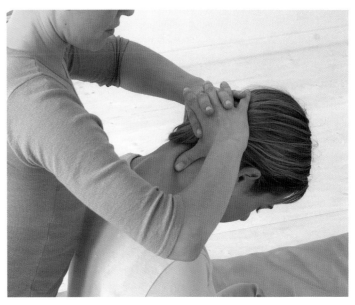

2 Palming the neck As with the butterfly squeeze (single leg sequence), interlace your fingers and, using the heels of your hands, gently squeeze up and down the back of the neck. Work from the shoulders up to the base of the skull. Be aware of how strong the pressure in your hands can be.

3 Thumbing the points on the neck Undo your clasp slightly and take your elbows wide, turning your thumbs face down. Use the pads of your thumbs to work up and down the muscular ridge on either side of the spine.

Head Massage

This is a simple but wonderfully releasing part of the sequence. Working into the roots of the hair stimulates blood flow to the scalp, resulting in healthy hair, and helps to relieve headaches and sluggishness, leaving your partner more alert and rejuvenated. The following techniques are simply suggestions – be playful and use your intuition.

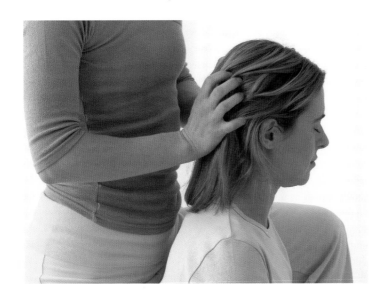

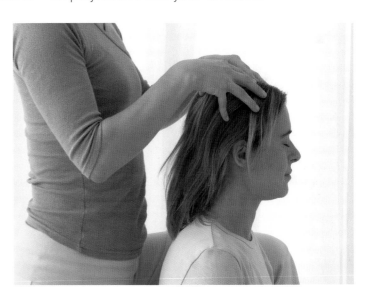

1 Shampooing Work right into the hair and rub the scalp vigorously with the tips of your fingers.

2 Plucking This technique is a little more specific. Place the pads of your fingers firmly against the skull and then briskly pluck your hands away. Repeat, covering the whole of the scalp.

People tend to either love or hate these kinds of techniques, so always check with your partner that they enjoy having their scalp massaged before you begin.

Getting it right

☒ Never work on wet hair, as it can damage the hair and also feels very uncomfortable.

3 Head Massage

Expanding the Upper Body

At this stage we move on to working with the whole of your partner's upper body. The sequence of exercises and techniques that follows involves some wonderful stretches that are aimed at integrating the flow of energy throughout the upper body. They should open up this whole area and help to release any held tensions. As a result, your partner should be left feeling fully relaxed and yet refreshed.

Stretch Sequence

This sequence features just some of the more expansive and opening exercises that can help to release energy which has become held deep inside the shoulder joints, the ribs, and the upper back.

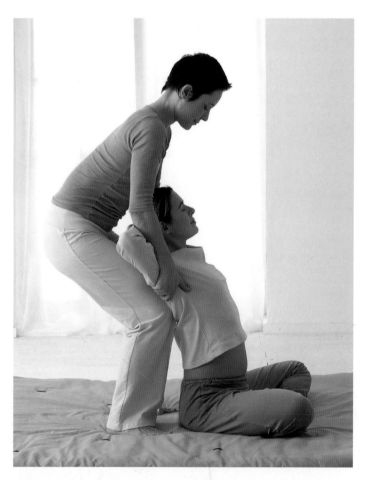

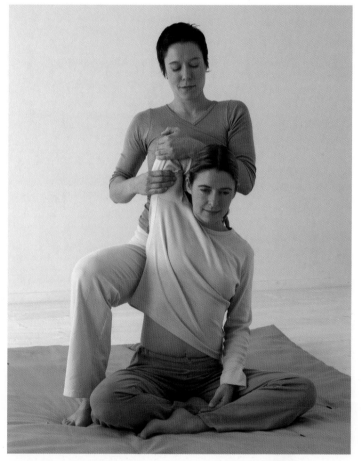

1 Hello world Stand close in behind your partner, but make sure that you leave a small gap between your knees and their back. Ask them to interlace their hands behind their head. Reach over and clasp around their upper arms, close to the armpits.

Let your partner lean back on to your knees. On the exhalation, lift their arms up and out. Encourage your partner to drop their weight into their hips as they open up through the front of their body. Repeat the stretch three times, making sure that you do not undo the position completely in between.

2 Opening the armpit Half-kneel behind your partner. Take their arm and lift the hand up to the ceiling to create space all the way through the side of the body. Drop their upper arm behind their head and, using your inside hand, support their elbow against your body. With your outside hand squeeze up and down the upper arm, from the armpit to the elbow, using the flats of your fingers. Change arms and repeat on the other side.

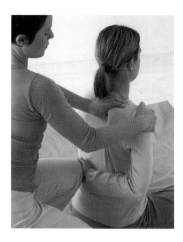 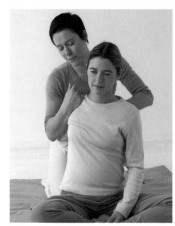

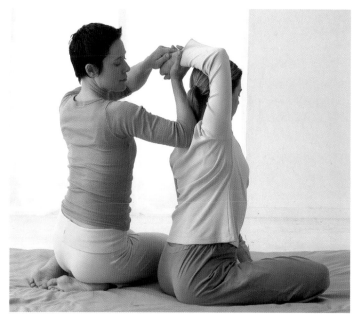

3 Finding your wings (above) This exercise opens up the hidden places behind the shoulder blade (scapula), and introduces a slight twist through the upper body. Take your partner's hand behind them and bring it across to the other side of their spine. Put your knee into their palm to fix their hand in place. This position helps to create space behind the shoulder blade.

4 (above right) Support the front of the shoulder joint with your outside hand. Place the thumb of your inside hand behind the shoulder blade and lean back. Release, reposition your thumb and continue working all around the shoulder blade. Repeat on the other side.

5 Spanish dancer This is a stronger opening for the shoulder and armpit, working into the little pocket of tension at the top corner of the shoulder blade. Kneel beside and slightly behind your partner, facing away slightly. Take their hand and circle it up and behind their head, maintaining its natural direction. Use your inside arm as the lever: hold their wrist and place your elbow in the small space between the spine and the corner of the shoulder blade.

As you sink your hips towards your partner, lean in with your elbow and away with your hands. Sink in and out of this stretch several times, repositioning your elbow very slightly each time.

Advanced stretch

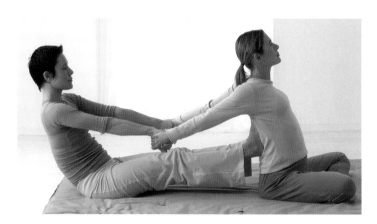

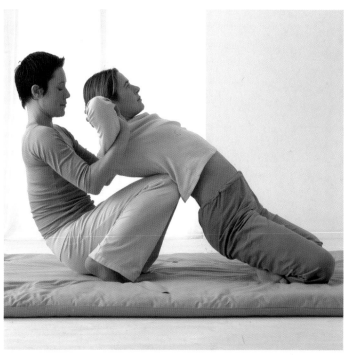

6 Back walk This is a lovely release for the back and provides a gentle stretch for the front. Sit far enough behind your partner so that you can almost stretch your legs out straight. Place your feet in their back, just either side of the spine, below the shoulder blades. Take hold of your partner's hands, clasping around their thumbs.

As you straighten your legs, encourage your partner to let their weight fall back on to your feet, opening fully through their chest. Push them gently back to sitting, reposition your feet slightly and repeat. Work up and down the back but don't take the feet too low, or your partner may feel discomfort in their lower back.

Above This pose, for advanced participants only, shows just how flexible and free your partner can feel in their spine towards the end of the massage.

Completing the Seated Sequence

The gentle sitting twist and forward bends that are shown below are aimed at consolidating the whole sequence of exercises that have been done with your partner in the seated position. These two exercises are excellent counter-poses for the back bends and chest-openers that have gone before. They integrate the energy, working through the whole length of your partner's spine. This should bring a feeling of completeness to the body and therefore prepare it properly for final relaxation.

Gentle Sitting Twist

This is a good all-round twist that is accessible for most body types.

Right Ask your partner to clasp their hands behind their head. Stand behind them, slightly to one side, and gently fix their thigh with your instep. Clasp their upper arms, close to the armpits. On an exhalation, encourage your partner to sink into their hips and allow their upper body to undo into a twist. Ease out of the twist on the inhalation and deepen into it on the exhalation. Do not force, but work gently with their breathing rhythm. Repeat on the other side.

Getting it right

X Avoid twists if your partner has any spinal problems.

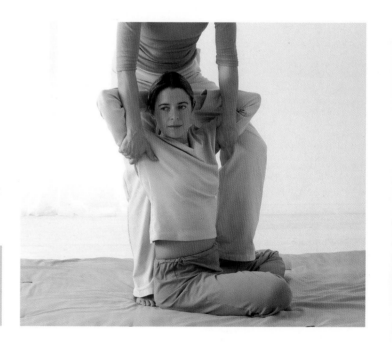

Forward Bends

These assisted forward bends help to bring your partner's focus inwards, preparing them for deep relaxation. The three variations provide options for different levels of flexibility. Find the one that gives your partner the deepest sense of release.

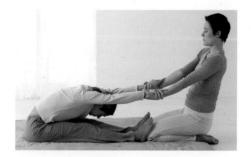

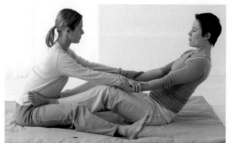

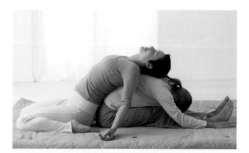

1 For average flexibility Rest your knees against your partner's insteps, as shown, and hold on to each other's wrists. As they inhale, lift slightly through the front of their spine. As they exhale, lean away, lengthening your partner's torso towards their feet. Repeat in and out several times.

2 For stiffer people With this variation, your partner needs to sit with wide legs and bent knees, so that their pelvis and the base of their spine feel free. Fix your insteps into the front of their hips. As your partner exhales, lean your upper body away and push into their hips with your feet.

3 Back-to-back This suits those who find version 1 comfortable. Both parties achieve release here: one in the back of the body, the other in the front. Kneel down sacrum to sacrum, with your feet either side of their hips. Relax totally. Slowly release your body weight along their back, feeling their spine lengthen.

Advanced position – the flying pose

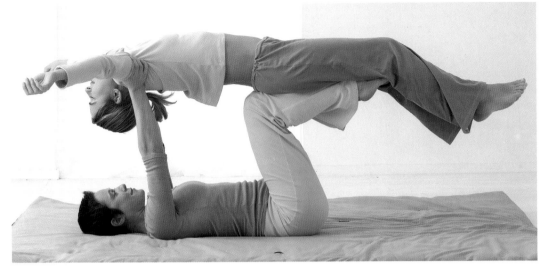

Left The flying pose is one of several advanced positions that facilitate a feeling of complete surrender at the end of a massage. Like all advanced positions, it should be done by experienced participants only, under expert guidance.

Review: Seated Sequence

Use the pictures below as a reminder of the main flow of the sequence performed in the seated position. Remember to keep checking that your posture feels comfortable and to maintain good communication with your partner.

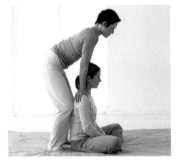

Palming the shoulders

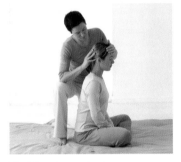

Working the occiput

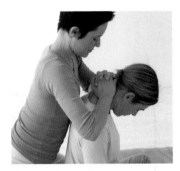

Palming the neck

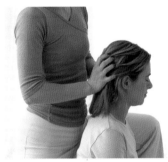

Head massage

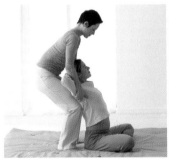

Hello world

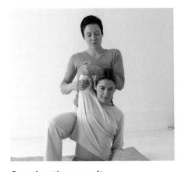

Opening the armpit

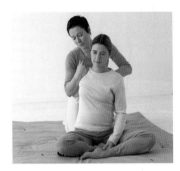

Finding your wings

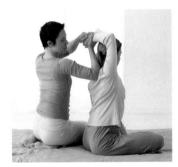

Spanish dancer

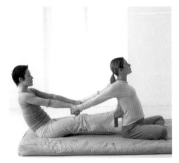

Back walk

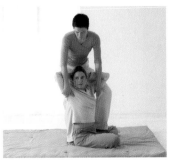

Gentle sitting twist

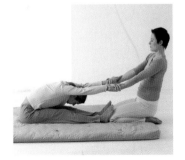

Forward bend

Caution

Once again, you must find out if your partner has any old or current injuries in their neck, shoulders or lower back before proceeding.

The Face

A face massage is a welcome and relaxing treat at any time. When it is given at the end of a full-body Thai massage, it is an opportunity for your partner to come to a point of stillness and quiet within their body and to release any tension that they may still be holding on to.

The face massage plays a similar role to that of relaxation after a yoga session. It is a time for the body to assimilate and consolidate the dynamic work that has preceded it. Make sure you leave a good ten minutes for the head and face massage; economizing on time here will leave your partner feeling unsettled, and the massage incomplete. Use this part of the treatment as an opportunity to let your instincts guide you and your creative juices flow.

Make sure that your partner is warm enough, since their temperature will naturally drop as they relax more deeply. Some people with lower back problems may need a little support under their knees at this point - you can use a bolster or a rolled-up blanket. Your partner may also want the support of a cushion or pillow under their head to help keep the back of their neck relaxed. Make sure that you are comfortable too – there is no point in ending the massage with an aching back. Place some support under your hips to help keep your upper spine free from tension.

Getting it right

☑ If your partner suffers from low blood pressure, then you may want to make the face massage more stimulating than relaxing. Also, remind your partner to get up slowly to avoid feeling dizzy.

☑ If you decide to use a little oil for the face massage, ensure that your partner doesn't have any allergies and that they like the smell.

☑ Make sure that your hands are clean, warm and dry. If you know they get a little sticky, use some talcum powder.

Using oils

Traditionally, oil is not used in Thai massage. However, massaging the face is a wonderful opportunity to introduce some essential oils to help relax or invigorate your partner. The oil is meant to enhance the quality of the face massage rather than dominate it, so use only a small amount. Apply the oil after you have done any acupressure point work, otherwise your hands will be slippery. Do not use essential oils neat on the skin. Always add them to a base oil such as sweet almond or grapeseed. Use organic oils wherever possible. For professional advice, however, consult a qualified aromatherapist.

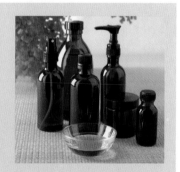

A few suggestions
- Calming/relaxing: lavender, chamomile, neroli, jasmine
- For stress: sandalwood, lavender, neroli, rose
- Grounding/supporting: lavender, frankincense, sandalwood, cedarwood
- Uplifting/refreshing: lemongrass, lemon, orange
- Comforting: rose, lavender, sandalwood
- Balancing: sandalwood, geranium

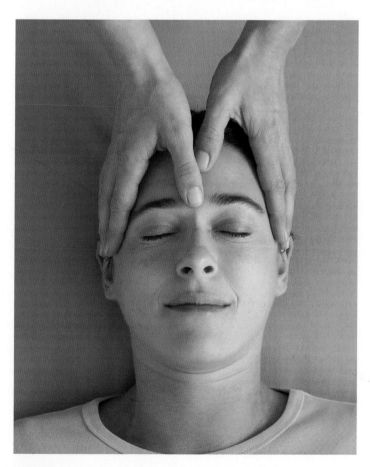

Above Simple, smooth, flowing movements are all you need for an effective and relaxing face massage.

Relaxing the Head and Neck

Start the face massage by encouraging your partner to bring their focus inwards and relax completely. Suggest that they close their eyes and listen to their breathing, letting their thoughts drift away and their body weight sink into the mat underneath them.

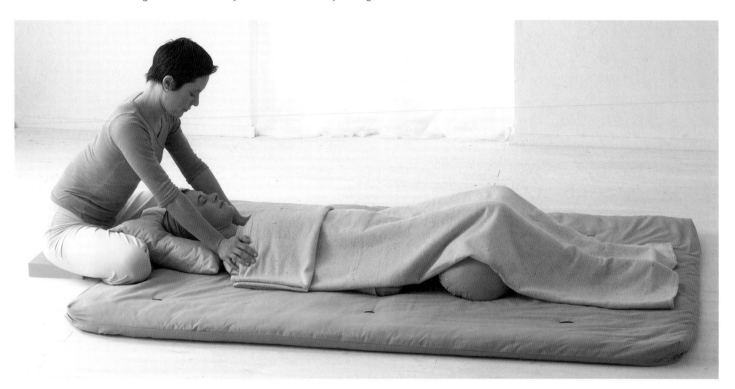

1 Relaxing the shoulders Sit down, on some support if necessary, positioned close to your partner just behind their head. Now alternately palm the shoulders, easing them away from the ears.

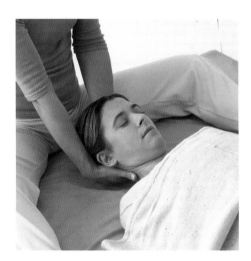

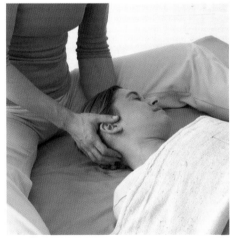

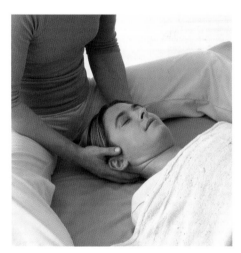

2 Neck lengthener Slide both your hands under the back of your partner's skull. Fix your palms against their occipital ridge. Now lean away, gently lengthening the back of the neck.

3 Cranial hold Simply supporting the weight of your partner's head in your hands can feel extremely comforting and facilitate a deep release throughout their body. To get your hands in the correct position, turn your partner's head slightly from side to side and place the flat tips of your fingers against the bony ridge of the skull. Now let your fingers and hands relax completely.

4 Keep the backs of your hands on the mat for support, as any feeling of effort or tension in your hands is quickly transferred to your partner's head. The less you do, the more effective this will be. Enjoy listening with your hands to the subtle movements and sensations in your partner's skull.

Working on the Face

As a rule, begin with repeated slow, broad, general strokes, then move on to the more focused work for the acupressure points. Work in either of two ways. For a deeply relaxing massage use slow, smooth, meditative sweeping movements. For a more stimulating massage, apply pressure with invigorating circles. The way you work depends on your partner's likes and dislikes and may also depend on what they have to do immediately after their massage. For example, if they have to drive a car or go back to a work environment, then it may be better to give them a more stimulating face massage.

Key to the pressure points

1 the third eye or ajna chakra

2 headache, insomnia, problems of the lower sinuses and dizziness

3 headache and facial paralysis

4 headache and facial paralysis

5 headache

6 facial paralysis and hypothermia

7 the temple – an important therapy point for headaches.

8 the tear ducts – therapy point for insomnia (use only gentle thumb pressure)

9–11 these small depressions next to the edge of the ear are good for treating deafness, ear pain and toothache

12 lower sinuses and facial paralysis

13 fainting, shock, sunstroke and respiratory failure

14 facial paralysis

15 migraine

USING PRESSURE POINTS ON THE FACE

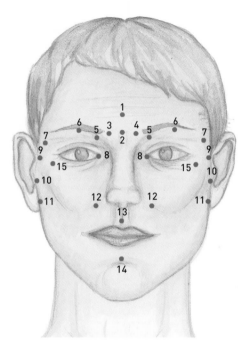

Above Thai massage stimulates a range of acupressure points. This shows a broad selection of useful ones.

Easy Massage Routine

The steps given below are just a suggestion of what you might want to try. Facial massage is an area where you can really enjoy exploring and experimenting with your own techniques.

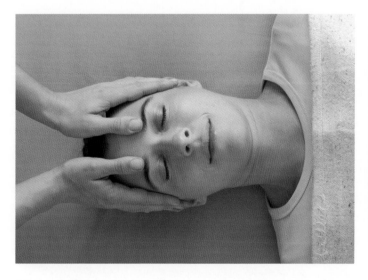

1 Brow sweep Place your fingers on your partner's temples, in order to stabilize your hands. Now use the flats of your thumbs to slide away from the centre of your partner's forehead towards their temples.

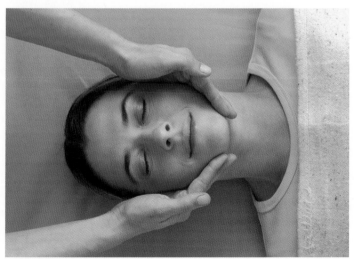

2 Jaw sweep Cup your hands around the cheeks and sweep up from the chin to the temples.

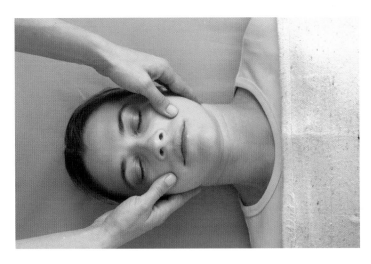

3 Cheekbone sweep Using your thumbs, sweep from the corners of the nostrils around the contours of the cheekbones and out towards the ears.

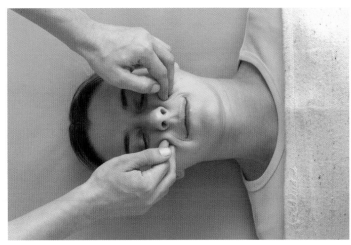

4 Sinus circles With the fingers together, circle around underneath the cheekbones.

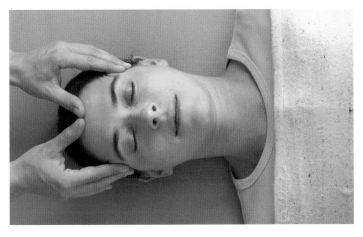

5 Temple circles With the thumbs supported on the forehead, circle gently with the flats of your fingers to ease tension from the temple area.

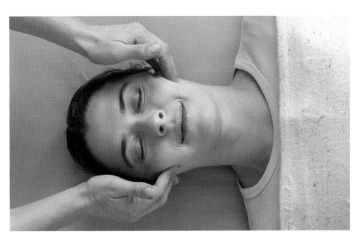

6 Jaw circles The jaw holds a surprising amount of tension. Check that your partner's jaw is relaxed and circle firmly all around this joint.

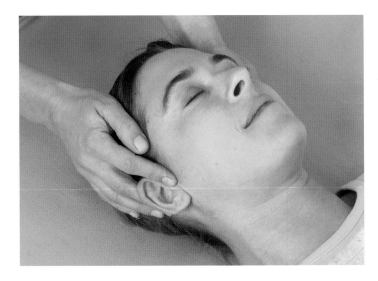

7 Ear circles Slide your fingers up either side of each ear and rub firmly around the front and back of the ear itself. There are several wonderfully releasing points around the ears and you can stimulate the whole area with firm, circular rubbing movements.

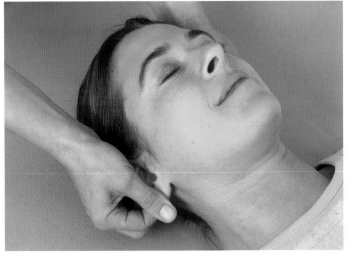

8 Stroking the earlobes The ears contain a multitude of acupressure points. Stroking and squeezing the earlobes, as well as pressing around the inside of the ear, is both soothing and stimulating.

Finishing the Full-body Massage

As the facial massage routine comes to a close, so too does the complete Thai body massage. These closing exercises can bring your partner to a place of complete rest. Never underestimate the power of stillness, of simply holding and listening. The very simple holds used to finish the facial massage will give your partner's physical and energetic body a chance to rest and rejuvenate. Enjoy this opportunity to sit and listen, without any expectation of your own or your partner's body.

The Final Holds

Make sure that you are comfortable and your shoulders and hands are free of tension. Observe your breathing rhythm and use it to check how relaxed you are in your own body.

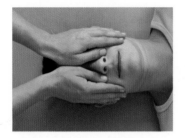 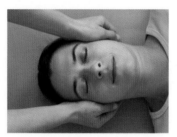 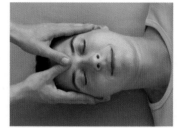 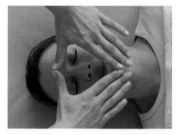

1 Eye hold (above left) Cup your hands gently over your partner's eye sockets, letting the heel of each hand rest on the brow and the fingers rest on the cheekbones.

2 Ear hold (above right) Cup your hands around your partner's ears. Shutting out external sounds helps to bring their focus inwards.

3 Third eye hold (above left) Place thumb over thumb on the ajna chakra (third eye point). This creates a focal point for the energy flow throughout the body. It helps your partner to become aware of the potential of infinite space within them.

4 Bodhi mudra (above right) A *mudra* is a yogic posture, in this case a hand gesture, that influences the body to function in a certain way. Using this mudra here enhances energy flow to the face and third eye.

Finishing Prayer

Just as you began the complete body massage with a prayer, with an intention of working with healing touch, it is important to complete it in a similar way, honouring the experience you have shared with your partner.

Right Taking care of your partner after a massage After you have completed the treatment, leave your partner to rest quietly for a few moments without interruption. It is often in the undisturbed moments, after the hands-on aspect of a massage has finished, that the deeper healing occurs. In addition, it can be a good idea to offer them a glass of water, as Thai massage can be strongly detoxifying.

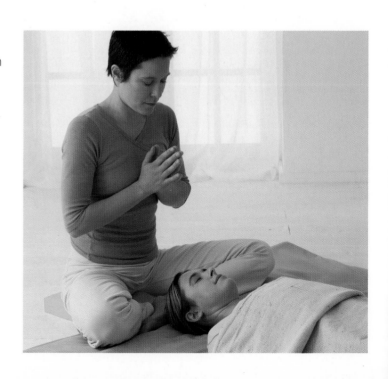

Review: the Face and Closing Holds

Use the pictures below as a reminder of the main flow of the facial massage sequence. As mentioned, the precise sequence for the facial massage is not crucial, but you may prefer to follow the order given until you feel confident enough to experiment.

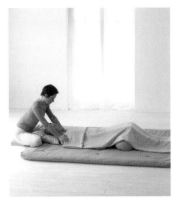

Relaxing the shoulders

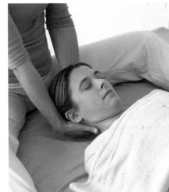

Neck lengthener

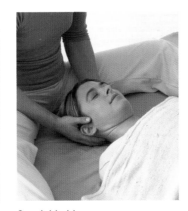

Cranial hold

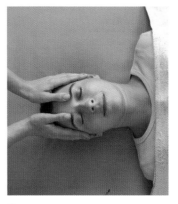

Brow sweep

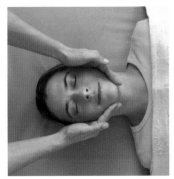

Jaw sweep

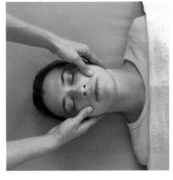

Cheekbone sweep

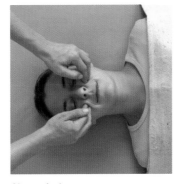

Sinus circles

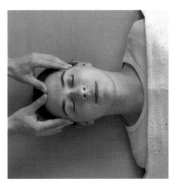

Temple circles

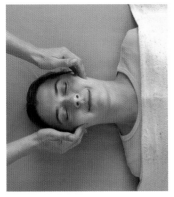

Jaw circles

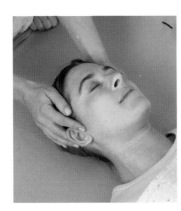

Ear circles

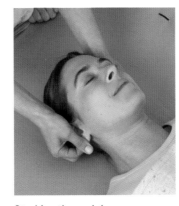

Stroking the earlobes

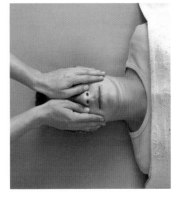

Eye hold

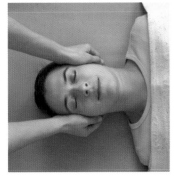

Ear hold

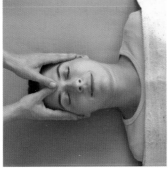

Third eye hold

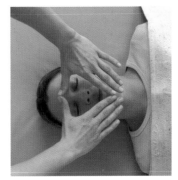

Bodhi mudra

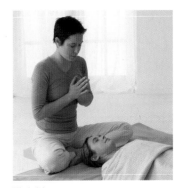

Finishing prayer

Recapping on the Full-body Massage

Use the pictures below to get an overview of the complete massage routine featured in the preceding pages. This is not intended as a comprehensive review but uses selected pictures to give an at-a-glance summary of the sequence presented in this section.

This overview is designed to give you a general feel for the range and balance of postures that are used in traditional Thai massage. It also demonstrates how one pose or exercise flows into another, creating the kind of "dance" to which Thai massage is often compared.

The Complete Routine: a Visual Overview

This ancient art uses an incredible variety of body shapes and positions, and having all these pictures together here starts to show how one pose supports, or provides a beautiful counterpoise to, another pose.

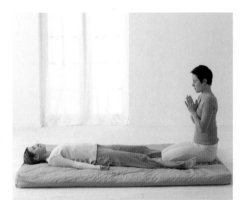
Opening prayer

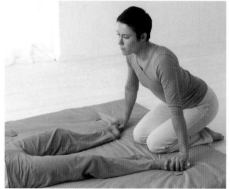
The feet

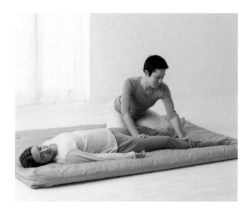
Palming the leg lines

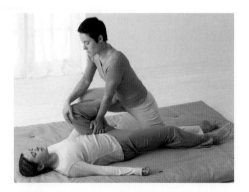
Hip opener

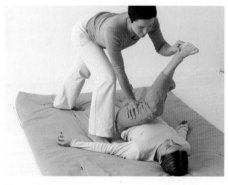
Hamstring yawn

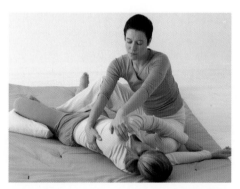
Spinal twist

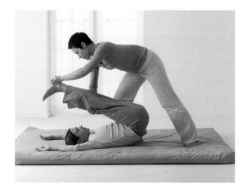
The plough

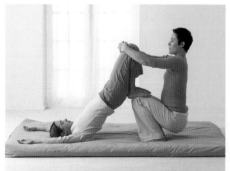
The bridge

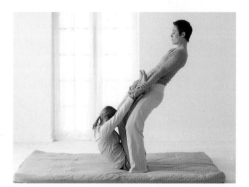
Forward fold

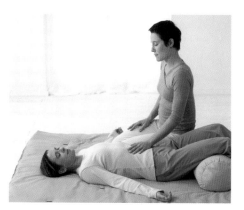

Relaxing the abdomen

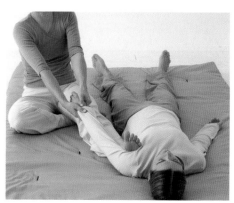

Arm stretch

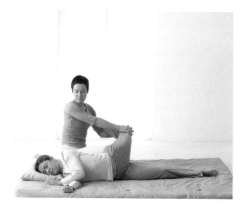

Shiva pose

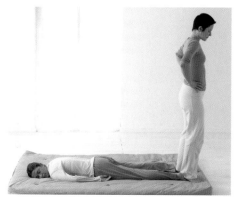

Walking on the feet

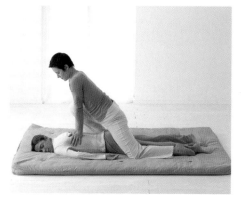

Palming the back lines

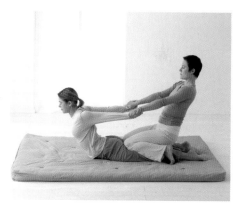

The cobra

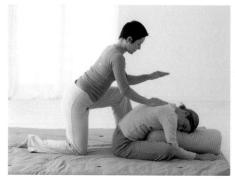

Percussion

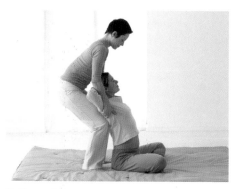

Hello world

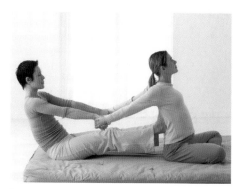

Back walk

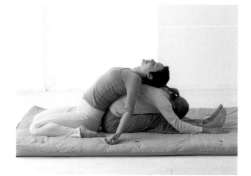

Forward bend

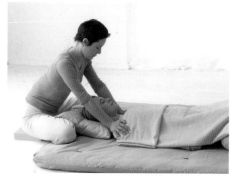

Relaxing the shoulders

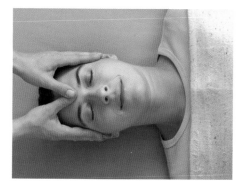

Face holds

Thai Massage and Pregnancy

Massage is a wonderful gift for mother and baby, both during and after pregnancy. A Thai massage given by an experienced practitioner can provide the space for deep rest and relaxation, supporting the new mother as she adjusts to the profound changes her body is going through in pregnancy.

Massage, or any form of nurturing touch, is extremely beneficial for pregnant women. But as a beginner in this field you should remember that it is not appropriate to try out the exercises shown in the main sequence on a pregnant partner. Instead, spend time with your partner offering gentle touch and loving attention, using some of the simple techniques shown below. They are adapted variations of what has already been covered in the main routine, so for more detail, refer back to the sequence focusing on that particular part of the body.

Getting it right

☒ If in any doubt, don't do it.

☒ Don't try any of the techniques shown here until after the first three months of pregnancy and the initial scan.

☑ Trust the mother to know what is right for her. Listen to her feedback and work attentively.

☑ Keep things simple so you can focus on your partner's feedback rather than your own technique.

☒ Do not press directly on the abdomen.

General Relaxing Routine

Make sure that your partner is comfortable. During the later stages of pregnancy most women will not want to lie on their back, so it is better to work seated or in the side position, using plenty of cushions as support.

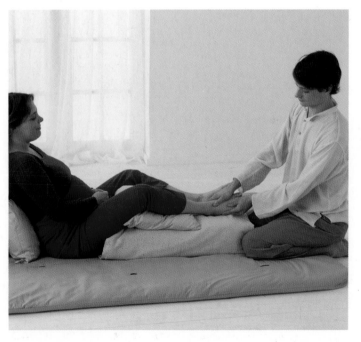

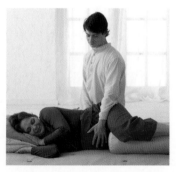

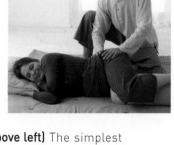

1 Grounding the feet Start by working on the feet. You may not be able to use all the techniques for the foot massage sequence directly, so adapt the less dynamic manipulations to suit working with your partner in a sitting position. Avoid pressing around the inside or outside of the anklebones as the points here are contraindicated during pregnancy.

2 Holding the front and back (above left) The simplest techniques are often the most soothing and powerful. Place one hand on your partner's lower back and cup the other gently around the belly and the baby. Just feeling additional external support can be deeply relaxing for a mother.

3 Working round the hip (above right) The hips can often feel very tight and under a lot of stress during pregnancy. As the pelvis shifts to accommodate the growing baby, the hips may feel in need of more focused attention. The side position is ideal for working round the hip joint as the body can be totally supported and relaxed.

Place the heels of your hands around the hip joint and work with rhythmic circular movements, covering the whole area and into the lower back.

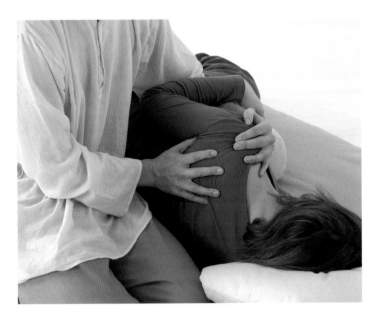

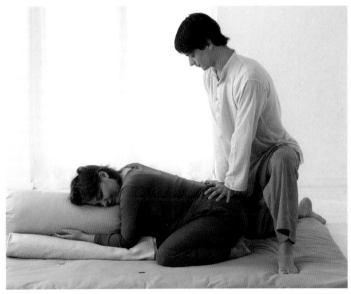

4 Easing the shoulders Kneel close behind your partner's upper back and encircle the front of their shoulder joint. Use your other hand to support behind the shoulder blade. Now encourage your partner to let go completely into your hands and begin to move the shoulder joint gently in circles, increasing the space with every repetition. Remember to work in both directions.

5 Child pose and sacrum press This is a lovely supported stretch that creates a feeling of space through the whole of the back. Ask your partner to roll on to all fours and place plenty of support under her chest and arms. Tell her to keep her feet together and her knees wide enough to accommodate her belly. Half-kneel behind her and place your hands on her sacrum. As she exhales, slowly and gently sink your weight down on to her sacrum, lengthening through the whole of the spine.

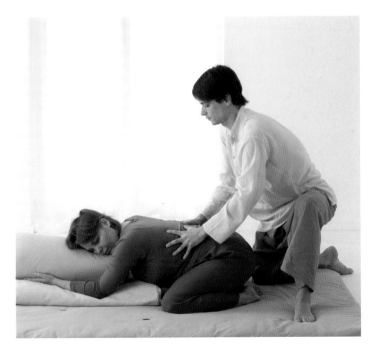

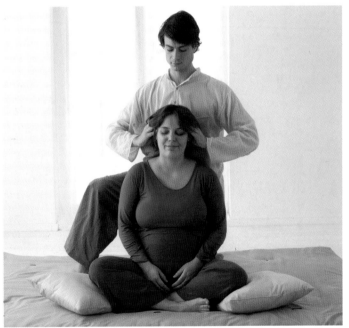

6 Sweep back Staying in the same position, sweep and smooth down the length of the back, stimulating the blood and energy flow from the shoulders to the hips. Begin at the shoulders and with brisk brushing motions sweep your hands down either side of the spine. Repeat several times.

7 Face and head massage Anything that helps relax the mind and ease away tensions and worries is going to have a relaxing effect on both mother and baby. If your partner is still comfortable lying on her back with support, give her a face massage from the traditional position. If she is more comfortable sitting upright, adapt your position accordingly.

Half-kneel behind your partner and let her lean back into your body for support. Work all around the scalp and face using the techniques described in the main sequence.

Thai Massage for Older People

Receiving massage is even more important later in life, as general wear and tear on the body starts to take effect. Thai massage is particularly supportive for an ageing body – maintaining joint mobility, easing aches and pains and helping you to feel more vibrant and active. The beauty of Thai massage is that even if your strength and physical stamina are not what they used to be, you can still benefit from its gentle motion and passive stretching without any effort or discomfort.

Massage is a lovely way of giving and sharing with parents or grandparents. Thai massage is suitable for any age or fitness level, as you can adapt treatments to suit your partner's needs. If they are very fragile or stiff, do more energy line work and use the gentle, easing stretches rather than the more demanding ones. There is no need to feel timid or over-cautious – just keep communicating with your partner and work with what feels good for their body. However, be sensible and don't choose an older body for your initial practice. Wait until you are more confident with the main routine before applying the adapted versions suggested below.

Getting it right

☒ Do not work on inflamed arthritic joints. With arthritis caused by wear and tear, gently ease through the joints when they are not inflamed.

☒ Never apply pressure on bone or try physically demanding stretches if your partner suffers from osteoporosis or softening of the bones.

☒ Avoid all inverted poses and over-stimulating exercises if your partner suffers from high blood pressure.

☒ Never press directly on any varicose vein.

☑ Check for heart conditions and work appropriately under the guidance of a medical professional.

☑ Have a good supply of cushions on hand for support.

Relaxing Routine

This sequence provides a selective but balanced massage routine. Make sure that your partner has all the padding support they need and is totally comfortable.

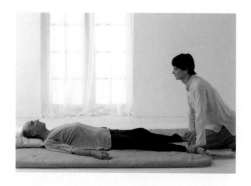

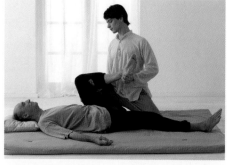

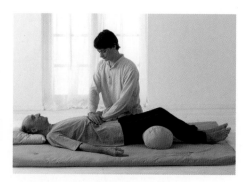

1 Feet – palming the instep Flexibility in all joints is affected by age. Any work that maintains an openness and flexibility in the feet and ankles will have a positive impact throughout the skeletal system. Work through as much of the foot sequence as your partner enjoys.

2 Leg circles Working all around the joints helps keep the hips well oiled and mobile, and can also help to relieve stiffness across the lower back. Make sure that you support your own body as you lift and circle the leg in both directions.

3 Relaxing the abdomen As the body ages, its natural rhythm slows, which can affect internal processes such as the digestion. Maintaining a healthy digestion means nutrients are better absorbed and ensures that the immune system is given adequate support. Start with general circling clockwise around the abdomen; proceed to the deeper work of palming and finger pressing if your partner feels comfortable.

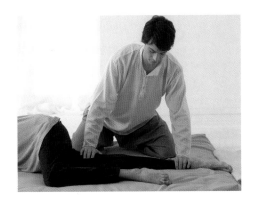

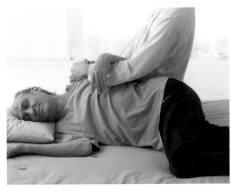

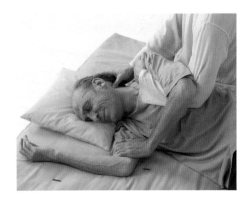

4 Leg lines in side position Your partner may not feel comfortable lying completely flat for very long so you can explore palming the leg lines in the side position.

5 Shoulder workout Help to maintain space in the shoulders and neck by spending some time slowly easing through the shoulder joint. Kneel behind your partner and make sure that their neck is well supported by cushions.

6 Neck release Focused work for the neck can be given in this reclining position, which is more relaxing than sitting. Keep the shoulder well supported from the front and use the hand at the back to work up into and around the occipital ridge at the base of the skull.

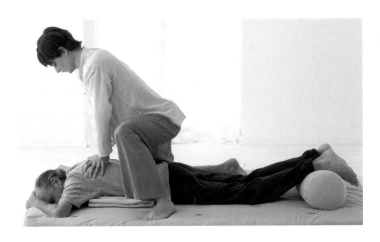

7 Working the back lines (left) Provide plenty of support for your partner's body when they lie on their front. You may need to put more padding under the fronts of their ankles to support their lower back and protect their knees.

Simple Seated Exercises

The versatility of the seated position comes into its own here. Not everyone is able to sit on the floor, so a low chair or stool can be used instead. The important thing is for your partner to feel comfortable so that they can relax more fully into the massage.

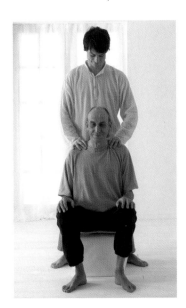

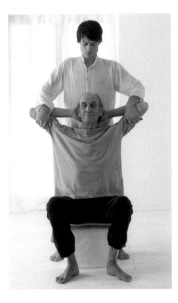

1 Relaxing the shoulders (far left) Work with gentle squeezing and milking techniques to release tension across the top of your partner's shoulders.

2 Hello world (left) (see section in complete body routine on expanding the upper body). Stand with a wide base directly behind your partner and come close in so that they can use your body as support. Ask them to interlace their hands behind their head and clasp around their upper arms. Work into the stretch on both the inhalation and the exhalation, exploring which feels most beneficial for your partner. Whichever way they breathe, encourage their opening to come from the solar plexus up through the centre of the chest and out through the armpits.

Easing Common Conditions

Thai massage is a whole-body treatment that works to rebalance the physical, energetic and emotional bodies. However, if your partner has a headache, back pain or stomach ache, for example, you may want to try easing them by using these short sequences as a guide.

There is no diagnostic tradition as such in Thai massage. Instead we work with the intention to support the body's natural healing ability by applying the techniques skilfully, appropriately and with awareness and understanding. There is no substitute for the complete rebalancing of energy experienced after receiving a full-body Thai massage. If you want to use massage to alleviate a long-term condition, such as migraine or back pain, the specific treatment should be incorporated within the full-body massage, by placing an emphasis on particular exercises or on energy line work. If you decide to work in this way you can refer to the energy line and point artwork so that you can start to integrate some basic theory into your practice.

The sequences below are not fixed plans but guides to help you ease some common conditions. They are shown in the order in which they would occur in a regular full-body massage. For more detailed technique descriptions, refer to the individual sections of the main routine.

Lower Back Pain

The main relevant treatment lines here are sen sumana, sen ittha and sen pingkhala. The lower back is supported in particular by work on the abdomen, the legs and the hips.

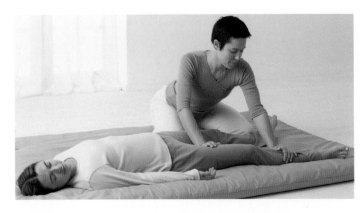

1 Work all the lines on the legs, focusing specifically on the third inside line of the legs (sen sumana).

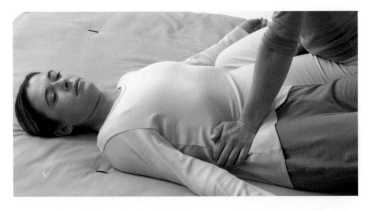

2 Focus on giving repeated abdominal massage. Pain felt in the lower back can often be caused by excess tension in the abdomen and may be relieved by a deep abdominal workout.

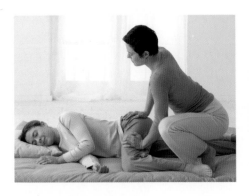

3 Work the third outside line of the leg (sen ittha and sen pingkhala), spending time around the hip area.

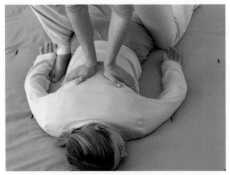

4 Palm and thumb both sets of back lines, especially the first back line (sen ittha and sen pingkhala). Focus on the lower back, rubbing around the buttocks and sacrum.

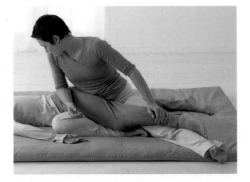

5 Use the forearm to work around the hips and buttocks in the take a break pose (in the sequence for the back of the body).

Knee Pain

Palming and thumbing the leg lines can help to ease knee pain caused by strain or overwork, but do not proceed if serious damage is indicated – if the kneecap is painful when you press directly down on it or move it alternately up and down.

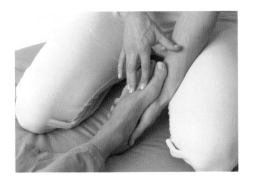

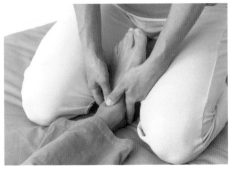

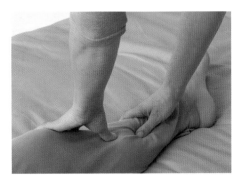

1 Work between the tendons of your partner's feet with your fingers. Use firm pressure but do not press too hard.

2 Work the knee pain point at the front of the foot. Use repeated pressure, but only hold it for as long as your partner can bear.

3 Palm and thumb all six leg lines, with particular emphasis on the first outside line (sen sahatsarangsi and sen thawari).

Sciatica

Tension in the lower back and hip can trap the sciatic nerve. This is often experienced as a sharp pain in the hip and down the leg. As well as performing the sequence below, you can also focus your work on sen kalathari.

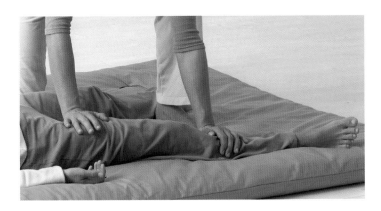

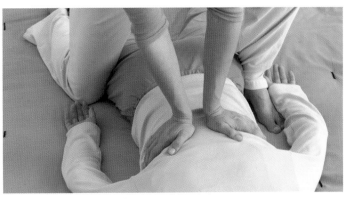

1 When palming and thumbing the leg lines, give particular focus to the second inside line (sen kalathari).

2 Work all around the sacrum, pressing hand over hand on to the bone with firm, gentle pressure, and also work the length of the first line of the back, including the area over the sacral bone, giving pressure in the small dips on either side of the bone.

3 Spend time massaging around the hip joint and buttock area to help soften the tissue and release the trapped nerve. Work the third outside line of the leg up into the C-shape around the hip joint.

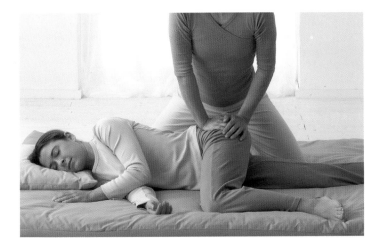

Sciatica: thumbing the foot points

Work the energy lines on the feet and focus on the point shown, where the fan-shaped massage featured in the foot sequence starts.

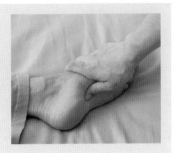

Headaches

These exercises can help a broad range of headaches. It may be best to use them when your partner is not in pain, as prevention rather than cure, as you can work more deeply. It is possible to work deeply if your partner has a headache, but check with them first.

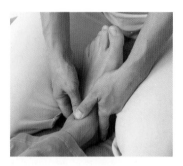

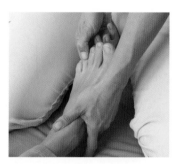

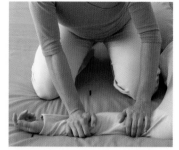

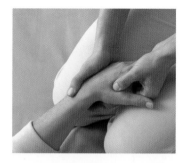

1 (above left) Foot massage can be very soothing, bringing your partner's energy away from their head back down to their roots. Work repeatedly into the knee pain and headache point (page 47).

2 (above right) Squeeze up to the sinus points at the tips of the toes.

3 (above left) Palm and thumb sen kalathari, to free shoulder tension – tension here and in the back are common causes of headaches.

4 (above right) Work the hands. Focus on the headache points and especially the hegu point (see the hands part of the total routine).

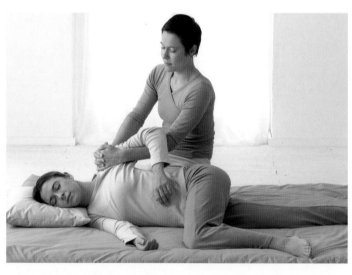

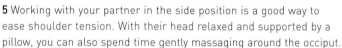

5 Working with your partner in the side position is a good way to ease shoulder tension. With their head relaxed and supported by a pillow, you can also spend time gently massaging around the occiput.

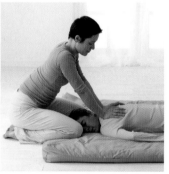

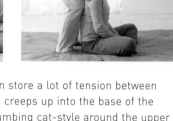

6 (above left) The upper back can store a lot of tension between the shoulder blades, which then creeps up into the base of the neck and head. Palming and thumbing cat-style around the upper spine and between the shoulders on lines 1 and 2 can be very effective for releasing tension.

7 (above right) Work the shoulder acupressure points in the sitting position with palming and thumbing techniques.

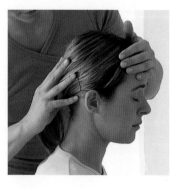

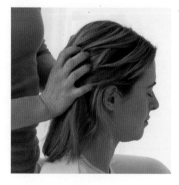

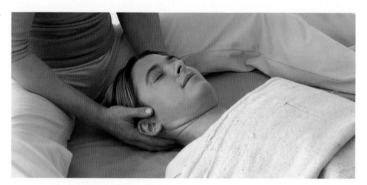

8 (above left) Work around the occipital ridge (see head routine) as this is where tension can become locked right into the neck, restricting vital blood and energy flow to the head area.

9 (above right) Nothing is more relieving for all kinds of headaches than a thorough head massage.

10 Finish off the sequence with a deep relaxing face massage. Start off with the cranial hold and focus on the temples and forehead. Let the eyes rest with the eye hold. Any essential oil that you use for the face massage could also be one chosen to help alleviate the headache. Try a blend of lavender, chamomile and geranium – a few drops of each in a tablespoon or so of carrier oil.

Coughs and Colds

If your partner is suffering from a cold or flu you would not want to give them a full-body Thai massage as it could overload an already compromised immune system. You may, however, find this short sequence useful for alleviating some of their symptoms.

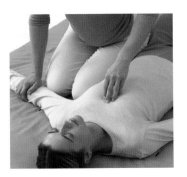

1 Circling the breastbone (sternum) will help boost and support the immune system and get the energy moving through the chest. General rubbing in this area may help to stimulate your partner's breathing if they feel congested and tight across the ribs.

The lung point
There is a reflex point for the lungs on the sole of the foot (right). Pressing and rubbing around this area can help to ease breathing and clear congestion.

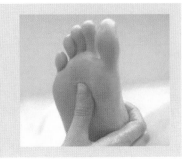

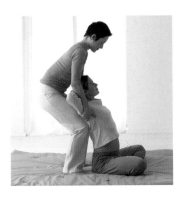

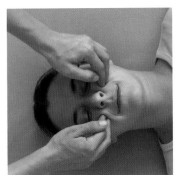

2 (far left) The "hello world" pose (see the Expanding the Upper Body section of the complete body massage routine) opens the lung cavity and encourages deeper breathing in cases of coughs or tightness across the chest.

3 (left) Pressing around the sinuses can feel incredibly releasing for congested head colds.

Constipation and Bloating

In cases of constipation or excess gas the main aim is to stimulate the digestion and release the trapped gases, which often cause a great deal of discomfort.

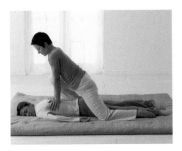

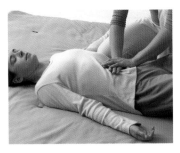

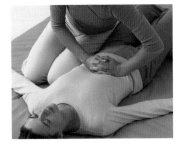

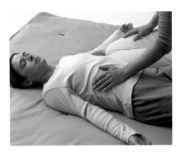

1 (above left) Initially, give your partner a repeated workout on the back lines, placing specific emphasis on line 1 (sen ittha and sen pingkhala) around the area of the lower back.

2 (above right) Relax your partner's belly and stimulate movement within the abdomen with a wavelike motion.

3 (above left) The wind-releasing exercise (page 69) is very relieving.

4 (above right) Work clockwise, following the natural direction of your partner's digestion, when palming and finger-pressing. If using oil, try three drops each of marjoram, lemongrass and rosemary in carrier oil, massaged into the belly and lower back.

5 (far left) Smooth and soothe an aggravated abdomen with some broad circling movements.

6 (left) The gentle plough (page 61) is a stimulating exercise that can help release wind trapped in the intestines. For a sluggish digestion the whole of the double leg sequence is recommended in order to help stimulate the digestive "fire".

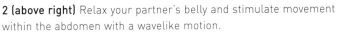

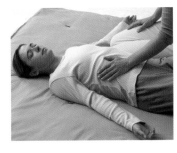

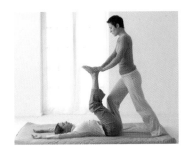

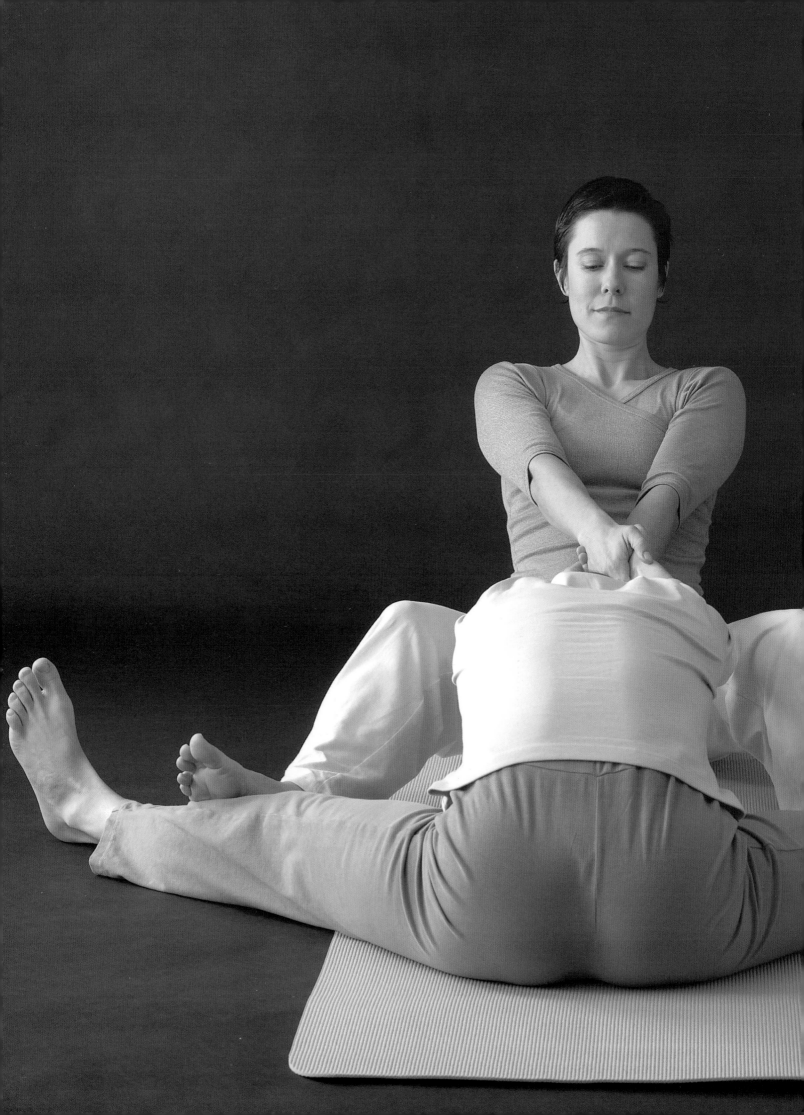

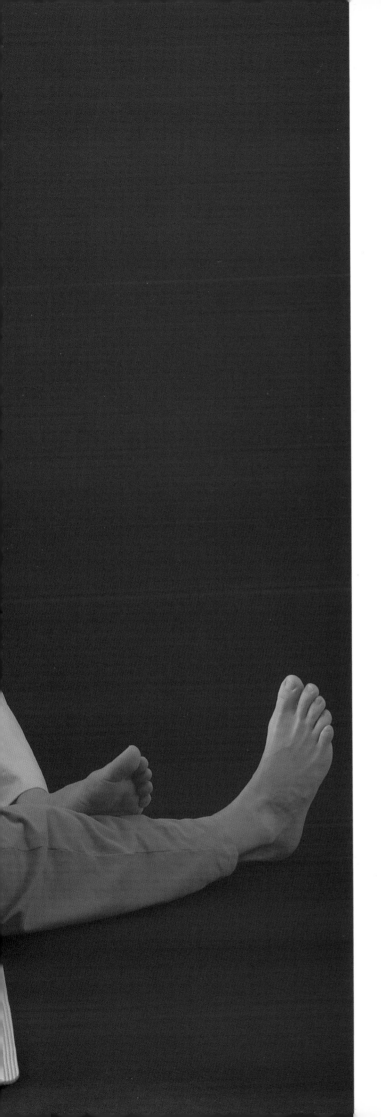

After a Massage

Well done! You have finished the sequence. When you have practised all the aspects of the body separately and feel comfortable with them, you can put the whole sequence together to give a full-body Thai massage. This intense level of working with another person's energy body can leave you in a heightened state of awareness and sensitivity.

While this is to be encouraged in your massage practice, it is important that you have the tools to ground, consolidate and contain this sensitivity after a session. Some simple guidelines will help you to integrate and ground this energy after giving a massage, ensuring that you remain in balance yourself.

Post-massage Routines

You can make use of these "post-massage" suggestions after any practice session – no matter how short – to give a sense of completion and containment. Remember to give yourself time for a longer relaxation after giving a full-body massage.

Thai massage is a dynamic and physical form of bodywork. It feels physical to receive and to give. While this aspect is obvious, you should keep in mind that you are also giving your partner an energy workout, and this can in turn stimulate your own energy flow. After a session you may experience heat or a buzzing feeling in your hands and forearms. This is the flow of prana or life energy that is stimulated when you set out with the intention to heal with touch, but it can also be an imprint or absorption of your partner's energy that you have picked up.

It is important to break this energetic connection with your partner, otherwise you can become very unclear about what you are experiencing – whether it is your energy, feelings and emotions or the residual energy pattern of your partner's feelings and emotions.

Below After the massage you need to return to a calm, quiet place – comparable, say, to still serene waters – to centre yourself.

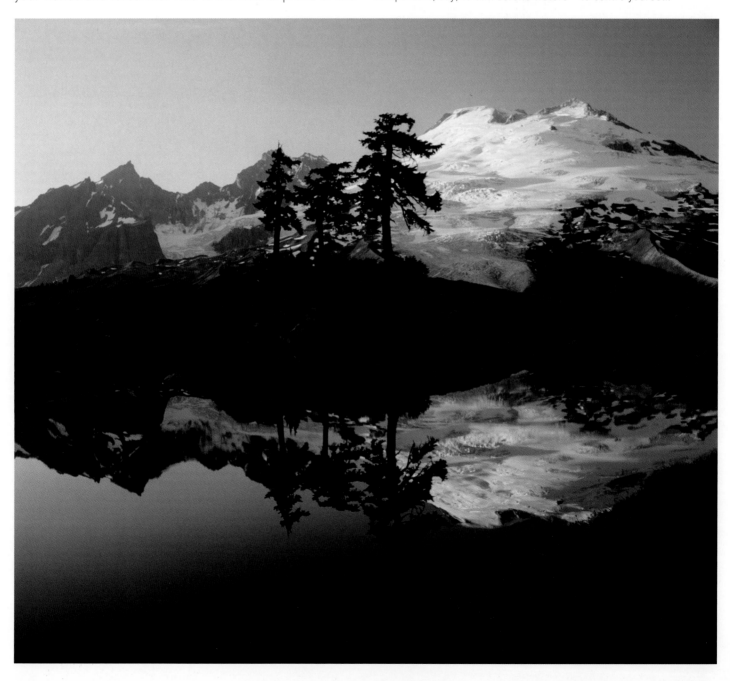

Clearing and Cleansing

Here are some easy techniques that you can employ immediately after massage, while your partner is relaxing. Completing a session in this way helps to establish an energetic boundary that separates the connection made during the treatment.

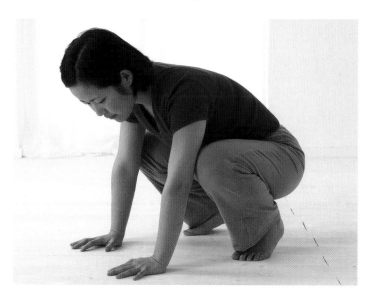

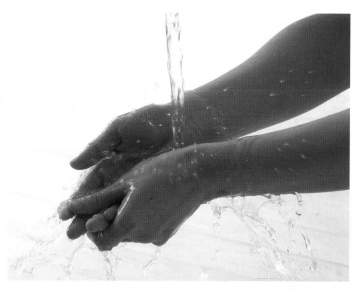

1 Grounding energy This exercise is very simple but highly effective. Just place your hands on the floor and mentally ask that any energy that is not yours, or that is no longer useful for you, be absorbed back into the earth. Stay with this feeling for as long as feels necessary for you. A few moments are usually enough.

2 Washing the hands This is a practical and hygienic thing to do after giving a massage, but it also has another purpose: flowing water is excellent for cleansing and clearing any residual energy felt in the hands and forearms.

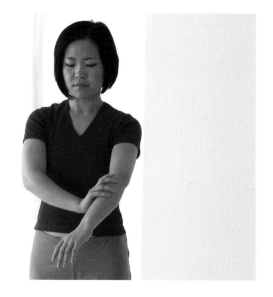

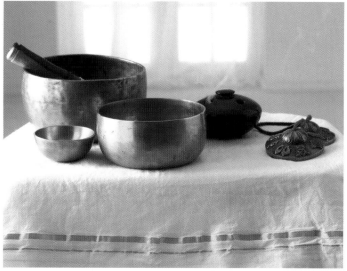

3 Sweeping the hands Sometimes it is not possible to wash your hands immediately after giving a massage. Another technique that is just as effective is to sweep excess energy from your forearms and hands.

4 Clearing with sound Sound is vibration, and vibration is energy that can be both heard and felt. Using chimes and singing bowls after a session not only produces beautiful sounds but can also be experienced as a soothing resonance in the body. You can use them to clear the energy in a room after a massage or to clear the aura around a person. Traditionally used in Tibet for ceremonial and healing purposes, singing bowls are made of several different metals, corresponding with the chakras, the seven energy centres of the body.

Relaxation Techniques

Just as you would take time for relaxation after any kind of yoga practice, it's a very good idea to take time for relaxation after giving your partner a Thai massage. Below are some suggestions for specific deeper relaxation techniques that allow for physical, mental and emotional release. To feel the full benefit of these techniques, make sure that you find a warm, quiet and comfortable place where you are certain you will not be disturbed. Don't be tempted to skip this stage – it is vital for your personal well-being.

Resting the Body

These gentle poses will alleviate any discomfort or strain in the hips and shoulders and are very relaxing counter-stretches for the half-kneeling and wide-kneeling working postures.

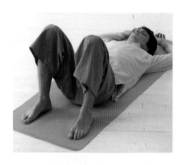 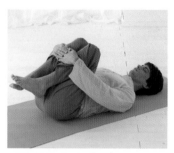 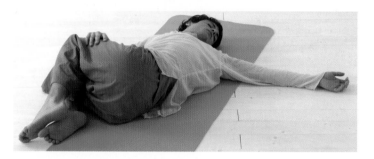

1 (above left) In this pose, your body is completely at rest, fully supported by the floor. Focus on letting your weight drop down through the back of your skull and pelvis.

2 (above right) Here, enjoy the feeling of your lower back and hips broadening and melting into the floor. Breathe, be playful, circle your knees or rock slightly from side to side.

3 With your knees still bent in towards your chest, take your arms out to the sides, palms up. As you breathe out, take your knees to one side and your head to the other; you might want to rest one hand on your leg, as shown. Keep the knees tucked up to protect your lower back. Relax the lower hip and ribs into the floor. Feel a release through the ribs and chest as you end your out-breath. Repeat on the other side.

Deeper Relaxation Techniques

For these two exercises, lie in savasana (corpse pose) with your legs and arms slightly apart, palms facing upwards. Remember to focus on your breathing as much as your movements. Let the breath pass smoothly in and out through your nostrils.

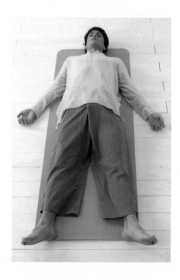

1 Tension and release (left) This quick and simple exercise is perfect if you have only five minutes for relaxation. The idea is to gather tension consciously in your body so that you are aware of when you have let it go. Begin at your feet and work through each part of the body until you reach the head and face.

Inhale and slowly tense your muscles in each body part for as long as you can hold your breath; don't strain. When you need to exhale, release the breath and all the tension at the same time. After working through the whole body, relax for a few moments.

2 Sun and moon (not shown) This visualization exercise helps to bring your right and left sides into balance and can be very rejuvenating. Be comfortable in savasana, close your eyes and focus on the rhythm of your breathing. As you inhale, imagine warm golden sunlight entering the toes of your right foot and then passing through the right side of your body and out through your head. As you exhale, imagine cool, silvery moonlight entering the top of your head and passing down through the left side of the body and back out through your toes. Repeat at least eight times.

Kaya Kriya

Kriyas are yogic cleansing exercises. Kaya kriya means body movement and this particular kriya is a very powerful cleansing technique in which you move the body simultaneously with your breath. Try to keep the in-breath and out-breath of equal length.

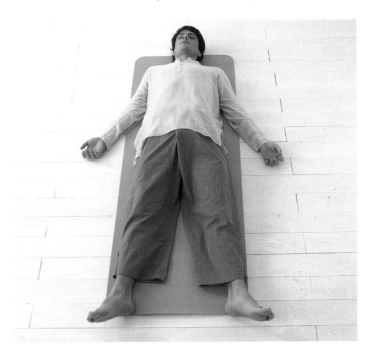

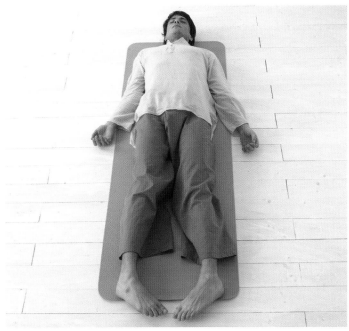

1 Start in neutral position. You will need to adapt savasana slightly, by taking your arms and legs a little further apart.

2 As you inhale, roll your feet inwards so that you feel the whole of each leg rotate right up into the hips. As you exhale, roll your feet outwards again and relax.

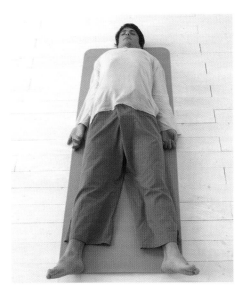

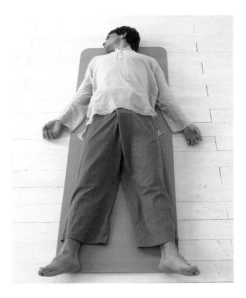

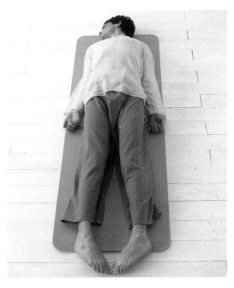

3 Turn your palms face down with your thumbs against your thighs. As you inhale, roll your arms out so that your hands rotate and your little fingers are now against the thighs. As your arms move, your chest will open and lift slightly, drawing your shoulder blades together. As you exhale, roll your arms back so that your chest drops and your palms come to rest face down.

4 As you inhale, slowly roll your head to the right and, as you exhale, roll your head to the left.

5 Practise each of the previous parts 8–12 times, and then practise all the elements simultaneously for a final 8–12 rounds. Allow the body to relax fully and your breath to flow naturally.

Energy Rebalancing Through Yoga

As practitioners of a profound healing art we have a responsibility to maintain our own physical health and build an awareness of our own bodies and minds that will make us more sensitive to the needs of massage partners. Maintaining a regular physical, energetic and meditative practice will help you to achieve this, and yogic practices such as this version of the classic *Surya Namaskar* routine may be the ideal route for you to try.

In ancient Indian culture, the sun symbolized spiritual awareness and was worshipped daily. Surya namaskar (*surya* means "sun" and *namaskar* means "salutation") is

an effective way of loosening, toning, stretching and massaging joints, muscles and organs, harmonizing movement with breathing and rebalancing energy flow within the body. Like Thai massage practice, the routine has its own form, works with energy rebalancing and is underpinned by a smooth and uninterrupted rhythm.

Ideal times to practise this sequence are at sunrise or sunset, but it can be performed at any time, as long as it is on an empty stomach. The full round works both sides of the body. Breathe in and out through your nostrils and let your breath guide you through each movement.

Surya Namaskar – Sun Salutation

Begin this exercise with your right foot, which will be the active foot through one half of the sequence. When you have completed all the postures on one side, repeat with the left foot as the active foot. Finish standing, with your hands in prayer position.

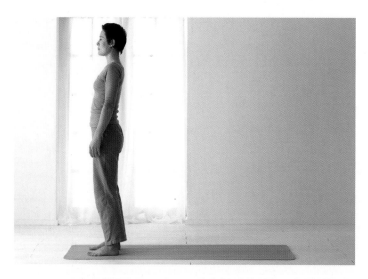

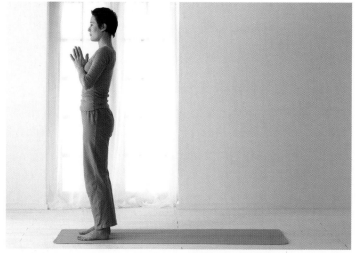

1 Begin with your feet hip-width apart, your body relaxed and your breathing easy. Take time to feel the contact with the earth beneath the soles of your feet. Feel yourself being rooted to the ground, with all the tension in your body flowing out through your feet.

2 Inhale and, as you exhale, bring your hands together in prayer position level with your breastbone, with elbows and shoulders relaxed.

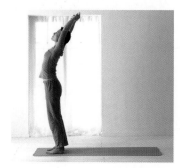

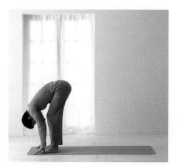

3 (far left) Inhale. Extend your hands straight up, feeling the opening come through the whole of the front of your body.

4 (left) Exhale. Release into a soft forward bend, making sure you fold from your hips, not your waist. Allow your knees to bend if they need to.

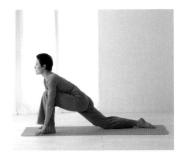 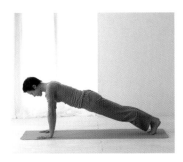

5 (above left) Inhale. Place your fingertips or palms on the floor and take your right foot back. Let your tailbone drop towards the ground. Keep your left foot flat on the ground. Feel the length come from the front of your pubic bone all the way up into the chest.

6 (above right) Hold your breath without straining. Take your left foot back, tuck the toes under and extend into your heels. Check your hips – your body should form a straight line.

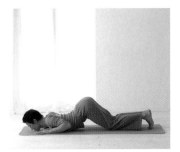 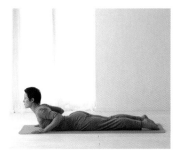

7 (above left) Exhale. Drop your knees, chest, elbows and chin to the ground. Keep your hips up.

8 (above right) Inhale. Slide your hips down and away. Flatten your feet against the mat. Sink your pubic bone into the mat and lift up through the front of your body. Check that your lower back feels comfortable – if not, you have come up too far. Keep your elbows tucked into the sides of your body and your shoulders relaxed away from your ears.

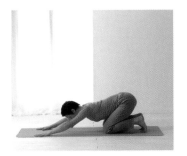 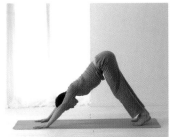

9 (above left) Tuck your toes under and, keeping your hands planted in front of you, drop your hips back towards your heels. Let your hips sink and feel your tailbone lengthen away from your head.

10 (above right) Exhale. With your feet and hands sinking into the mat, let your hips fly up and away towards the sky. If necessary, allow your heels to stay slightly off the mat in order to keep freedom of movement in your hips.

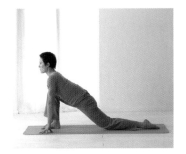 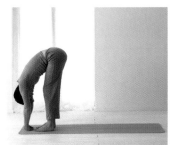

11 (above left) Inhale. Bring your right foot forward in between your hands. Let your tail drop down and the front of your body open.

12 (above right) Exhale. Bring both your feet together and come into a soft forward bend.

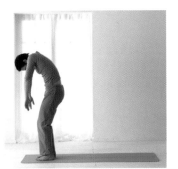 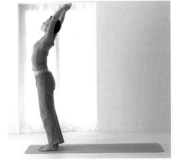

13 (above left) Inhale. Gently roll back up to standing.

14 (above right) Continuing the inhalation, unfold fully, extending your hands up towards the sky.

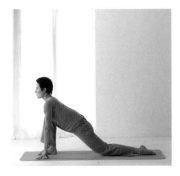 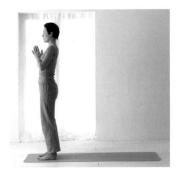

15 (above left) Repeat the sequence, exhaling into forward fold again. This time take your left foot back to continue the movements on the other side.

16 (above right) Complete one whole round, working both right and left feet. Finish in prayer position. Repeat at least six times and then relax in savasana.

Meditation in Motion – Qi Gong

It is very important for the Thai masseur to maintain a sense of balance within their body, and there is a wide variety of energy practices that you can use to achieve this. A particularly beautiful way to experience the subtle flow of energy around the body is by practising the Chinese tradition of *qi gong* – meditation in motion – on which the exercises shown below are based. Qi (or chi) is life energy and gong refers to work or exercise that requires both study and practice.

You can perform these movements after a massage, as a way of calming and grounding the energy stimulated during the session, or even beforehand, as preparation for giving massage.

BUILDING MOVEMENT AWARENESS

These exercises help to cultivate a soft, flowing quality of movement in the body. They can build greater awareness of how the flow of breath is linked with the flow of life energy and how it can permeate through the body to re-energize us. This type of internal exercise is more subtle than the Sun Salutation featured earlier, which is a more dynamic way of balancing internal energy through exercise. Explore both approaches and see which suits you best. Different forms of energy work may suit you better on different days. Try not to become fixed about which practice you adopt, but be sensitive and attentive to your inner cues.

Warm Up

These general movements are an excellent way to stimulate the movement of energy
in all of the joints. This brings greater mobility and freedom throughout
the whole of the body.

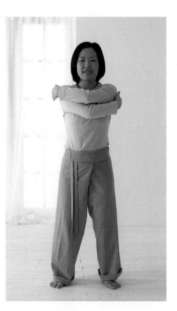 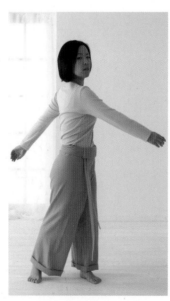 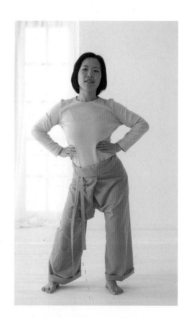 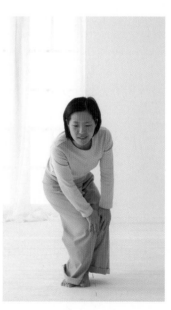

1 (above left) Let your arms swing out and then wrap around your shoulders or ribs in a hugging action. Allow your arms to build their own momentum. Alternate the upper and lower arm.

2 (above right) This is a similar movement to the previous exercise but this time swing both arms to the side, letting them wrap around your body, then swing the other way. To protect your knees, allow your heel to come away from the ground as you swing.

3 (above left) Place your hands on your lower ribs. Looking straight ahead, slowly circle the hips repeatedly in both directions. Try to keep your upper body completely still and move only your hips.

4 (above right) This exercise opens the knee and ankle joints. Bring your feet and knees together. Bend your knees slightly and cup your palms over your kneecaps. Circle your knees in both directions, bringing your heels off the ground if you need to.

Moving Energy

This energizes the hands, arms and chest, bringing lightness to the upper body. Keep your movements quiet, gentle and light as you move between positions. Be attentive to your breath and feel the sensations in your body.

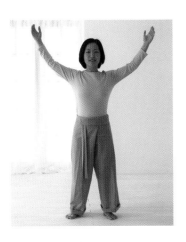 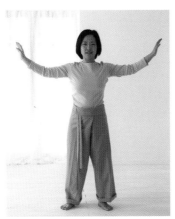

1 (far left) Stand with your feet a comfortable distance apart. Check that your legs are straight without the knees being locked. With your arms hanging by your sides, turn your palms to face the sky. Inhale and slowly raise your arms away from your sides to bring the palms up above your head. Keep your shoulders relaxed and don't overstretch the arms.

2 (left) Exhaling, turn your palms to face downwards and sweep the arms back down to rest either side of your body.
  Repeat each movement several times, for as long as feels good to you.

Connecting Heaven and Earth

This re-establishes your link with the earth and the sky. Feel as if you are raising a ball of energy from the ground up the front of your body and releasing it to the sky, then receiving a new ball of energy from the sky and bringing it down the back of your body to the earth.

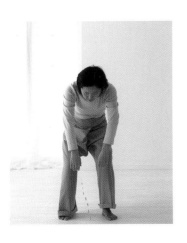 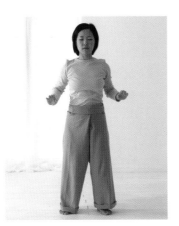

1 (far left) Bend forward, and, as you inhale, draw your hands up from the ground, mirroring the contours of the front of your body without actually touching it. Now continue to extend your arms above your head so that your fingertips are pointing skywards.

2 (left) Exhaling, bring your hands down, mirroring the contours of the back and sides of your body and legs, until you come all the way down to the ground. Continue this cycle of energy from earth to sky and from sky to earth, experiencing your body as a conductor of qi.

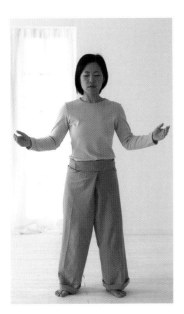 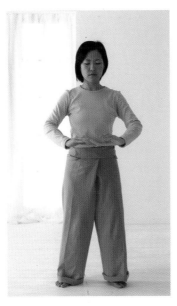

Returning to Your Centre

This grounding exercise works with a small range of circular movement. It focuses on building energy around your abdomen, the body's energetic centre.

1 (far left) As you inhale, turn your palms up to face the sky. Lift your hands up, bringing them no higher than your shoulders. Keep your shoulders completely relaxed and your elbows soft.

2 (left) Exhaling, turn your palms to face downwards and then bring the palms back down until they are level with your abdomen. Repeat this movement several times until you feel that the two halves of the movement have become one continuous flow.

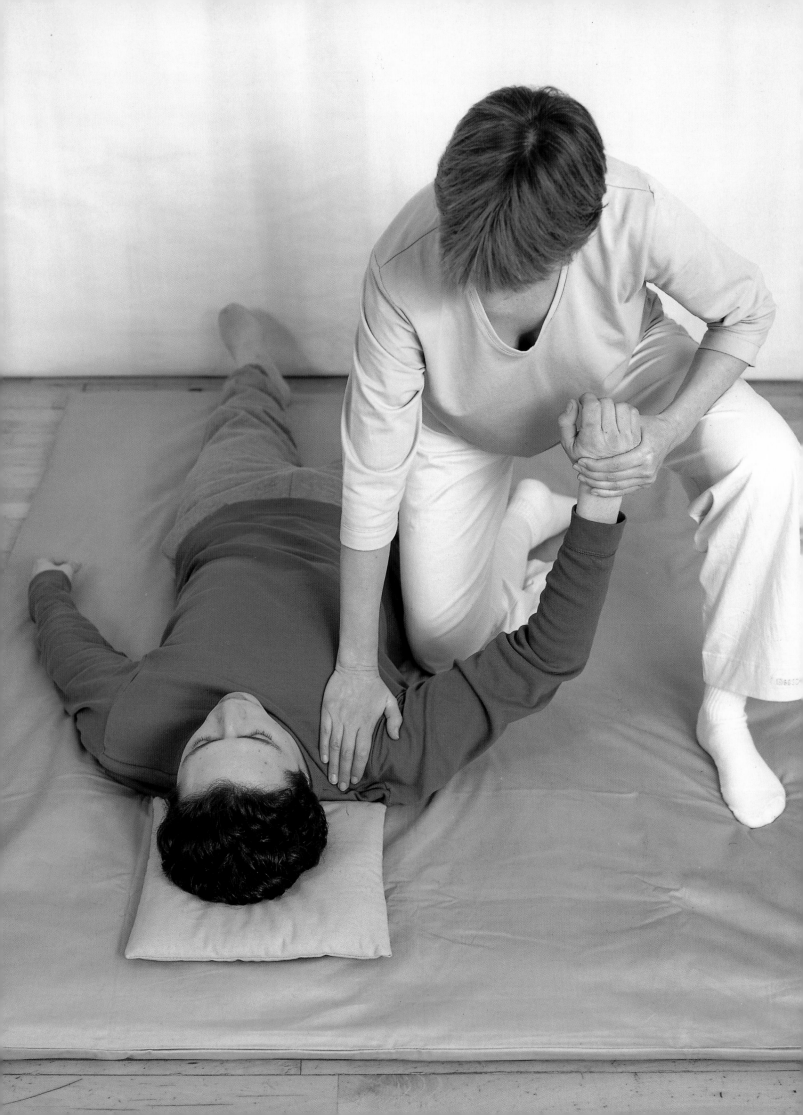

Shiatsu

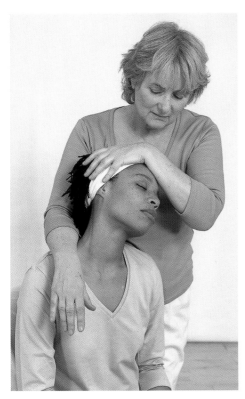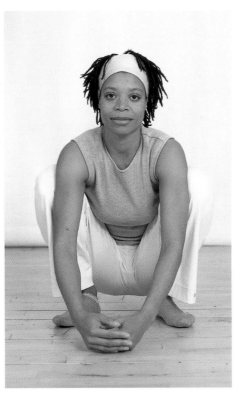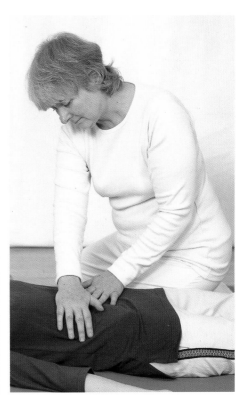

What is Shiatsu?

Shiatsu is a traditional healing art from Japan, using touch and pressure to release and rebalance the energy of the body. It is both a form of physical therapy and a means to greater integration of body, mind and spirit. Based on traditional Eastern principles, Shiatsu works on the energetic system of the body, through energy pathways, known as meridians, to bring balance and harmony on a mental, emotional and spiritual level.

The power of Shiatsu is in the use of touch – maybe the oldest form of healing there is. Touch is a comfort, seen every day when a child falls and hurts itself and is soothed by the mother "rubbing it better", or when a hug is shared between friends in times of emotional stress. Touch is as essential a nutrient as food and water for both physical and mental health, nourishing a feeling of trust and of security and belonging. A baby needs to be held to develop a sense of safety and of being loved, and in the same way in adulthood touch can be soothing, healing, and provide an effective method of letting go.

The Japanese word Shiatsu literally means "finger pressure" and a Shiatsu practitioner will use pressure with the thumbs or palms on pressure points and energy channels of the body to induce deep relaxation. Sometimes the practitioner will use elbows, knees and feet to apply pressure and can give a more dynamic treatment with stretches, massage and mobilization techniques. Receiving Shiatsu brings about a release of tension and leaves the receiver with a sense of being deeply touched and brought back into a state of balance.

The art of Shiatsu depends on the quality of touch of the practitioner, through communication and responsiveness to the client's needs. The practitioner

Below In Japanese, the term Shiatsu means finger pressure. Traditionally, Shiatsu was used as both treatment and as a preventative to encourage good health.

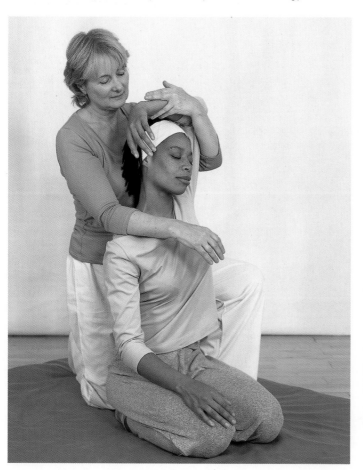

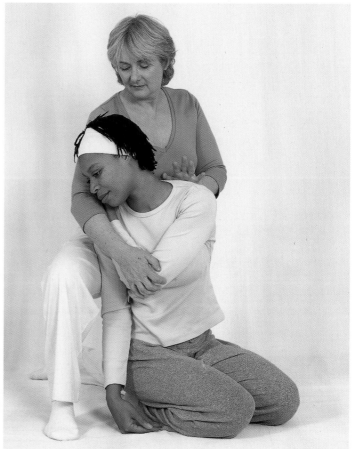

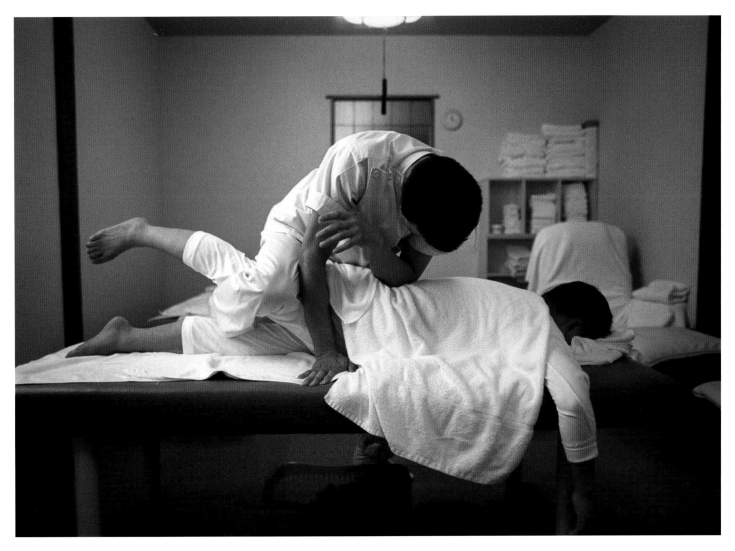

Above The practitioner will use elbows, knees and feet, as well as the fingers and palms, to apply pressure and give a more dynamic treatment of stretches and mobilization techniques.

will use deep, slow holding techniques to work on areas of weakness, and more vigorous techniques, such as rubbing or rocking, on more stiff or tense areas. The practitioner will use their sense of touch as well as observing a person's face, posture, actions and lifestyle to assess how energy may be out of balance and how to bring it back into harmony. Shiatsu combines physical techniques with a finely developed intuition and an understanding of the principles of Eastern medicine, especially the movement and interactions of different energies around the body. These principles supply a framework from which the practitioner can observe and assess the receiver's condition and give an appropriate treatment.

Shiatsu treatment is given with the client lying on a futon mattress on the floor, allowing the practitioner access from all sides and the ability to apply pressure using their body weight with plenty of surrounding space. No massage oils or lotions are required as the practitioner does not move along the body surface, but gives pressure through loosely fitting, comfortable clothing.

Conditions treated

These are some of the more common conditions that a Shiatsu practitioner can treat. Make sure that you advise your practitioner if you would like the treatment to focus on a specific problem or body part.

Traditionally used as both a treatment and a form of preventative medicine, Shiatsu can also be used as part of a healthcare programme or as a form of general relaxation, to rest and recuperate spirit and body.

Headaches	Circulatory problems
Back pain	Anxiety
Neck tension	Depression
Shoulder tension	Stress-related
Stiff muscles	problems
Pulled muscles	Tension headaches
Knee problems	Sleeping disorders
Sports injuries	Tiredness
Digestive problems	Irritable bowel
Menstrual problems	syndrome
Asthma	Childbirth
Insomnia	Pregnancy (not first
Fatigue	trimester)

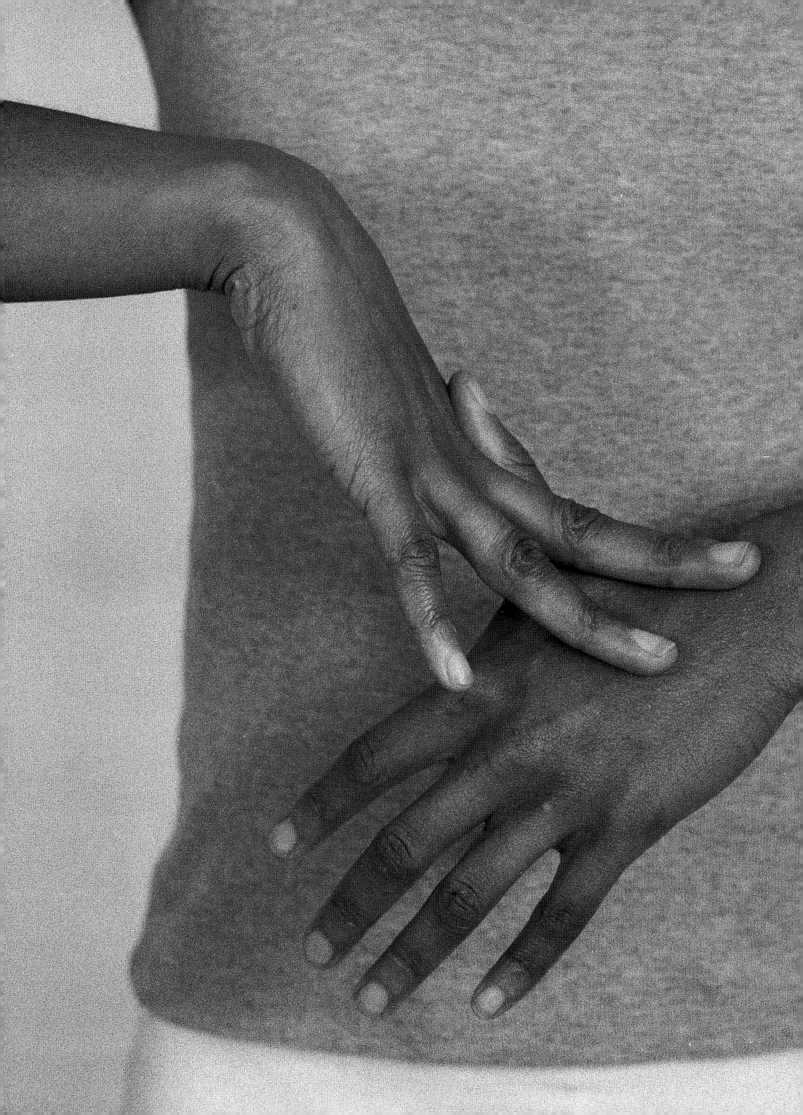

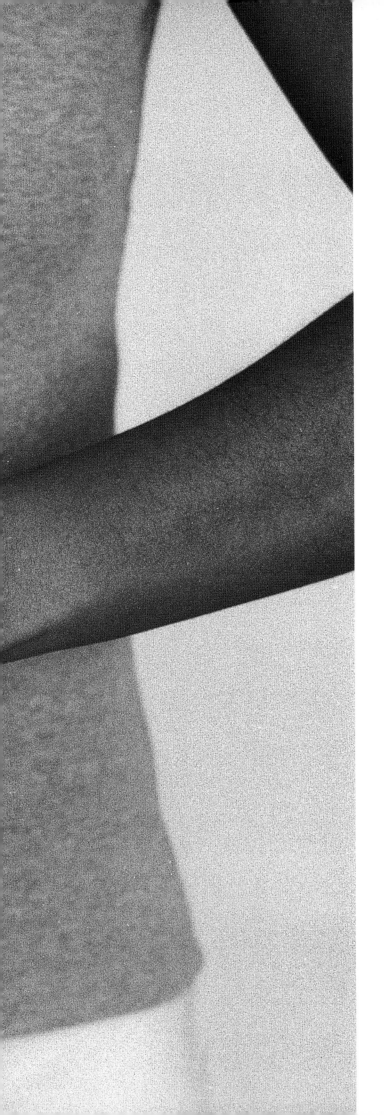

The Beginnings

Fundamental to Eastern medicine is the principle of vital energy flowing through the body, known as chi. The smooth and balanced flow of this energy is thought to be essential to good health and longevity.

Shiatsu works on this vital energy and through the simple application of touch can restore a harmonious balance to the chi flow. Blockages or energy imbalances can be caused by physical, mental or emotional problems and Shiatsu aims to uncover how these factors affect the chi and the treatment needed in order to re-establish balance. Shiatsu will strengthen the body's own innate healing power and will improve health, vitality and well-being.

Understanding the origins and some of the principles of Traditional Chinese Medicine forms the first step to learning and appreciating the art of Shiatsu and discovering how it can help you in everyday life.

The History of Shiatsu

Shiatsu is a uniquely Japanese form of therapy, but its roots date back to ancient Chinese philosophical ideas. Four classical approaches to medicine were developed in China. In the south, herbal remedies were readily available. In the east and north, acupuncture and moxibustion were practised, the latter applying heat on chosen points of the meridians. In central China, physical techniques, such as massage and breathing exercises, were used.

In Japan, as travel and trade with China increased during the 10th century, Chinese thought and philosophy, and with them Traditional Chinese Medicine, were becoming more influential. The traditional Chinese form of massage, known as *anmo* (*anma* in Japanese), combined rubbing and pressing on stiff and sore areas and included self-massage

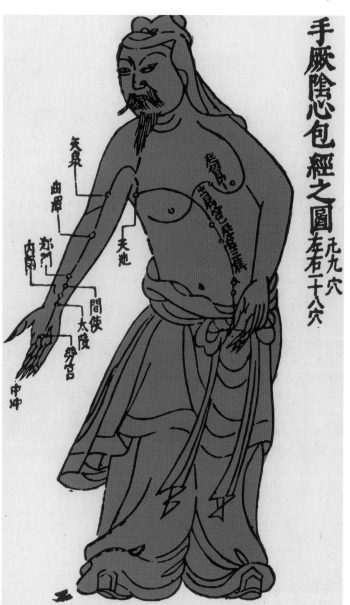

手厥陰心包經之圖 左右一十八穴 元九穴

天泉
曲澤
郄門
內關
間使
太陵
勞宮
中衝

and exercises for detoxification and rejuvenation. By the 17th century Chinese medicine was firmly established in the Japanese culture and the use of anma became widespread. However, over time it lost its medical status and became predominantly a therapy for meditation, relaxation and pleasure.

In the early 20th century, an anma practitioner, Tamai Tempaku, wrote a book called *Shiatsu Ho*, combining anma, *ampuku* (abdominal massage) and *do-in* (self-massage), signalling the birth of the modern-day Shiatsu practised around the world today.

He greatly influenced another practitioner, Tokujiro Namikoshi, who opened the first Shiatsu Institute of Therapy in Hokkaido in 1925. Namikoshi's focus was the legal recognition of Shiatsu in Japan, achieved through acceptance by Western scientific and medical theory. Consequently, all mention of meridians, energy or traditional theory was removed from his work. In its place he required a thorough knowledge of the musculo-skeletal structure and the nervous system, emphasizing neuro-muscular points. He was a popular and charismatic figure in Japan, the author of the book *Do It Yourself – 3 Minute Shiatsu*, which became a best-seller. He appeared on television to promote his technique, using the catchphrase "All you have to do is press". By the 1950s, he had established Shiatsu as an officially recognized and much practised therapy with standard qualifications.

BACK TO BASICS

It was one of Namikoshi's pupils, Shizuto Masunaga, who integrated Shiatsu back into the traditional principles of Eastern medicine, emphasizing the meridians and the Five Element theory (see pages 16–19), which describes the different energy qualities. He was a student of Western psychology and Traditional Chinese Medicine, and was fascinated with the spiritual, psychological and emotional aspects of individuals. He developed his own Shiatsu

Left This Chinese acupuncture chart showing the meridian points dates from AD1031. It indicates the specific medical conditions that can be treated by using each particular point.

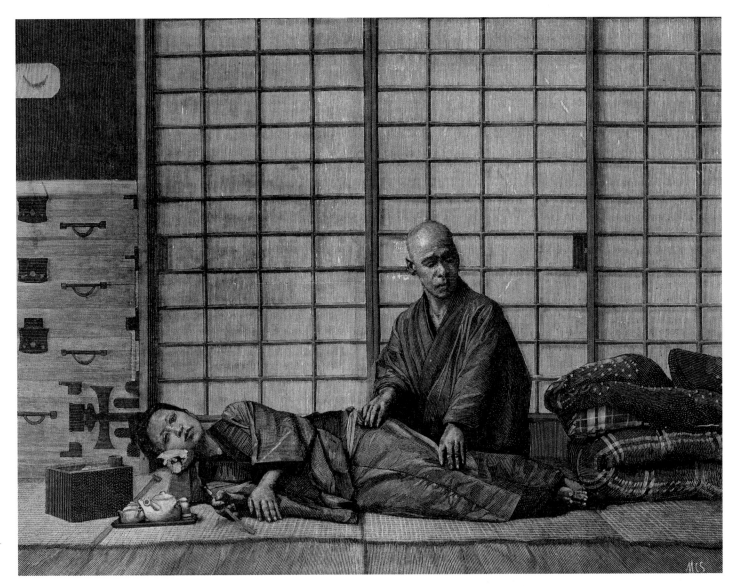

Above This engraving dates back to 1896. It depicts a traditional scene with a woman receiving therapeutic massage treatment from a professional Shiatsu practitioner.

bodywork system, later called Zen Shiatsu. Masunaga also developed a form of abdominal diagnosis known as the Hara diagnosis, and extended the traditional acupuncture meridians to include supplementary ones. He established a school in Tokyo called the Iokai School of Shiatsu. His focus on the practitioner's awareness and technique made his system unique and more accessible to the West. He stressed the practitioner's intention, attitude and observation in influencing the treatment, and the importance of using two hands to provide support and connection, creating a more nurturing and less painful experience.

Both Namikoshi and Masunaga came to the West but Masunaga has had the most important influence on Shiatsu today, encompassing more traditional principles and the integration of the psychological and emotional aspects of Eastern medicine. During the late 1970s, one of his students, Wataru Ohashi, brought Masunaga to the United States where he founded Zen Shiatsu, producing a book in English on the subject in 1976. This was the first step towards global popularity. Ohashi describes Namikoshi as the showman of Shiatsu, with his television appearances and popular books, whereas Masunaga was more the intellectual. He attributes Masunaga's popularity in the West to the growing interest in the 1960s and 1970s in all things Eastern and spiritual, whereas Namikoshi was more popular in Japan where the focus was on Western developments and medical advances.

Zen Shiatsu

A sect of Buddhism, Zen focuses on the training of the mind through meditation. The purpose of Zen is to achieve total enlightenment through the discovery of one's basic nature. Its principles and approaches can be applied to numerous human endeavours, including archery, aikido, judo and other martial arts, gardening and architecture, tea ceremony, calligraphy and haiku (Japanese poetry). In the case of Shiatsu, touch is used to balance the body and to reach inner peace. This is achieved through bringing a deep energetic awareness, focused through meridians and points to the part of the body being treated. Emphasis is placed on the inner perception of both giver and receiver.

Chi and the Life Force

The theoretical foundation of Shiatsu uses the concept of the healthy flow and balance of energy, or chi. This idea of energy balance is applied through the body, externally in our environment, and holistically in the way in which we live our lives. Most Shiatsu training involves learning these principles of energy, and understanding how they relate to one another; this enables a much deeper benefit from the Shiatsu experience.

Around the 6th century BC, the Chinese philosopher Lao Tsu wrote the Tao Te Ching, outlining a personal, political and philosophical treatise on a way of living. The Tao, meaning "the way", is an explanation of how the universe came into being. Lao Tsu taught that all straining and striving is counterproductive. One should endeavour to discern and follow the natural forces – to go with the flow of events and not to pit oneself against the natural order of things. This concept underpins all concepts behind Traditional Chinese Medicine. Lao Tsu wrote:

The Tao begat one.
One begat two.
Two begat three.
And three begat the ten thousand things.

CHI ENERGY FORCE

"The Tao begat one" in Lao Tsu's philosophy refers to the chi energy force. Chi, also known as ki or qi, can be translated as "energy" in its widest sense – it manifests in an infinite variety of forms, in air and food, in rock and vibration. It is the source of all movement and change within the universe. Chi never disappears, it just changes form, continually transforming over time. It is essential to life and contained within all living things. Every cell of our body is alive with chi. It is the life force.

Disease, tension and pain are a manifestation of an imbalance or blockage of chi within the body. The work of the Shiatsu practitioner is to bring the chi back to a balanced state through the use of applied pressure on certain areas of the body, based on a correct diagnosis.

The concept of chi is central and is incorporated in many Japanese words: *genki* (good flowing chi) means healthy, while *byoki* (blocked chi) means disease.

YIN AND YANG

Lao Tsu's "One begat two" refers to yin and yang. Over a period of several hundred years, Chinese philosophers differentiated the chi of the Universe into two forces, yin and yang. In Taoist philosophy, the yin and yang symbol represents the two forces that pervade everything in the universe, describing how the universe works, and everything within it.

Chi exercise
In a kneeling position, hold your hands in front of you at elbow height, palms facing each other, about a hand's width apart, as if you were holding a ball. Breathe slowly and attentively. Gently move your hands towards and away from one another several times. Can you feel anything?
Do you experience "something" pushing or pulling between your hands? This feeling or energy can be described as chi.

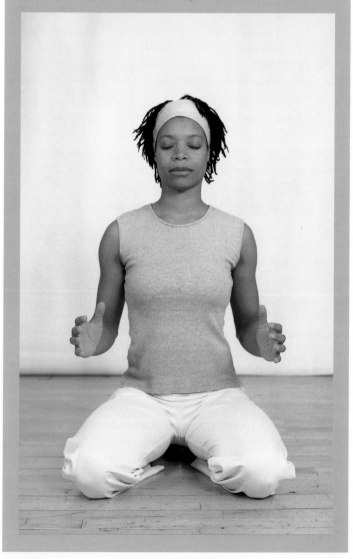

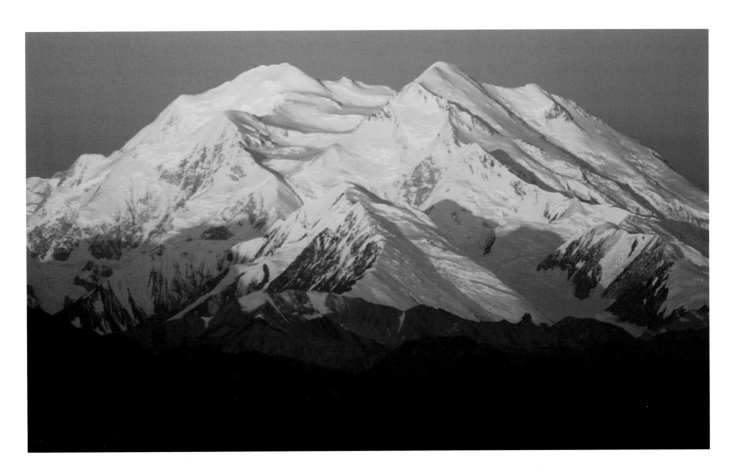

The Chinese used the observation of nature to describe aspects of the world, and the original meanings of the Chinese symbols of yin and yang were the "dark side of the mountain" and the "light side of the mountain". As the sun was seen to move in the sky so the light and dark side of the mountain changed until what was dark became light and light became dark, as all things transform from yin to yang and back again. Things are yin or yang only in relation to other opposite, or balancing, things, such as dark and light, night and day, earth and heaven, front and back, down and up, cold and hot.

Above Mountains were used to describe the qualities of yin and yang; the movement of the sun makes the dark side of the mountain light, as yin becomes yang.

THE YIN/YANG SYMBOL

- The outer circle symbolizes the wholeness and infinity of the cosmos. It contains the yang (light) and the yin (dark).
- Yin and yang are divided by a curved line that represents the movement and constant flow of yin into yang and yang into yin.
- Within the largest portion of each colour there is a dot of the opposing colour. This shows that everything contains the seed of its opposite within it. All things contain both yin and yang energies. There are no absolutes.
- The two colours are in equal proportion, equally balanced. If there is more of one aspect, then there is less of the other, a state of being yin or yang.
- One cannot exist without the other, and all things contain elements of yin and yang.
- All matter, substance and things in the universe are made up of both yin and yang, although at times they may appear to be more influenced by either yin or yang.

The nature of yin and yang

YIN is the quiet, female, intuitive, receiving force, associated with earth. The earth is the source of life, it provides us with what we need to survive. Associated with: earth, down, dark, passive, material, female, front, intuition, interior, autumn and winter, stillness, moon and cold.

YANG is the strong, male, creative, giving force, which is associated with heaven. The heaven above us is always in motion and brings about change. Associated with: heaven, up, light, active, vibration, male, back, intellect, exterior, spring and summer, movement, sun and hot.

The Five Elements

The five elements – wood, fire, earth, metal and water – are the basic building blocks and fundamental components of the universe. Everything in existence contains all five elements but one element will always predominate. The five elements describe the different qualities of chi energy – the five different ways in which it manifests itself in the universe. They represent the cycles in the change from yin to yang and yang to yin.

The origins of the five elements spring from the observation of nature, particularly the cycles of nature. The five elements do not refer to physical elements alone, but to cyclical movements. The name "five elements" can be misleading as it suggests an association with static, immutable properties. Sometimes the theory is referred to as the Five Transformations, which gives a more accurate picture of the fluidity of the cycle.

The theory comprises two aspects. The first is the grouping together of things or phenomena with a similar energy quality, and there are lists of correspondences illustrating this. Listed below are just a few of the major correspondences, which relate to both the natural world, for example the seasons, and the human world, for example tastes and emotions. So you find birth, green and muscles under the wood element and compassion, ideas and humidity under the earth element. The important point is that things that relate to human activity and the activity of nature are woven together when describing the elements.

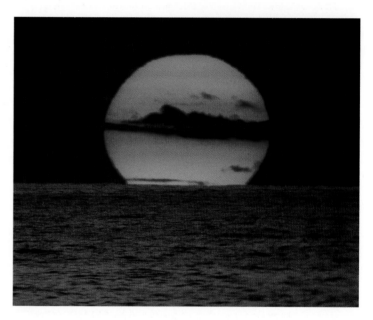

Above The sun provides the fundamental fire energy for the world, affecting the seasonal cycles and the balance of the five elements.

The five elements correspondences
Each of the five elements is imbued with a lengthy list of characteristics, from their colours to the season and body parts and organs. These are used in all practices of Traditional Chinese Medicine to diagnose, harmonize and provide treatment for any imbalances within the system, be it in Shiatsu massage or in feng shui or T'ai Chi. There is an extensive table on pages 246–7.

ELEMENT	WOOD	FIRE	EARTH	METAL	WATER
Season	Spring	Summer	Late Summer	Autumn	Winter
Process	Birth	Growth	Transformation	Harvest	Storage
Climate	Windy	Hot	Humidity	Dryness	Cold
Colour	Green	Red	Yellow/Brown	White	Black/Blue
Yin Organ	Liver	Heart	Spleen	Lungs	Kidneys
Yang Organ	Gall Bladder	Small Intestine	Stomach	Large Intestine	Bladder
Tissue	Muscles	Blood Vessels	Flesh	Skin	Bones
Sense	Sight	Speech	Taste	Smell	Hearing
Taste	Sour	Bitter	Sweet	Spicy	Salty
Sound	Shouting	Laughing	Singing	Crying	Groaning
Emotion	Anger	Joy	Compassion	Depression	Fear
Capacity	Planning	Spiritual	Ideas/Opinions	Elimination	Awareness

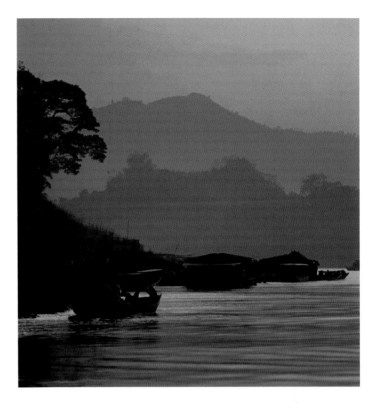

The second aspect of the five elements theory looks at the flow of energy between the elements in a defined sequence. There are two cycles that describe this interaction of the five elements. They are the Creative (Shen) Cycle and the Control (Ko) Cycle.

THE CREATIVE (SHEN) CYCLE

This cycle describes the interaction of the five elements where one element precedes and gives rise to the next one. It illustrates how the energy flows in a circle from yin to yang. Sometimes called the Supporting Cycle, each preceding element, which can be described as the mother, nourishes or supports the following element.

This cycle is clearly manifested in the external world by the seasons. Wood-spring (birth) feeds the fire of summer (maturation) creating the earth-late summer (harvest). Out of earth comes metal-autumn (dying back, letting go) continuing on to water-winter (death, hibernation), which then completes the cycle to regenerate as wood-spring (rebirth). In Traditional Chinese Medicine treatments, a weakness in one part of the body can be treated by boosting the key element for that body part, such as metal for the lung, and also by increasing the element that creates metal, which is earth.

THE CREATIVE CYCLE

One of the two cycles that describes the interaction of the five elements, the Creative Cycle – also called the Shen Cycle – explains how the five elements support and create one another. Each element springs, or is created, from the previous one, as the seasons transform from one to another: spring (wood) turns into summer (fire), which mellows into late summer (earth), then autumn (metal), which finally flows into winter (water).

WOOD produces FIRE
A material that burns easily, without wood there could be no fire. Wood grows upward (growing yang) and generates fire (extreme yang). As spring turns into the bright and dry summer, wood becomes parched, giving way to fire.

WATER produces WOOD
Trees and plants give life and without water the trees would die. Water (yin) flows into wood (becoming more yang). The end of winter feeds the beginning of spring, with the flow of water into new shoots and trees.

METAL produces WATER
When metal is heated it transforms into a liquid, giving rise to water. As metal turns to fluid it becomes more yin. Late autumn it freezes over and becomes the extreme yin of the cold winter months.

FIRE produces EARTH
As the fire burns out it leaves behind the ashes, which fall and unite with the earth. Fire turns to ashes and settles into earth (yang begins to change to yin). Natural energy flows out of the sun and into the soil as summer dies giving way to the late summer harvest.

EARTH produces METAL
Metal comes from the earth and without earth there would be no metal. Earth condenses (becomes more yin) and becomes metal. As late summer transforms into autumn, with the decay and enrichment of the land, metal becomes dominant.

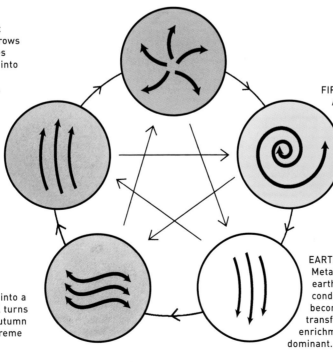

THE CONTROL (KO) CYCLE

The second cycle that describes the interaction of the five elements is the Control Cycle; this provides a check on the indefinite growth of the Creative Cycle. This is the opposite of the Creative Cycle in that it expresses a relationship where one element exerts control, leading to a suppression that inhibits another element. For example, a metal knife can cut wood and therefore will shape or control it. The Control Cycle is used to prevent one element from draining energy from another. For example, the lung problem that has been treated with Metal (the base element for that part of the body) and Earth (the element that creates Metal) can also be treated by reducing Fire, Metal's controlling element, and allowing Metal to flourish.

The Creative Cycle and the Control Cycle provide a balance that is essential for normal growth and development and also describe the natural balance of chi in the universe. However, when this balance is disturbed the cycles can become distorted. Sometimes the controlled element is too strong or the controlling element too weak and therefore the "natural" order is temporarily reversed. For example, if a fire is fierce and out of control and there is not enough water to suppress it, the water evaporates away.

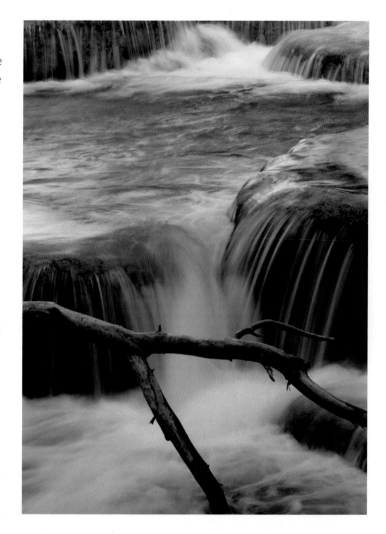

Right Water is the most yin element, representing winter. It flows into wood, in the same way that winter turns gradually into spring.

THE CONTROL CYCLE

This cycle – also called the Ko Cycle – explains how the elements control and reduce the power of one another. If an element becomes too strong, it will cause an imbalance in the whole system. While it will help to create the element next to it, as explained in the Creative Cycle, it will also harm the element after the next, reducing its energy and preventing equilibrium.

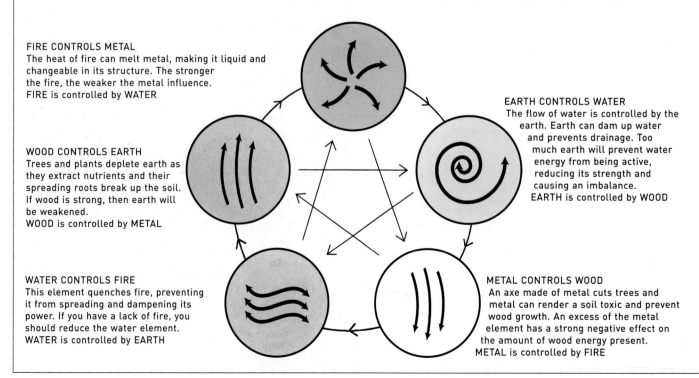

FIRE CONTROLS METAL
The heat of fire can melt metal, making it liquid and changeable in its structure. The stronger the fire, the weaker the metal influence.
FIRE is controlled by WATER

WOOD CONTROLS EARTH
Trees and plants deplete earth as they extract nutrients and their spreading roots break up the soil. If wood is strong, then earth will be weakened.
WOOD is controlled by METAL

WATER CONTROLS FIRE
This element quenches fire, preventing it from spreading and dampening its power. If you have a lack of fire, you should reduce the water element.
WATER is controlled by EARTH

EARTH CONTROLS WATER
The flow of water is controlled by the earth. Earth can dam up water and prevents drainage. Too much earth will prevent water energy from being active, reducing its strength and causing an imbalance.
EARTH is controlled by WOOD

METAL CONTROLS WOOD
An axe made of metal cuts trees and metal can render a soil toxic and prevent wood growth. An excess of the metal element has a strong negative effect on the amount of wood energy present.
METAL is controlled by FIRE

Some common elemental imbalances

IMBALANCE	MEANING	SYMPTOMS
Wood over-controls Earth; Earth becomes weak	Liver (Wood) excess is invading Spleen (Earth) and making it weak	Irritability, diarrhoea, abdominal distension, alternating between diarrhoea and constipation, irritable bowel syndrome, tiredness
Too low Metal cannot support Water	Lung (Metal) is weak and weakens Kidney (Water), grasping Lung chi	Shortness of breath, cough, asthma, lower back ache
Water is weak; Fire out of control	Weakness in Kidney (Water) allows Heart (Fire) to become too hot	Feeling agitated, insomnia, thirsty, high blood pressure, red face
Earth is low; unable to support Metal	Weakness in Lung (Metal) or Spleen (Earth) adversely affects the other	Tiredness, loose stools, weak voice, breathlessness

TREATMENTS USING THE FIVE ELEMENTS

The nature of Traditional Chinese Medicine is holistic – it encompasses the whole life and environment surrounding a person rather than focusing on a specific part of the body. Therefore, when a physical problem occurs, it is viewed as a symptom of a deeper energy imbalance involving the five elements, and is categorized alongside other considerations, such as emotional issues, environmental disharmony or social problems.

The treatment of a disorder is achieved by rebalancing the five elements. As mentioned earlier, this can be done through a variety of therapies, from herbal medicine to the movement therapies of T'ai Chi and Chi Kung. In Shiatsu, meridian pairs relate to each specific element, and by treating these meridians and related points, the flow of the elements can be brought into balance. It is important, when deciding on the meridians to treat, to consider the relationships between the elements according to the Shen and Ko cycles as well as looking at the signs and symptoms in relation to the five elements correspondences.

By looking at the supporting and controlling cycles you can decide which is the element or elements to be treated. For example, if the cause of the condition is weakness in the mother element in the Creative Cycle (as in the example above where Earth is low and unable to support Metal) there will be signs and symptoms in both elements. Earth symptoms are loose stools and tiredness; Metal symptoms are breathlessness and a weak voice. It will be important to treat both mother and child elements to restore balance.

A combination of using the correspondences to see into which element the signs and symptoms fit, and looking at the relationships according to the cycles, can provide a treatment plan to restore health and well-being.

The mother-child analogy

There is a saying in Traditional Chinese Medicine: "If the child screams, treat the mother". The Creative Cycle – also referred to as nurturing – is traditionally seen as the mother-child dynamic. The root cause of the symptoms in the child can be a weakness in the mother where the mother is unable to nourish the child in a wholesome and balanced way. In this case it is important to treat the mother first, as well as treating the child. The Control Cycle is seen as the grandmother-grandchild relationship, where the elders traditionally control the family and keep the young ones in check. If the grandmother is too strict this can lead to a stifling of the child; if she is not strong enough the child may be out of control.

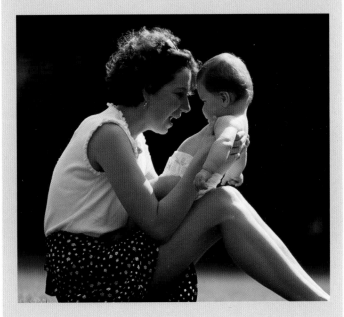

Meridians

Chi energy flows through the body in a similar way to blood, following twelve special invisible pathways or channels that are known as meridians. When chi is flowing freely and in balance through the meridians then a person is healthy. Each of the meridians relates to an organ or organ function. In contrast to Western medicine these are seen as having an emotional as well as a physiological aspect.

The body contains six pairs of vital organs or organ functions corresponding to the twelve meridians, and these perform all the functions of nourishment and sustaining life.

The meridians either carry energy to the organs or carry the energy that the organs produce to other areas of the body. Thus the meridians stretch all over the body, linking apparently unrelated areas such as ears, arms or feet to the vital organs in the centre of the body. In this way, the energy of all parts affects the whole. In meridian theory, chi runs from one meridian to the next in a continuous loop or circuit. The connections between the channels ensure that there is an even circulation of chi, creating a balance of yin and yang. Each meridian pair has a yin meridian and a yang meridian, the yin on the front and the yang on the back.

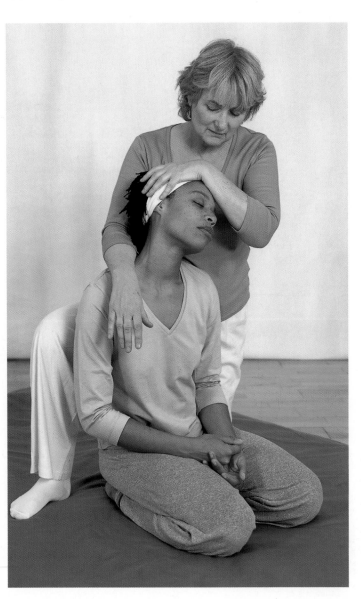

Six pairs of vital organs

Lungs Take in chi during respiration. Symbolizes openness, enthusiasm and positivity.

and Large Intestine Processes food and eliminates waste. Symbolizes ability to "let go".

Spleen Transforms food into energy. Symbolizes plenty and nourishment.

and Stomach Receiving and ripening ingested food and fluids. Symbolizes security.

Heart Governs blood. Houses the mind and emotions. Symbolizes joyfulness, calmness and communication.

and Small Intestine Controls blood and tissue quality. Symbolizes emotional stability, calmness and assimilation.

Heart Protector Protects the Heart, acting as a physical and emotional buffer. Symbolizes harmonious relationships.

and Triple Heater Maintains homeostasis and symbolizes integration and harmony throughout the body.

Kidney Controls the hormonal system. Symbolizes vitality, courage and the will to move forward in life.

and Bladder Transforms and excretes urine. Symbolizes qualities of will power and determination.

Liver Stores and distributes blood. Symbolizes creativity, ideas and organization.

and Gall Bladder Stores the bile. Symbolizes decision-making, flexibility of thought and movement.

Left Shiatsu makes use of stretches, as well as pressure, to release blockages and help the smooth flow of chi through a meridian.

THE FRONT OF THE BODY

The meridians found on the front of the body are the yin meridians (except Stomach, which is yang). They are considered to have a more important role than their yang pair and tend to be more often used in treatment. The front of the body is deep and more to do with maintaining core stability.

Key to the yin meridians

— Lung

— Spleen

— Stomach

— Heart

— Heart Protector

— Kidney

— Liver

(The remaining meridians are shown on the following pages.)

Pressure points

There are specific points (called *tsubos*) along the meridians where the chi can be more easily accessed, in a similar way to switches on an electrical circuit. These points can be used to help the flow of chi along the meridian, or they can be used to treat specific areas or sets of symptoms. For example, points on the shoulder on the Small Intestine meridian can treat shoulder problems. There are over 700 *tsubos* in the meridian system, each numbered according to the meridian.

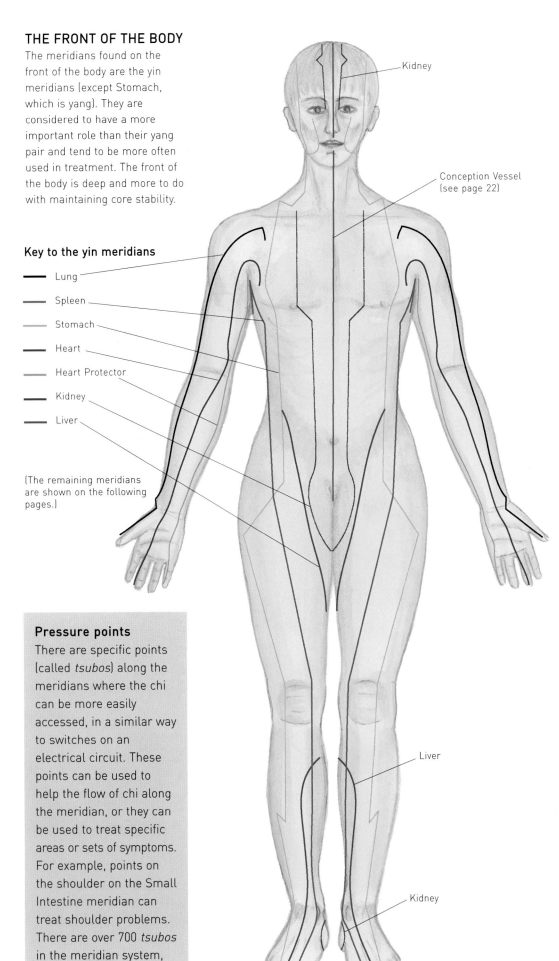

Kidney

Conception Vessel (see page 22)

Liver

Kidney

Useful pressure points on the front

The pressure points illustrated below and on the next two pages are a selection of important points on the meridians. There are more points illustrated on pages 68–101, provided in the context of the meridians.

Sometimes points can be used to alleviate specific symptoms and the usage given here follows this approach.

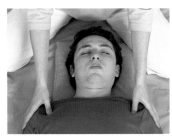

Lung 1
Location: Between the first and second ribs, below the middle of the collarbone.
Usage: Good for coughs, colds and sore throats. Can also help with sinus problems.

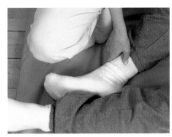

Spleen 6
Location: Four finger-widths above the tip of the inside ankle bone, just behind the shin bone.
Usage: Good for lower abdominal pain, especially period pains. Good for insomnia. Contraindicated during pregnancy.

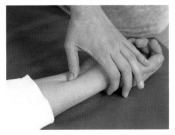

Heart Protector 6
Location: Three finger-widths above the wrist crease on the inside of the lower arm, between the two tendons.
Usage: Good for nausea, especially morning sickness, post-operative nausea and travel sickness.

THE BACK OF THE BODY

The meridians found on the back of the body are yang meridians. The spine is the major structure in the back and represents movement. It is supported by the Bladder meridian and its yu points – major points that relate to each of the body's organs. The yang meridians are more active, transforming, digesting, moving and excreting.

Key to the yang meridians

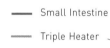

— Large Intestine
— Small Intestine
— Triple Heater
— Bladder

Triple Heater

Governing Vessel

Large Intestine

Governing Vessel and Conception Vessel

These two channels run through the centre of the body and govern all the yin and yang meridians. The Governing Vessel on the back is called the "Sea of yang", and points on this channel can be used to stimulate the yang energy and to benefit the spine. Points on the Conception Vessel, known as the "Sea of yin", can be used to nourish the yin and help with fertility. They are not used in treatment but they do have important points.

Useful pressure points on the back

These points can be used individually for specific problems or conditions. Apply steady, perpendicular thumb pressure.

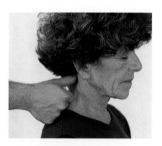

Gall Bladder 20
Location: Below the base of the skull, midway between the mid-line and the prominent bone behind the ear.
Usage: Relieves headaches coming from neck tension and neck pain.

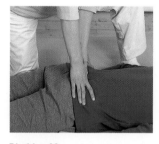

Bladder 23
Location: At the back of the waist between the 2nd and 3rd lumbar vertebrae, one thumb width either side of the mid-line.
Usage: Relieves lower back ache – can be tender, so go in slowly and hold for a while. This point is an important point for the kidneys (known as Kidney Yu point).

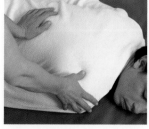

Small Intestine 11
Location: In the centre of the shoulder blade in the depression (you will know when you are on it because it is always a painful point).
Usage: Helps stiff, painful or frozen shoulder, especially at the back of the shoulder.

THE SIDE OF THE BODY

Many of the twelve meridians pass through the side of the body. Gall Bladder, a yang meridian, is the predominant meridian running down the side of the body with important points on the major joints such as shoulder, knee and hip. Joints reflect flexibility and the ability to change direction. Gall Bladder is important in the decision-making process, requiring flexibility and adaptability.

Key to the meridians

— Large Intestine

— Small Intestine

— Triple Heater

— Kidney

— Liver

— Gall Bladder

Movement and the meridians

The meridians in the front of the body, especially the Spleen and Stomach, give stability and support. The meridians at the back, especially Bladder, provide the impetus for movement and spontaneity. A big contributor to back problems is the confusion of these two distinct functions – support and impetus. Shiatsu stresses the importance of strength in the belly or hara to provide support for a healthy spine.

Triple Heater

Small Intestine

Liver

Useful pressure points on the side

These points can be used individually for specific problems or conditions. Apply thumb pressure for one or two minutes.

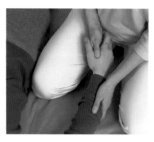

Large Intestine 4
Location: On the back of the hand in the depression where the two bones of the thumb and index finger meet.
Usage: Good for constipation or diarrhoea (known as "the great eliminator"), can relieve toothache and can be used to increase general vitality. Contraindicated during pregnancy.

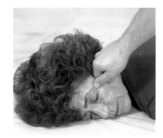

Gall Bladder 1
Location: About one thumb width outwards from the outer corner of the eye in the depression.
Usage: Can relieve headaches behind the eyes and revitalize tired eyes.

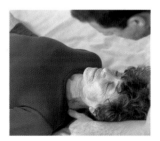

Gall Bladder 21
Location: Midway along the shoulder on the highest point.
Usage: Good for stiff, painful or frozen shoulder, especially on the top of the shoulder. Contraindicated during pregnancy.

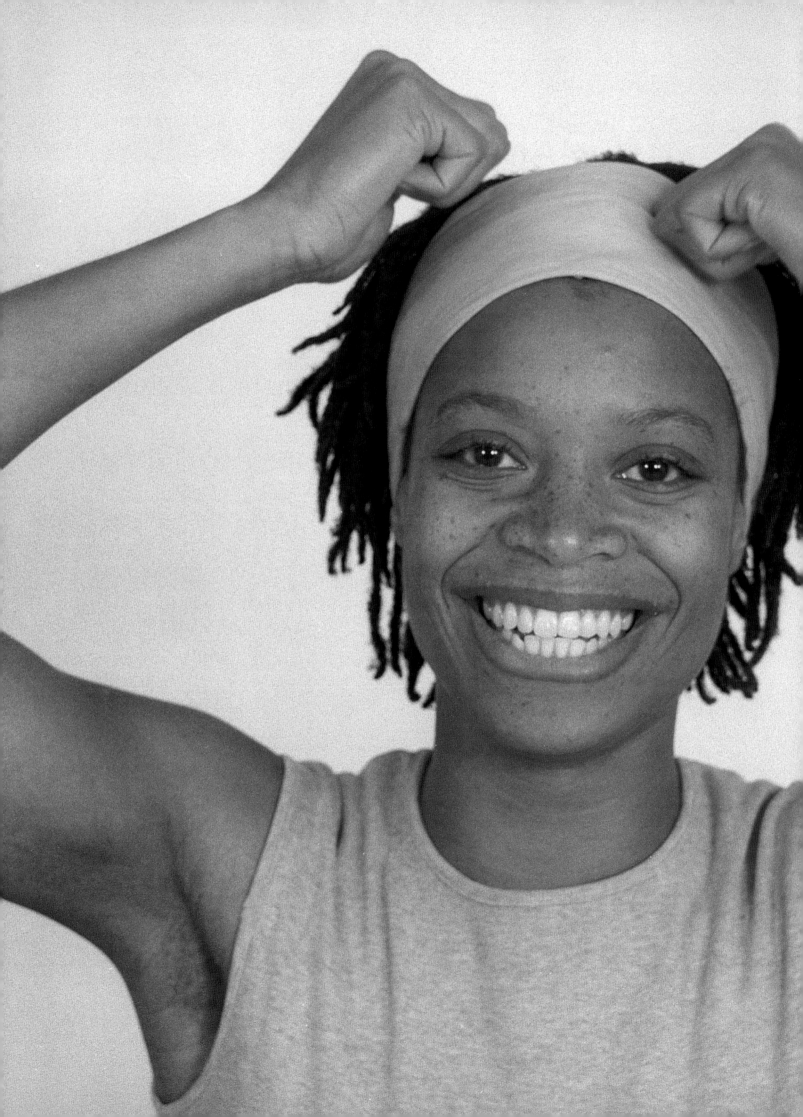

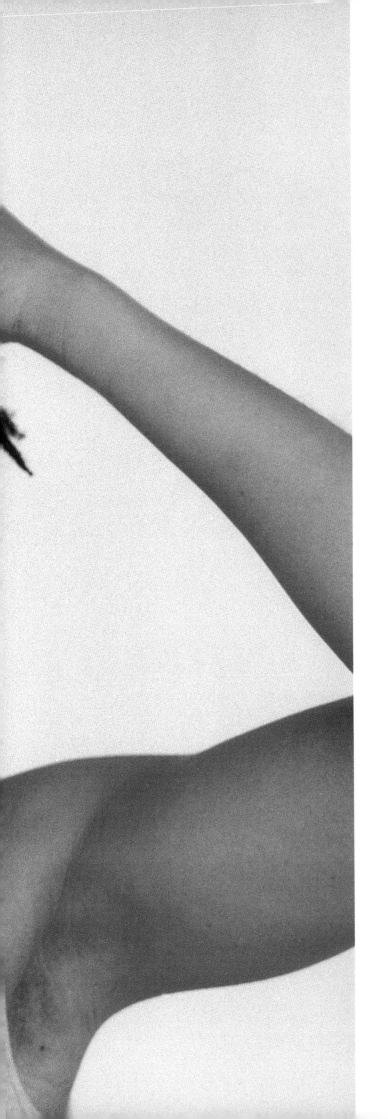

Do-In

Do-in, meaning self-massage, is a set of exercises used to strengthen energy or chi in the meridian systems of the body and in the abdominal area known as the hara. These exercises help to restore balance throughout the whole body, ensuring that the chi is flowing easily and correctly. Do-in includes meridian-stretching exercises, percussion or tapping techniques and breathing meditation.

You can combine the exercises relating to do-in in this chapter – including hara development, energy awareness, self-Shiatsu and makka-ho – to significantly improve your physical and mental well-being. Create your own exercise routine, customized to your own level of fitness and health, to build up strength and awareness. One of the reasons that many people want to learn Shiatsu is to encourage self-healing. This chapter shows you how to develop your body and mind so that your practice of Shiatsu will become easy and enjoyable.

The Practice of Do-In

The following exercises are grouped under different headings and are designed to help in specific areas. Exercises to develop the hara focus on methods of using the breath to centre chi in the hara, as well as exercises to develop hara-centred posture. Energy-sensing exercises use basic techniques to develop an awareness of energy. Self-Shiatsu massage and makka-ho stretches are designed to stimulate the flow of chi throughout the body.

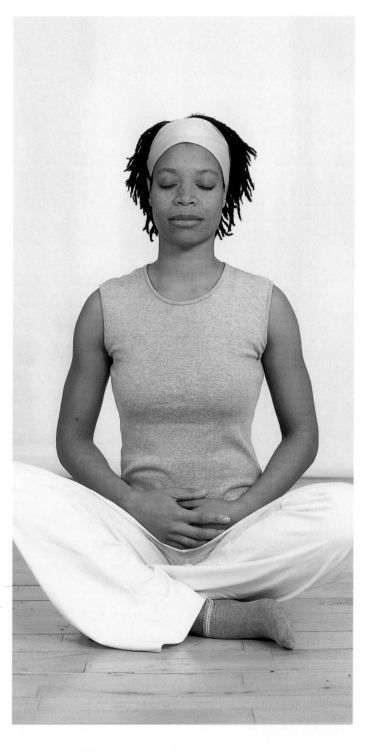

THE HARA

The Japanese word hara literally translated means "belly". The hara usually refers to the abdomen, bordered by the ribs above and the hips and pubic bone below. The centre of the hara is called *tan den*, situated just below the navel, and is also referred to as "one point". The hara is the body's centre of gravity. Energy is stored in the hara, where it is heated before spreading a warm glowing feeling throughout the body.

Hara is an important concept in Japanese culture. To have a good hara is to be healthy. The term for the Japanese tradition of ritual suicide is *hara kiri*, literally meaning "to cut off the hara". The popular sumo wrestlers are incredibly nimble, despite their weight and size, displaying agility and flexibility. The seat of strength is in the big belly, or the hara. In martial arts, the hara is the power centre from which the fighter moves and creates stability and strength.

In Shiatsu the hara is the centre from which we move. The practitioner will allow the body weight to come from the hara. A person with a good hara will stand upright, firm and collected, and will be able to relax their shoulders and be firmly rooted to the ground. With good hara, a person remains balanced both in action and in stillness. There is a sense of security and peace both in body and mind. When based in the hara, we can allow intuition to flow throughout our lives.

In Western cultures people are encouraged to hold the belly in, creating tension and cutting off the free flow of energy in the hara. It helps if you view your belly as the centre of your power. You may find it empowering to think that you have boundless potential energy stored in your hara, and can draw upon it in times of need. It can provide a sense of stability and confidence in everyday life.

Left One of the simplest ways you can develop a sense of hara is by living at floor level. Try moving all the furniture out of the living room, leaving just cushions to sit on. This will increase your flexibility and encourage your centre of gravity to sink. It will also have other benefits, such as helping the digestive system.

Right When you are standing and walking, learn to feel your hara and the energy that it creates. Allow the weight of the belly to drop into the feet and see how stable you become. Feel your hara generating more energy, fuelling your balance and well-being.

ENERGY-SENSING EXERCISES

Shiatsu emphasizes the importance of the vital energy that flows throughout the body using the meridian channels. The energy-sensing exercises in this chapter help practitioners become attuned to their energy flow and initiate the process of rebalancing the body to achieve a freer movement of energy.

SELF-SHIATSU MASSAGE

Self-Shiatsu exercises are a series of massage techniques to restore the flow of chi along the meridians. The exercises in this chapter involve tapping, squeezing, rubbing and pressure to the whole body.

MAKKA-HO STRETCHES

These are a series of six stretches, all of which are similar to yoga postures, stimulating and rebalancing the chi along the twelve primary meridians in the body. The stretches encourage the body to elongate using the breath to let go of tension rather than by forcing the movement. These exercises are frequently used by Shiatsu practitioners to prepare the body for the practice of massage. Using makka-ho stretches will quiet the mind, relax the body, focus attention and improve concentration.

Practising Shiatsu "from the hara"
The art of giving Shiatsu lies within the practitioner's ability to generate chi and move it from the hara. Hara-based work distinguishes Shiatsu from ordinary massage. Here are some benefits of working from the hara.

- The practitioner uses body weight, not muscle power
- The practitioner can relax and physical energy is saved
- There is less risk of injury such as RSI, or "burn out"
- The practitioner uses the whole of their body through the hara to make contact
- The receiver will feel deeply contacted
- The receiver will be more able to relax
- The practitioner will be more in contact with their intuition
- The treatment will flow more smoothly

Before a treatment session, while the receiver is lying on the mat, the practitioner can sit for a few minutes to focus and breathe into the hara to build up chi, let the energy drop to the ground, relax and come up into the body.

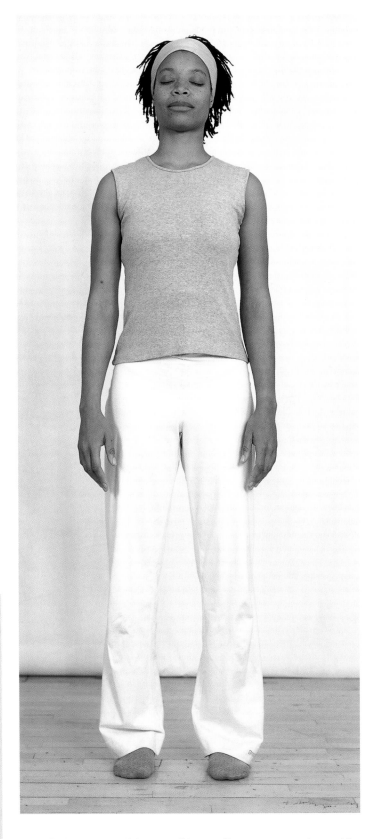

A Shiatsu practitioner will usually recommend specific do-in exercises to individual clients to encourage the flow of energy and to help a particular condition or energy blockage. Practising these Shiatsu exercises will require the ability to move comfortably at floor level. Knees, hips, ankles and wrists should be flexible and shoulders relaxed. Physical strength is not necessary as Shiatsu is given with body weight, but a certain level of stamina and fitness is helpful.

Hara-based Shiatsu

The hara lies deep in the core of your abdomen and acts like a burning flame that brings energy to the rest of your body. Building up the energy in your abdomen by connecting with the hara plays a key role in the warm-up to every Shiatsu session.

Developing the Hara

The exercises that follow are designed to fire up your energy. Close your eyes and focus on your hara, feeling the heat expand through your body. When you feel a tingling, warm sensation in your abdomen, chi is building up and you are ready to begin Shiatsu.

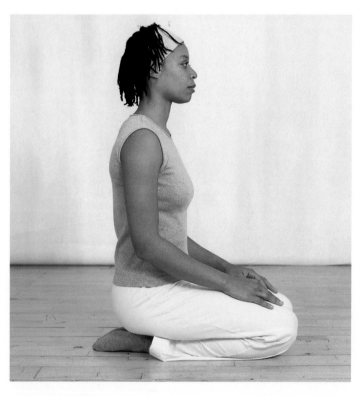

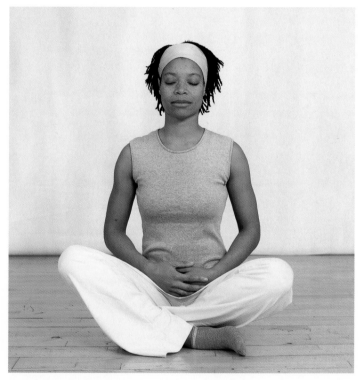

1 Sitting in seiza To adopt the kneeling position, sit on your heels. If this is uncomfortable you can place a cushion between your calves and your thighs. Relax your shoulders and allow the weight to drop to the floor. Gradually increase the time that you sit in seiza until you can sit comfortably for about ten minutes or more.

In Shiatsu, seiza position is used when working on a person's hara, and a wider seiza position is used for other Shiatsu techniques. It is important to be comfortable in this position and feel relaxed while remaining upright.

To focus on your breathing, sit in seiza or cross-legged if you find it more comfortable. (If you are cross-legged you may need to sit on a cushion so that your back is straight.) Close your eyes and relax your shoulders. Observe your breathing calmly and without trying to change it.

2 Breathing into the hara After a few minutes, allow your focus to come to the hara – you may want to place your hands on your belly to help the focus. Gradually encourage your breathing to move down into the abdomen, expanding the belly as you breathe in and contracting it as you breathe out. Imagine your belly is filling with chi as you breathe in and this is dropping to the bottom of the belly. You are getting heavier and your weight is sinking. The belly is filling with chi as you breathe in and you are expelling stale chi as you breathe out. You can imagine the chi as a white light if this helps. Breathe like this for about five to ten minutes, and then gradually allow your focus to come back to the room. Open your eyes and remain sitting for a while. Observe any sensations in your hara – a feeling of warmth, perhaps, or feeling more grounded or heavy.

3 Shifting weight from the hara

Come on to all fours with your hands underneath your shoulders and your knees below the hips. Keep your arms straight. Breathe again into the hara, expanding the belly as you breathe in and contracting as you breathe out. Feel the weight drop evenly between your hands and knees.

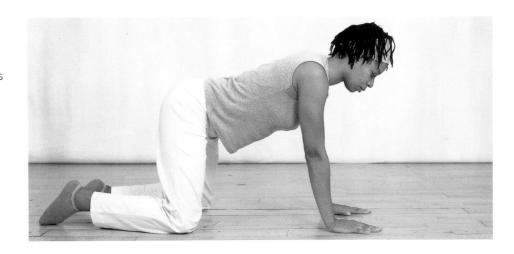

3a Shifting weight from the hara

When you have established your breathing, on the next out breath move your belly forward so that the weight comes more on to the hands. Breathe in and come back to the centre position. Breathe out and this time shift the belly back so that the weight comes more on to the knees. Repeat these two movements.

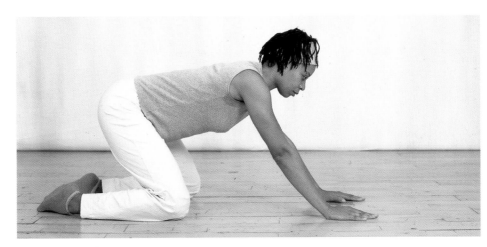

3b Shifting weight from the hara

Begin to make circles with your belly so that the weight shifts first to one hand, then the other, back to the knee on the same side and then the other. Coordinate with your breathing. Repeat a few times and then circle in the other direction.

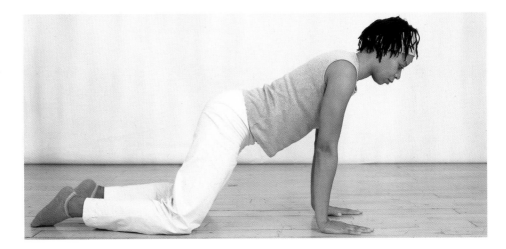

3c Shifting weight from the hara

When you have practised the circling a few times, come back to the central position and breathe again into the hara, feeling the weight drop into your hands. See if you can feel a connection between your hara breathing and the energy in your hands. Come back to seiza, with your hands over the hara.

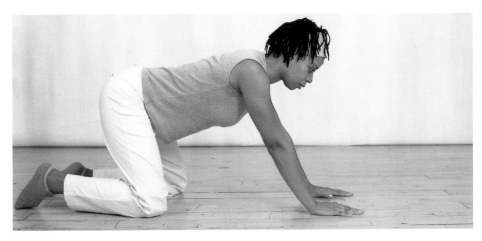

▷

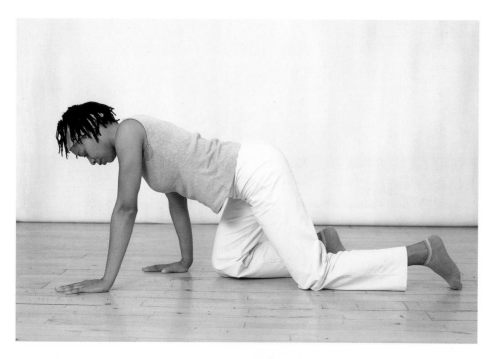

4 Crawling Stay on all fours and crawl around the room as if you were a baby. Move from your hara rather than the hands. Keep your centre of gravity low and concentrate on your hara as you move. Focus on your breath, breathing out as you shift your weight on to your hands. Practise crawling backwards and sideways moving from the hara.

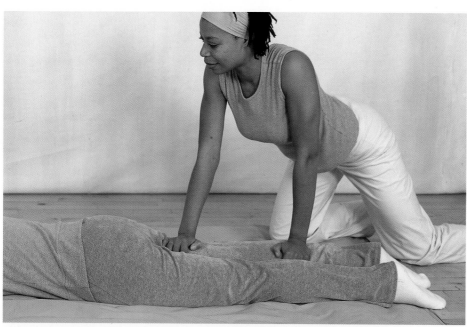

5 Shifting weight with a partner Ask your partner to lie face down on the floor in prone position. Starting from the feet, crawl your palms on to the back of the feet and legs, letting your weight drop into your hands. Work your way up the body on to the back, avoiding direct pressure on the back of the knees and the spine. Make sure that you maintain a relaxed posture, staying open so that the weight always comes from the hara.

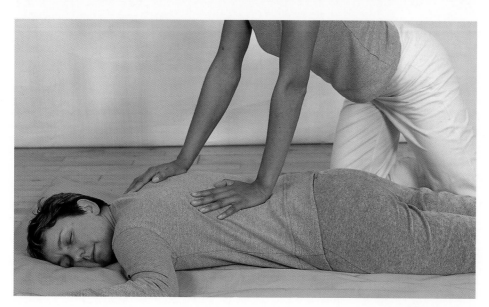

6 Moving your weight Placing your hands in the centre of the back, allow your weight to settle, then shift your weight back and forward by moving your hara in a circular pattern. Slowly crawl your hands down the body, moving your hands down the spine. Don't forget to breathe with your movements, ensuring that the energy is coming from your hara.

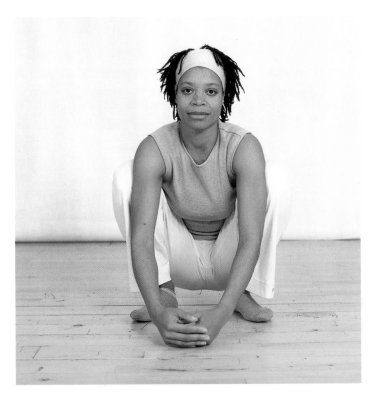

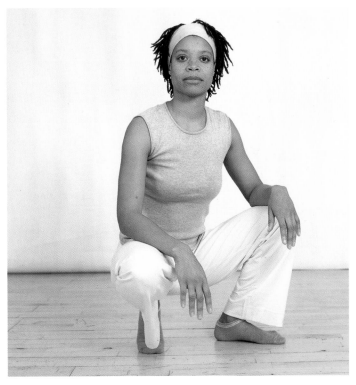

7 Squatting This is a good exercise to increase flexibility in the hips, knees and ankles. While squatting, be aware of your hara and let your weight drop into the feet from the belly. Practise squatting regularly, increasing the time you stay in the position until you are comfortable.

9 Knee-walking (right) This is an aikido exercise that enables the practitioner to move around the client without standing up while remaining in hara. Start in the half squat position. Make sure your stance is not too wide. Let the raised knee drop down and at the same time bring the other foot forward so that you reverse your position. You should find that you move forward. Knee-walk around the room, changing direction. It is better to do this on a carpeted floor or on a padded surface or Shiatsu mat.

8 Half squats This position is a very common one used in many Shiatsu techniques. Squat on the ground with both feet on the floor. Now shift from one side to the other, by lifting one heel then the other. Again be aware of the weight dropping. Practise this exercise regularly.

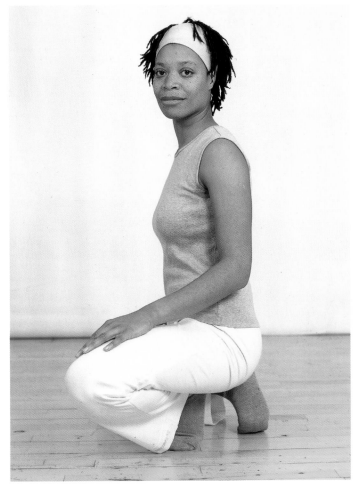

Crawling
Babies naturally use their hara when crawling. It is thought that a person is naturally aware of the power of the hara from a very young age, and in later life may lose this sense. Next time you see a small baby notice the crawling motion and the use of the belly in the movement. Consider this when you practise on your own.

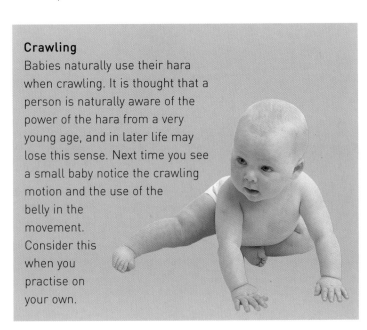

Energy Awareness

Witnessing the flow of energy from the hara to other regions of your body can be both empowering and invigorating. If you have a problem in a specific area, imagine the chi energy flowing in, bringing energy and nourishment.

Tuning in to your Energy

These exercises give you guidance about relaxing and breathing, and about finding the energy in your body. The magnetic energy that you should feel is visualized as an energy ball in your hands; the ball, or rather the chi, is eventually absorbed by the body.

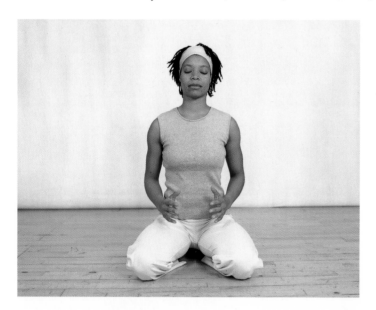

1 Relax and breathe Sitting comfortably in seiza or cross-legged, relax your shoulders and straighten your spine. Bend your elbows and bring your hands in front of your belly, with palms facing. Close your eyes and breathe into your hara, imagining chi filling your hara as you breathe in.

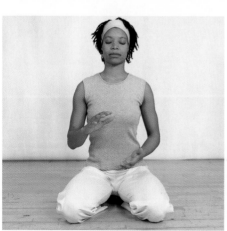

2 Finding the energy Take time to build up energy between your hands. You may be aware of a magnetic sensation on bringing your hands together or pushing them apart. Imagine that this energy is a ball and, keeping your hands on either side, move it around and play with it.

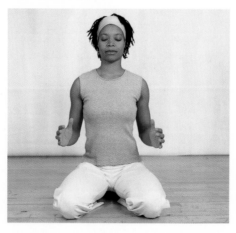

3 Push your hands apart Bring your hands and the energy ball back into the original position and as you breathe out allow the chi to push your hands apart. Gradually, on each out breath, the chi will force your hands to drift apart.

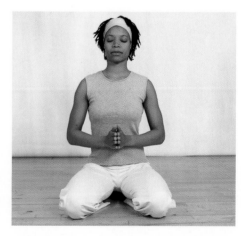

4 Draw back your hands As you take a breath in allow your hands to be drawn back towards each other as if by a magnetic force. Eventually your hands will come back together as the chi disperses between your palms and enters your body.

Self-Shiatsu Exercises

Do these exercises in the morning, when you want an energy boost, or in the evening to physically and mentally relax and encourage a good night's sleep. The routine should take around forty minutes, although a shortened version can take from five to twenty minutes.

Preparation

Aim to maintain a natural posture and steady breathing and try to keep your mind empty, free of disturbing thoughts. Many people like to focus on their breathing, feeling the air passing in and out of the chest right through to the tip of the nose.

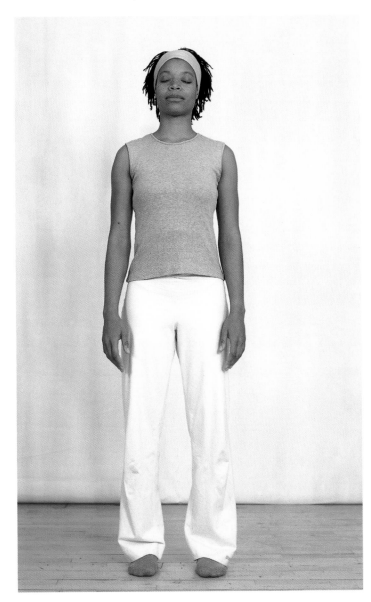

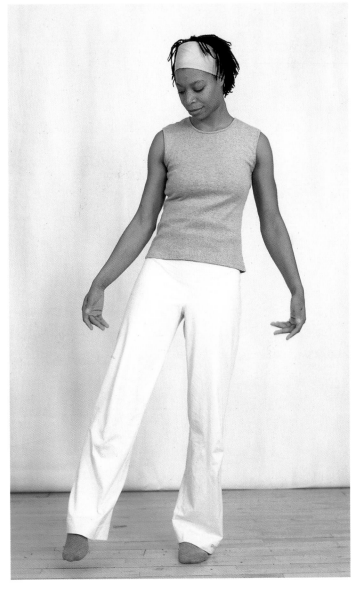

1 Tuning in Stand with your feet shoulder-width apart, knees slightly bent and spine straight. Stand for a few moments, eyes closed, and get in touch with how you feel, being aware of any discomfort in your body and mind.

2 Relax the joints Gently shake out your arms and hands, legs and feet to relax the joints. If you have time, shake out each part of your body separately, starting from your fingers and working down your arms and trunk to your legs.

The Head

Bringing chi to the head is important for waking up the brain and increasing mental clarity. These are good exercises to do first thing in the morning so that you start the day alert. Releasing tension in the neck increases blood flow to the head.

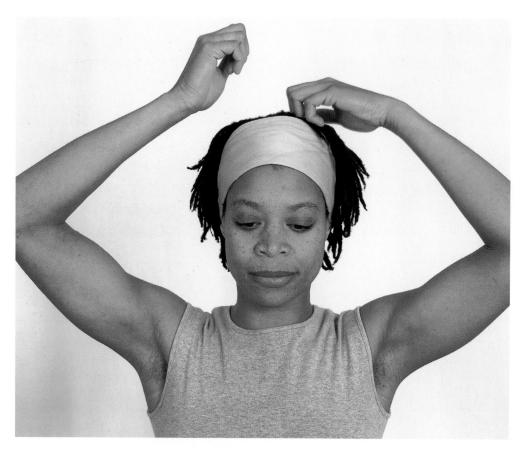

1 Tapping all over the head
Use loose fists to tap all over the head, especially at the base of the skull. This wakes up the brain, stimulating blood and energy flow around the brain and helping you to feel alive and fresh. You can gauge how hard or softly to tap, using your fingertips for a more gentle approach if necessary. Ensure that you tap all over the head, including behind the ears, the top of the head and the base of the skull.

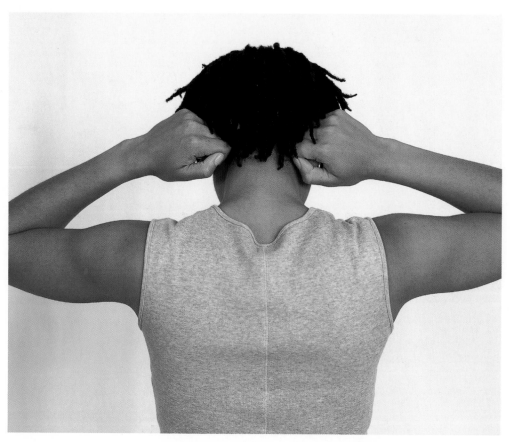

2 Tapping down the back of the neck Open the back of the neck area by lowering your chin down as far as you can, but without over-stretching. Reach your arms right back before you start tapping, opening your chest out and feeling the chi from your hara flowing freely into the head and neck area. Then tap gently all over the area, moving up and down the sides of your neck, avoiding direct pressure on the central vertebrae.

The Arms and Shoulders

Tension in the shoulders and upper arms can prevent the proper circulation of chi around your whole body, and especially into the head area. Make sure that your arms and shoulders are feeling loose by performing the following exercises.

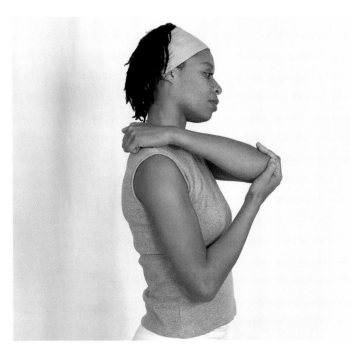

1 Tapping across the shoulders Tap across one shoulder at a time, starting at the base of the neck and moving out to the outside edge, working along the trapezius muscle. Support your elbow with the other hand so that you can reach as far as possible along the back of the shoulder. Spend some time here, tapping away any tension.

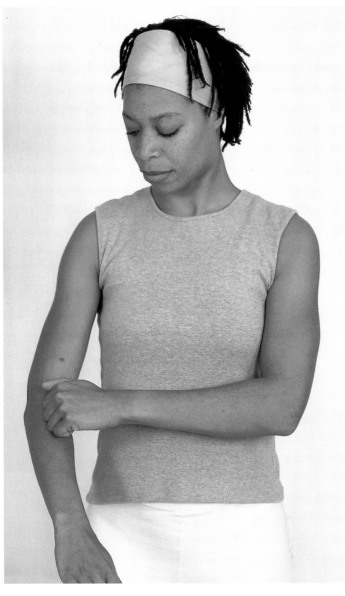

3 Tapping up the back of the arm Tap from the wrist up the back of the arm to the shoulder. This will stimulate the meridians on the back of the arm – Large Intestine, Triple Heater and Small Intestine – which all start on the fingers. Repeat on the other side.

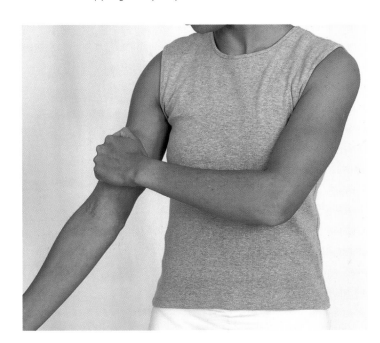

2 Tapping down the inside of the arm Open the arm with palm up and starting from the top tap down towards the hand. This will be stimulating the meridians on the inside of the arm – Lung, Heart Protector and Heart – which all end on the fingers.

Visualization

You can visualize the chi flowing through the body during this exercise. Imagine the energy or chi flowing freely through your arms as you stimulate the meridians. Feel the chi flow down the inside of the arm and up the back of the arm as you tap. Picture the pathway of each arm meridian, changing the line of tapping each time, from outside edge to middle and inside edge, to release any blockages.

The Hands and Wrists

Spend some time working on your hands; these are your Shiatsu tools, so take care of them. Here are a few exercises to do daily and before giving Shiatsu. They will bring chi to the hand by activating the meridians and increasing flexibility.

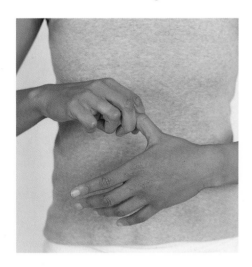

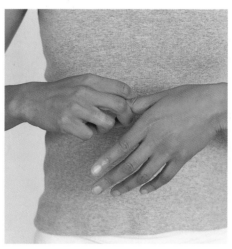

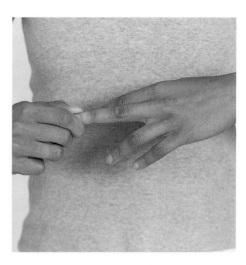

1 Rotate the fingers Rotate and flick the thumb and fingers. Rotate the thumb first one way and then the other. Repeat on the rest of your fingers.

2 Flick the thumb With your thumb and forefinger flick either side of the thumb to the edge of the fingernail. The movement should be performed quickly.

3 Flick the fingers Do the same with each finger, stimulating the beginning and end of each of the meridians that begin or end in the hands and fingers.

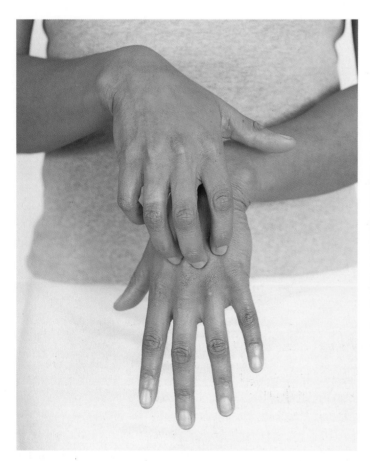

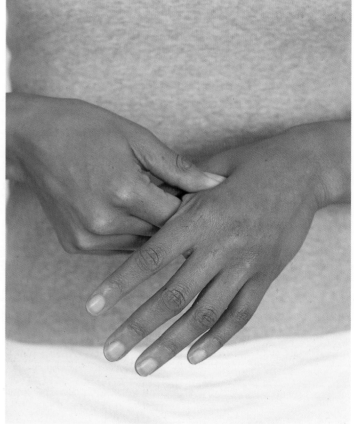

4 Loosen the back of the hand Massage the back of the hand between the metacarpals (the main bones that run through the back of the hands). Work in between the bones of the hands with your thumb and fingers and the tips of your fingers, making space and loosening between the bones.

5 The Great Eliminator Find the point LI 4 (located in the web between the thumb and index finger). This point on the Large Intestine Meridian is called the Great Eliminator and is good for increasing vitality and treating headaches, constipation and diarrhoea. Caution: Do not use LI 4 during pregnancy.

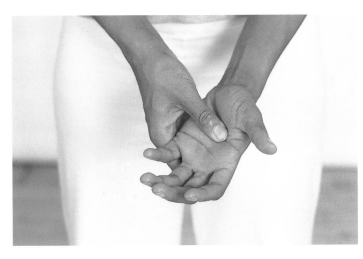

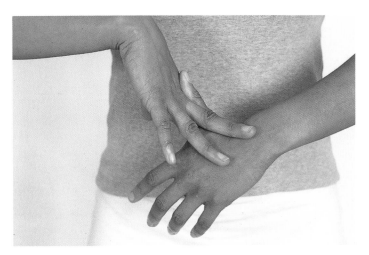

6 Massage the palm Use your thumb to massage HP 8, "the Palace of Anxiety", a good point to calm anxiety and nerves. To find the point, fold your fingers into the palm: the point is where the middle finger touches the palm.

7 Stretch the fingers Using the "V" between two fingers of the other hand as a lever, stretch each finger and the thumb backwards. This will help to increase the flexibility of the hand, making it more adept at performing Shiatsu.

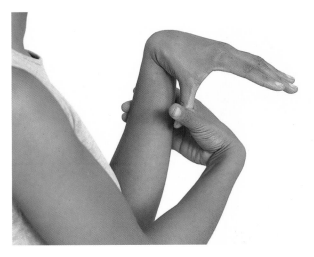

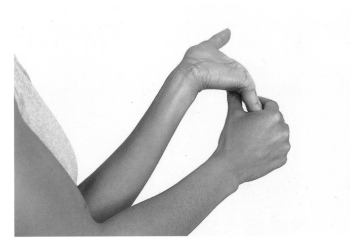

8 Flex and stretch Flex the wrist and stretch the thumb towards the wrist, using the thumb of the other hand. It is important to develop strength and flexibility in the thumbs.

9 Open up the wrist Stretch the wrist open. Bend the wrist back using the fingers of the other hand to exert pressure and open up the wrist. Make sure that you do not overstretch.

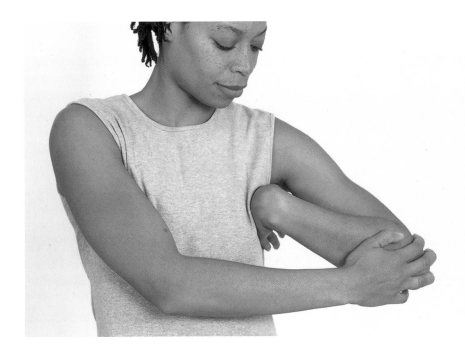

10 Full stretch Stretch the wrist forward. Tuck your hand under the armpit and pull the elbow towards you with the other hand to stretch the wrist forward.

Comparing sides
Do all these techniques on one hand first. Take a moment to compare the hand you have worked to the one you haven't. Notice how it feels. Is it lighter, warmer, more tingling? Find your own words to describe each side. Then repeat all the techniques on the other hand, being aware of the difference between the sides.

The Back and Legs

Loosening the back and legs is a great way to feel energized and increase the flow of chi around your system. Try to reach up your back as far as possible for greatest effect, covering as much area as you can without straining.

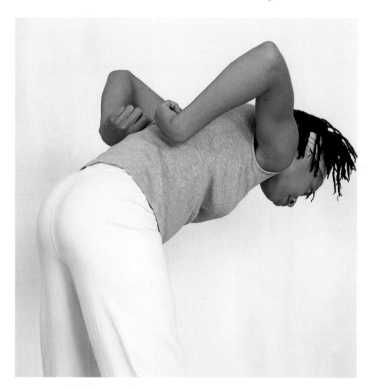

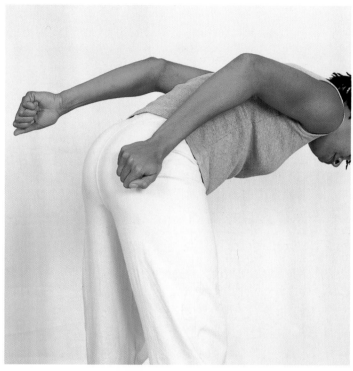

1 Tapping down the back I Bend forward and with loose fists tap down both sides of the spine from the top down to the lower back and then on to the buttocks.

2 Tapping down the back II This process works on the Bladder meridian, the longest meridian, which helps to relax the nervous system and the spine, promoting energy flow.

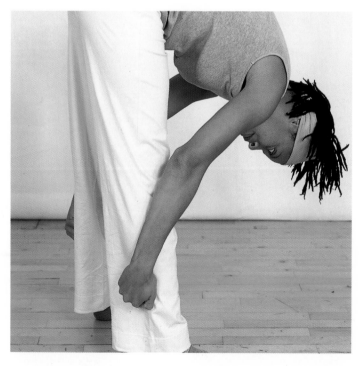

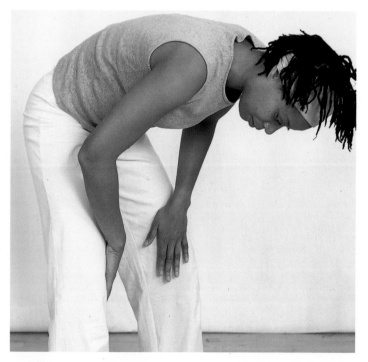

3 Back and sides of legs Tap down the back and outside of the legs and up the inside. Open your feet a bit wider and tap down the back of the legs from the buttocks to the heel, continuing down the Bladder meridian. Bend legs if necessary.

4 Outside and inside of legs With loose fists tap down the side of the legs, then with flat palms tap up the inside of the legs from the ankles to the groin area, paying more attention to the inner thighs – where energy can become sluggish.

The Hara

Releasing tension throughout the hara region allows the chi energy that is generated there to grow larger and become less constricted. Focus on your hara as you apply pressure, feeling the chi energy warming the rest of your body.

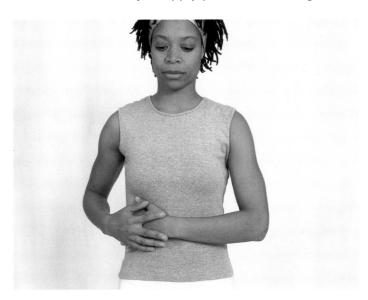

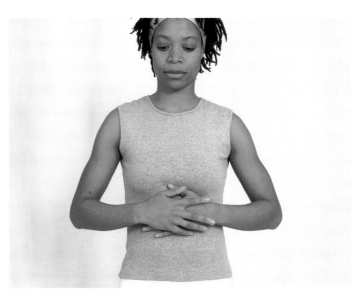

1 Stroke round the hara Finish this Do-in sequence by standing up again with relaxed shoulders and knees. Gently stroke around the hara in a clockwise direction.

2 Stroke the abdomen Use both hands, one placed on top of the other, and stroke around your abdomen clockwise. This follows the direction of the intestines and helps digestion.

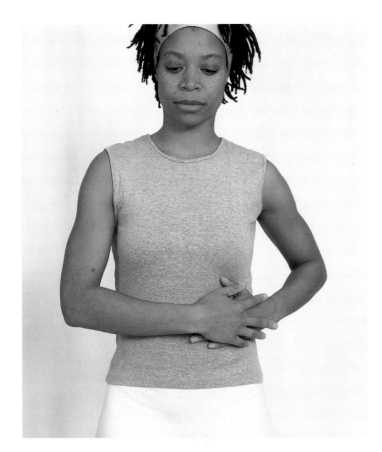

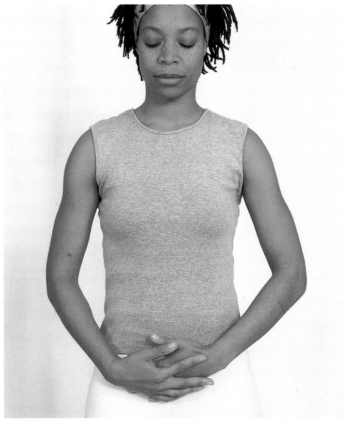

3 Assess changes As you rotate your hands around your hara, take a few moments to get in touch with how you feel now and notice any differences from how you felt at the start of this sequence. Do you feel energized? Did you notice any particularly tense or stiff parts of your body?

4 Stand with both hands on your hara Close your eyes and maintain a relaxed posture, placing one hand over the other and both over the lower part of your hara. Focus your mind on to your hara, imagining it glowing with positive energy and fuelling your whole-body energy system.

Makka-ho Exercises

Each of the makka-ho exercises balances and activates a meridian pair. They can be used as a daily exercise system, and the ease with which you do each stretch also monitors your meridian functioning. A practitioner might recommend a particular stretch to a client based on his or her condition. Start with an in breath and move into the stretch on the out breath. Stay in the position for three or four breaths and on each out breath relax a bit more into the stretch.

The Lungs and Large Intestine

This stretch helps to open up the chest, aiding breathing as well as improving the function of the Lung and Large Intestine meridians. Breathing is a crucial element of good chi circulation. Feel the chi enter with every breath.

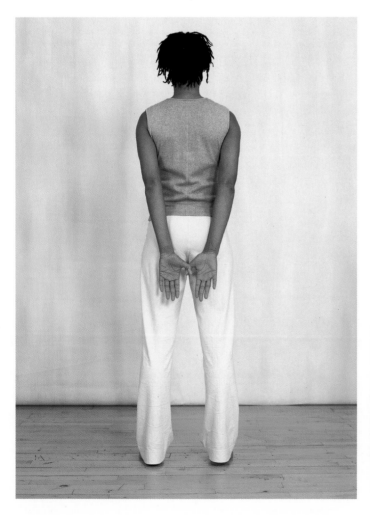

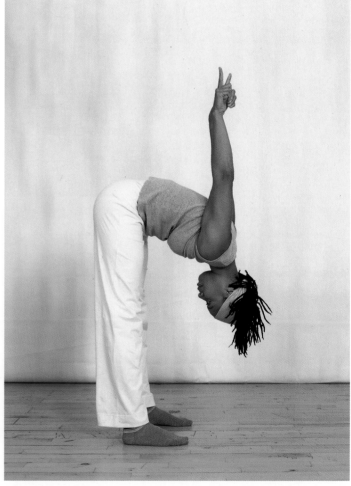

1 Stand and link thumbs Stand with feet hip-width apart. Bring the hands behind your back and link thumbs.

2 Forward and arms up As you breathe out bend forward, bringing your arms up behind you as high as possible and keeping your back and neck straight. Stay for 3–4 breaths, relaxing as you breathe out and feeling your chest open. Come up slowly on the in breath. Repeat with thumbs the other way round.

The Spleen and Stomach

This stretch helps to activate the Stomach meridian on the side of the thighs and helps with digestion. Take care not to overstretch your back and thighs with this exercise. Go down in stages and only go as far as is comfortable.

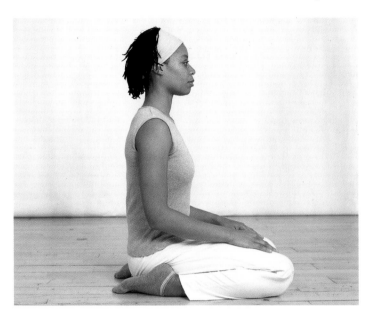

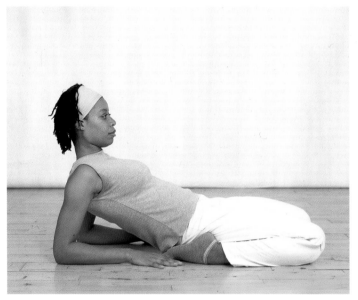

1 Seiza Sit in seiza with your heels on either side of your body, if you can. (If necessary, you can sit on a cushion to ease the hip, knee or ankle joints.) Start with your hands gently resting in your lap, your elbows bent and your shoulders square and upright, looking directly forward.

2 Lean back on your elbows Place your hands behind you, with arms straight, breathe out, lean back and relax. If this is far enough for you, stop here. As you next breathe out, lean back on to your elbows. If this is far enough for you, stop here and breathe into this stretch.

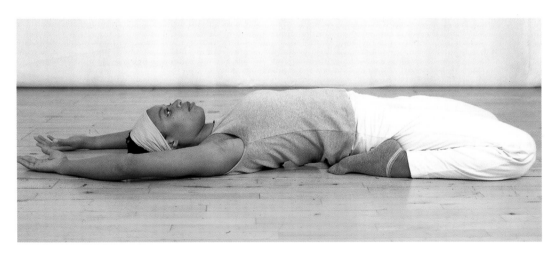

3 Back to floor Breathe out and go all the way back to the floor, raising your hands above your head. Stay here for a few breaths, relaxing into the stretch. If your knees or your lower back come off the floor in this stage come back to the previous position.

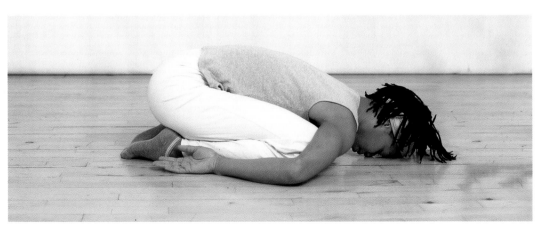

4 Counterbalance stretch Come back out of the stretch in the stages with which you went down. When you are back up, lean forward to counterbalance the stretch. Relax and breathe deeply, resting your forehead on the floor in front of you.

The Heart and Small Intestine

Heart and Small Intestine are part of the Fire element and govern the emotions. This stretch helps to bring the emotions into balance and to feel centred and calm. It opens the hips and pelvis.

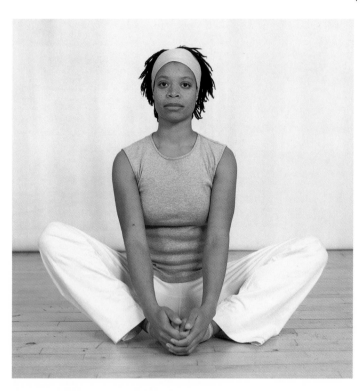

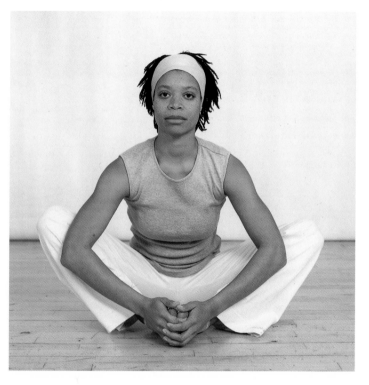

1 Feet together and face forwards Sit with your knees apart and feet soles together. Clasp your feet, keeping your back upright and your shoulders and face pointing forward.

2 Leaning forward On the out breath lean forward, bending from the hips and keeping the back straight. After 3–4 breaths relax into the stretch. Come back up on the in breath.

Heart Protector and Triple Heater

These two meridians associated with Secondary Fire have no Western equivalent. Heart Protector shields the heart and Triple Heater governs the peripheral circulation. They are responsible for a healthy and balanced emotional state.

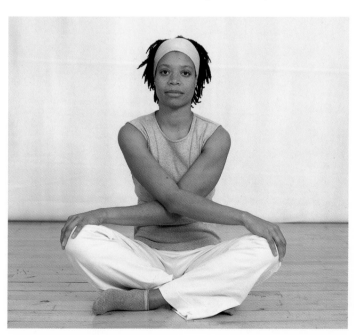

Crossing arms and legs As the photograph to the left shows, sit in cross-legged position with a straight back and cross your arms. Bring the hands on to the knees. On the out breath bend forward, keeping the back straight. Stay in this position for a couple of breaths, stretching the hands away from each other to get more of a stretch in the arms. Come back up on an in breath and repeat, crossing the arms and legs the other way round.

The Kidney and Bladder

This stretch opens up the back and activates both the Kidney and Bladder meridians. These meridians are ruled by Water, helping balance the water in your system, and can treat retention, bloatedness and dryness of the skin and hair.

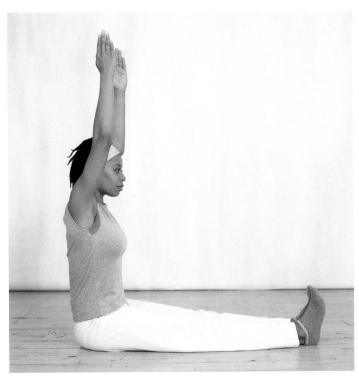

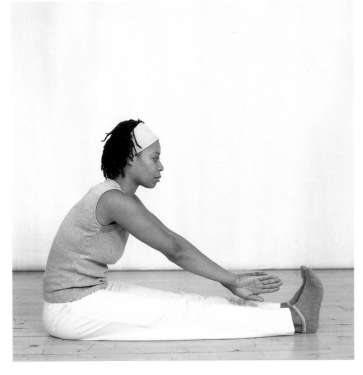

1 Bend from the hips Sit with your legs straight out in front of you. Lift your arms above your head and, breathing out, bend forward from the hips, keeping your back straight.

2 Hands between feet Bring your hands towards the feet, pushing the hands, with little fingers up, between the feet. If you can't reach your feet, hold your ankles or shins.

Gall Bladder and Liver

These meridians are associated with Wood. Gall Bladder is important in the process of decision-making and Liver governs the smooth flow of chi throughout the organs. It also provides flexibility and the ability to change direction when needed.

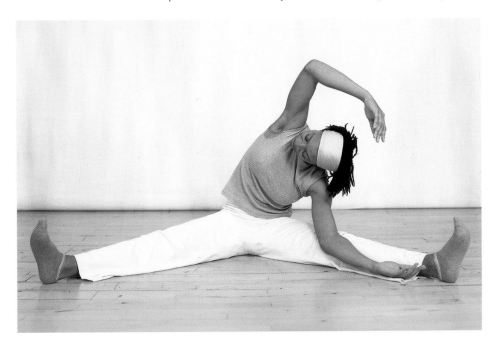

Lean over stretching your waist This exercise shows how to stretch open the meridians on the side of the body, especially affecting the Gall Bladder and Liver meridians. Sit with your legs straight and apart. Point your toes upwards and stretch your heels and ankles back, feeling the muscles in the back of your thighs as you go. Raising your arms over your head, lean your body over to one side, stretching your waist and the side of your chest. Make sure that you keep your body facing forward, and only bend sideways, not forwards.

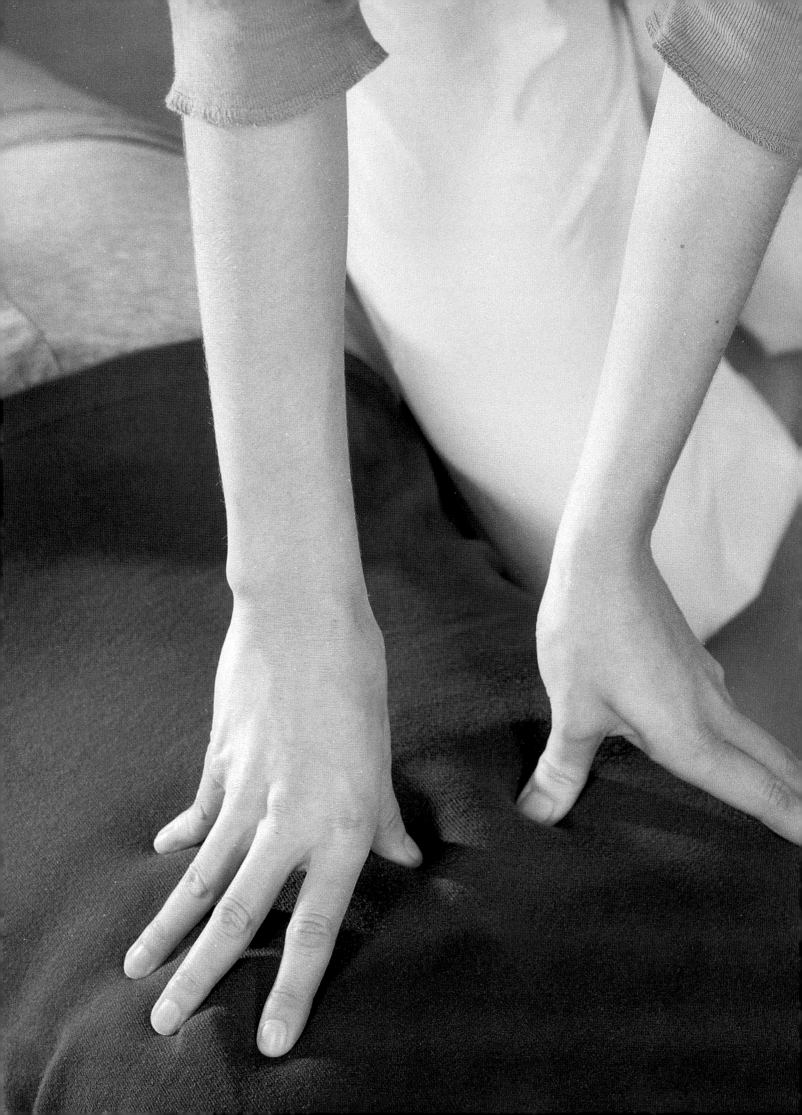

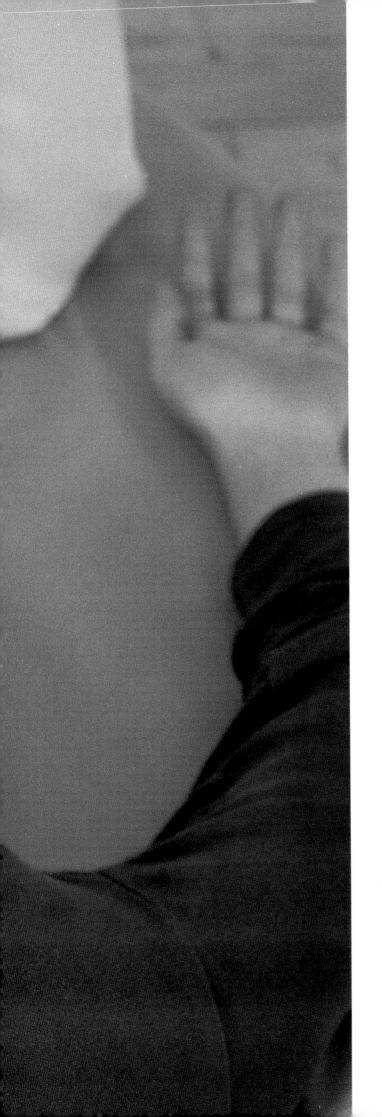

The Basic Framework

By following the step-by-step Shiatsu framework described in this chapter you can start to practise what you are learning by working on others. The framework shows a clear progression around the body, starting with the back and finishing with the feet, covering all parts in a smooth and flowing way.

This basic treatment, once mastered, can be used as a basis for designing a whole treatment, paying special attention to the appropriate meridians. If, for example, your receiver needs special attention to the back, you should proceed through the entire basic frame, but spend more time on the back. Practise this step-by-step process on any willing friends and family until you can give an entire treatment without having to think what to do next.

Preparing Yourself

Although the treatment that follows is suitable for most people, you should check with the contraindications listed on the page opposite if your receiver has any medical conditions. You also need to organize an appropriate location as well as clothing and equipment, and ensure that you are physically prepared for a session, taking particular care of your hands and fingernails. Finally, you need to prepare yourself mentally.

TREATMENT ROOM

A Shiatsu session should be performed in a warm, light room, preferably one that is simply furnished and clutter-free. Avoid using harsh or bright lights. Use a thin futon with a cover or a clean cotton sheet for the receiver to lie on, or alternatively two or three blankets covered by a sheet. You will also need some small cushions to make your partner comfortable and a blanket to cover them if they get cold or to cover them at the end of the treatment.

CLOTHING

Both you and your partner should wear loose, preferably cotton, trousers, top and socks so that you can both stretch and move around easily. Shiatsu is given through the clothes and it is better if your partner wears clothes with long sleeves and socks. Use a soft cotton cloth to work through where the skin is exposed. Shiatsu should not be performed on the skin.

PHYSICAL AND MENTAL PREPARATION

Make sure that your hands are clean and your fingernails are short and smooth. It is important to look after your hands regularly, because they are your Shiatsu tools. Do the preparation exercises for the hands on pages 160–1 to warm them up and increase flexibility, feeling the chi energy in your hands after you have done the exercises. If you have poor circulation or your hands are always cold, do the hand exercises every day.

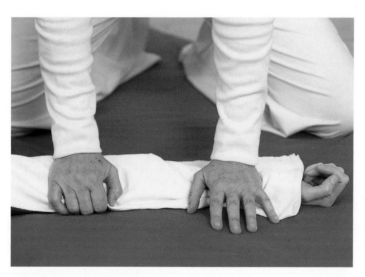

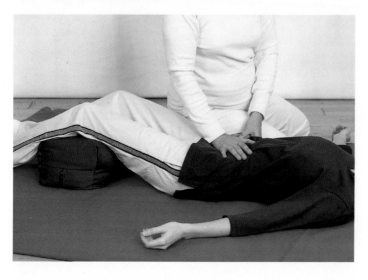

How to start treatment

- Check that your partner is sitting or lying comfortably, and use supporting cushions if necessary
- Be calm, centred and sensitive, with hara breathing and a good posture, taking your time
- Focus for a few minutes, sitting quietly, meditating or exercising
- Observe your partner, noting anything that attracts your attention
- First contact should be gentle and reassuring, as you become "as one" with your partner
- Synchronize your breathing with your partner's, keeping your mind empty and receptive to your partner's energy

Above left If your partner has short sleeves, or other exposed areas of skin, lay a soft cotton cloth over the area and work through the cloth.

Left A cushion can be placed under the knees if the receiver has a stiff back. A cushion under the head or neck can help the neck and upper back.

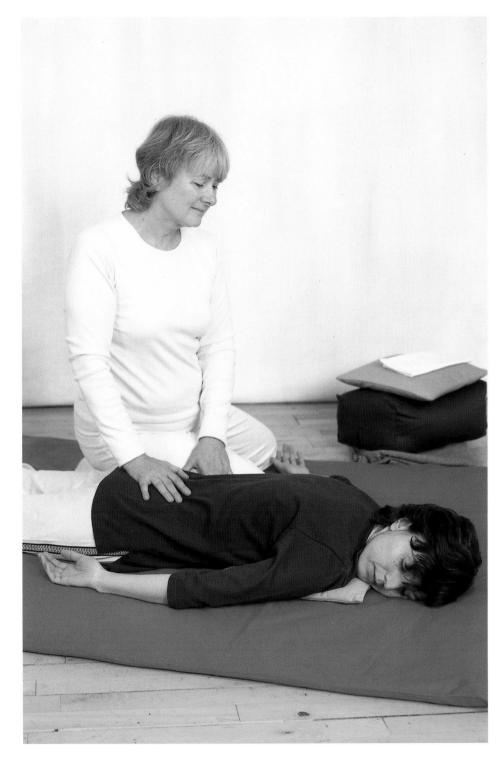

Above When the receiver is lying on his or her front, cushions can help to support the body, especially in sore or stiff areas. A cushion may be placed under the chest if the neck is stiff or the breasts are sore. Some people can feel more comfortable with a small cushion under the ankles as this relaxes the legs and feet.

Shiatsu should not be given or received by someone who has just eaten a large meal, so wait several hours before giving or receiving Shiatsu and advise your partner to do the same. This is because lying down with pressure applied to your torso after a full meal would feel uncomfortable.

Having the right frame of mind is crucial, so ensure that you relax and remain focused before you give a Shiatsu treatment.

Practise the preparation exercises outlined in the Do-in chapter (see pages 148–67) before starting your treatment; this will increase your flexibility and comfort in working around the floor.

Care and contraindications

As with every therapeutic treatment, care must be taken if one or both of the participants have medical conditions. There are some contraindications, meaning conditions in which you wouldn't give treatment, to giving Shiatsu both for giver and receiver. If you are treating someone for the first time, check down the following list beforehand:

- As a beginner, do not give a Shiatsu if your receiver has a serious condition such as cancer, a serious heart disease (although mild heart disease or angina can benefit from Shiatsu) or has had recent major surgery. If in doubt your partner should check with their doctor.
- It is advised not to give Shiatsu to someone in the first trimester of pregnancy and some contraindicated points (GB 21, LI 4 and SP 6, shown on pages 213, 188 and 199), should not be used at all in pregnancy.

Do not give Shiatsu if your receiver:
- Has a high fever
- Is intoxicated or has taken non-prescribed drugs
- Has just eaten – wait two hours after meals
- Has a serious contagious disease
- Has varicose veins, broken bones or recent scar tissue – although you can work around these areas

Do not give Shiatsu if you:
- Are fatigued or upset
- Are intoxicated
- Have a serious contagious disease

Remember your level of skill and ensure that your partner knows that you are not giving orthodox medical treatment. If you find a serious problem, refer your partner to a doctor. Ensure that they understand that a healing "reaction" such as tiredness or headaches can occur as the body adjusts to a better level of health. If in doubt ask an experienced practitioner.

How to Give Shiatsu

During a Shiatsu treatment it is important for both giver and receiver to remain relaxed and connected and not to overstretch the body. Here are the basic guidelines: remember them every time you give or receive Shiatsu in order to ensure a beneficial treatment. With practice it should become instinctive, so that you won't need to think about the guidelines consciously, but you may still need an occasional reminder.

RELAXATION

A comfortable physical and mental condition is essential for Shiatsu. Your whole body should be relaxed, especially hands, arms and shoulders, and your posture upright. Change your position if you feel tension in your back or shoulders. The receiver will relax more deeply when you are relaxed.

TWO-HANDED CONNECTEDNESS

Contact with the receiver's body is maintained at all times. The mother hand, or more passive hand, keeps constant contact while the other hand can move along the meridian. When contact is maintained the receiver can relax without worrying about where the practitioner is going to touch next. This is a function of the autonomic nervous system (ANS). The sympathetic mode of the ANS assesses, distinguishes

and tries to work out if the touch is hostile. When connection is maintained, the ANS is able to relax into the parasympathetic mode, where healing and deep relaxation occurs.

MERIDIAN CONTINUITY

The focus of Shiatsu is to treat an entire meridian, rather than individual points or regions, and this is called meridian continuity. The aim is to bring the whole meridian back into balance by encouraging the free flow of chi, opening blockages and balancing energy.

CHI PROJECTION

You need to use chi projection throughout your Shiatsu treatments. Although we talk about pressure points and Shiatsu techniques using pressure, the practitioner will

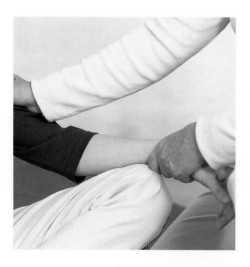

Hugging and palming Always use a hugging hand to increase relaxation by softening your hand when palming. Practise working down the arm as if you were hugging the arm with your hand. Remember how it feels to give and receive a hug, when the whole of your body softens. This is just the same feeling that you need to create when giving Shiatsu.

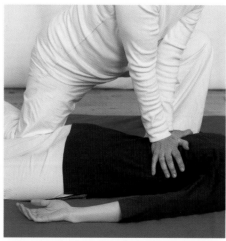

Body weight Position your body so you can use body weight to give pressure, rather than muscle power. Always move from your hara, using the knee-walking shown on page 155. Use a wide, stable stance, with your knees apart, to transfer your weight into the move. Keep your centre of gravity low and place yourself so that the area you are working on is in front of you and close to the hara.

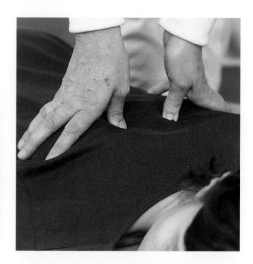

Perpendicular penetration Pressure is always perpendicular, at 90 degrees to the body surface. Rather than movement across the surface, Shiatsu involves penetration at each point. Treatment involves simple, inward-directed hand movements, and not rotation, back-and-forth, or wiggling movements. Even when the body is not parallel to the ground, maintain perpendicular pressure.

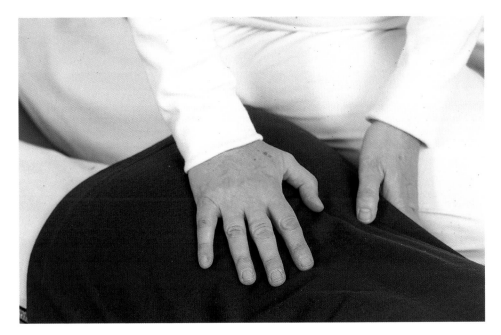

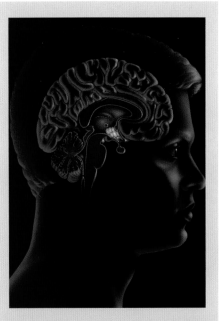

actually project his or her chi when working on a point or meridian. The result will be greater penetration, and this is an entirely different experience for the receiver than just pressing.

KYO AND JITSU

These Japanese terms, roughly meaning empty and full, are used to describe the state of energy as observed in the body. Energy can manifest in three different ways. There can be too little energy, a kyo situation, which results in a weakness or depleted function. There can be too much energy, a jitsu situation, which can manifest as tension or pain. Or energy can be stuck as a result of either fullness or emptiness. In a kyo case this will result in an empty pocket through which no energy can pass. In jitsu this is often an area of fullness that can't move anywhere, becoming stuck or stagnated. Kyo and jitsu are used to describe the quality of energy, for example a kyo area will appear lacklustre whereas jitsu may be stiff. The type of treatment required will then be based on this assessment. Generally a more kyo area will be

Kyo is empty, hidden, the cause, hollow and soft.
Jitsu is full, obvious, the effect, raised and hard.

Above There is always a mother (passive) hand (the hand on the right) and a hand that moves around the meridians (the hand on the left). Instead of the sweeping, stroking movements common to other massage techniques, Shiatsu pressure is perpendicular and uses chi projection.

Above right The hypothalamus, a control centre of the autonomic nervous system.

treated with tonifying techniques such as holding and slower, calmer work. Jitsu areas will be treated with more dispersing techniques such as rubbing, rocking and faster work, with the aim of redistributing the energy and moving blockages. In a treatment, kyo will pull you in and not resist, while jitsu will push you back out and make you bounce back. Kyo is considered to be the underlying cause of a condition and jitsu its effect. For the most effective treatment you need to look for the kyo and work with that. When the kyo is addressed, then the jitsu can relax.

GETTING FEEDBACK

Ask your partner how comfortable they feel with your pressure – they should always feel relaxed. Never overstretch or force movement so that your partner experiences pain or resistance. You may not want to keep asking for feedback, as talking could disturb them out of deep relaxation, but make it clear at the beginning that they should say if anything feels uncomfortable.

Autonomic nervous system (ANS)
The autonomic nervous system (ANS) deals with the automatic functioning of body systems, such as the digestive system, the heartbeat and water metabolism. It is the ANS that makes our organ functions start up and stop or change automatically when they are needed, without us being conscious of this happening.

There are two branches of the ANS: the sympathetic branch and the parasympathetic branch. The sympathetic branch controls the "fight and flight" mechanism, deciding when the body needs to go into action to deal with stress, by stimulating the production of adrenalin and increasing the blood supply to muscles, shutting down any unnecessary organ functions. The parasympathetic branch has the opposite function, of helping the body to relax and recuperate by slowing down the heartbeat, relaxing the muscular system, stimulating the digestion and encouraging the conservation of energy in the body.

In Shiatsu massage, the aim is to relax and calm the body, bringing the parasympathetic branch to the fore. This approach is designed to bring a deep relaxation that helps to replenish vital energies.

The Back

The back is one of the most satisfying areas of the body to treat and also to receive treatment upon. The basic routine starts with the back due to its importance in relaxing the nervous system and therefore the energy balance of the whole body.

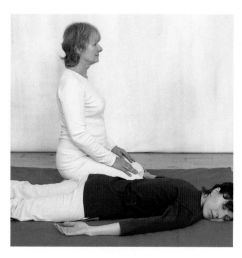

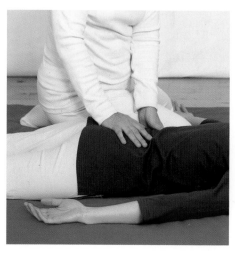

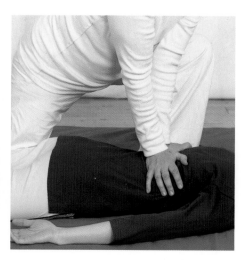

1 Prepare and breathe Start by sitting in seiza next to your partner who is in prone position (lying on their front). Sit with the outside of your leg in contact with your partner's left side. Take some deep breaths into your hara – you can close your eyes if you wish for complete concentration – and focus your attention into your hara. Open your eyes slowly and observe your partner's back.

2 Rest your hand Gently place your hand palm down on to the sacrum at the base of the spine. Be aware that this is your first contact with your partner. Notice how their body feels under your hand – it may feel hot or cold or you may feel a tingling sensation. Let your hand rest here for a couple of breaths while you "tune in to your partner". It will help if you match your breathing with your partner's.

3 Lean your weight Come into position with one knee up and one down. Starting one hand's width below the shoulders, place both palms either side of the spine and lean your body weight into your hands as you breathe out. Ask your partner to breathe out slowly with you as you apply pressure. Shift your weight back and move your hands down a little and lean in again.

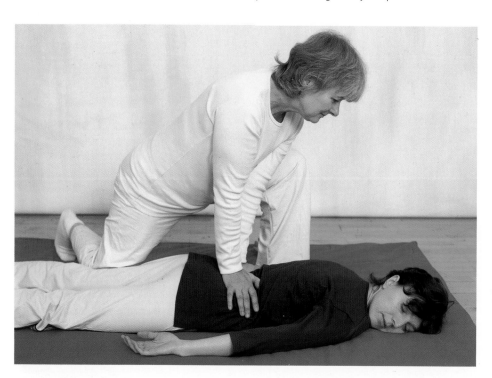

4 Move down the spine Continue down either side of the spine until you reach the sacrum, which is the base of the spine. You may have to move your legs back as you get further down the spine so that you are still comfortable and using your body weight. Check with your partner that they are comfortable with your pressure.

The sacrum

When your hand is on the sacrum, what do you feel? Do you feel hot or cold? Is there a tingling? Do you have an image? Try and find a word or a picture to describe it. Observe if some areas are looking more full or empty than others. Notice if there is a difference between the right and left sides of the body. Notice differences in the shoulders or feet or places of tension.

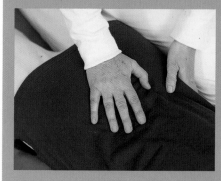

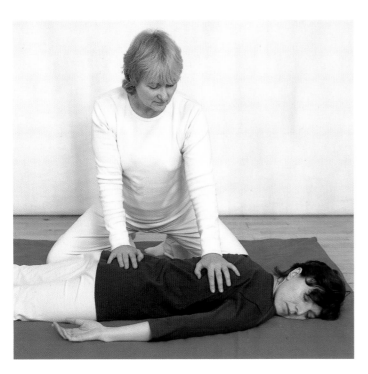

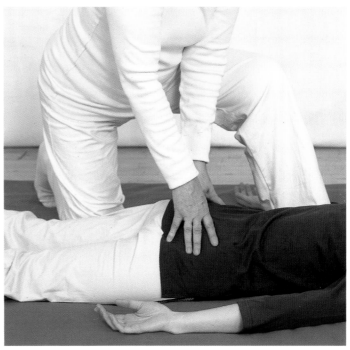

5 Rock the body Change your position so that you are facing the body from the side with both knees on the ground but wide. Place one hand on the sacrum and rock the body gently from side to side, using your body weight to maintain a rhythm. With the other hand, work down first one side of the spine then the other, maintaining the rocking rhythm with both hands and your body weight. Let the movement come to a gradual stop.

6 Lean in to apply pressure Change your position back to one knee down and one knee up (as in step 3). Starting at the top of the spine, one hand's width below the shoulders, thumb down either side of the spine on the Bladder meridian. Work with straight thumbs, two finger-widths from the midline of the spine, leaning in with your body weight to apply pressure. Work down the back slowly, moving a little way down each time.

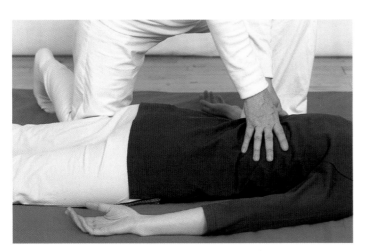

7 Move down to the sacrum

Continue to work down with your thumbs until you reach the sacrum. There are three natural depressions in the sacrum which your thumbs will fit into. Notice if there is a difference in the depth of penetration as you go down the spine. Check with your partner that they are comfortable with the pressure.

Thumb positioning

It is important to keep the thumbs straight as you work, otherwise you will put strain on the joints of your thumbs.

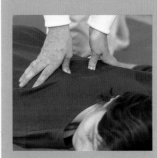

Use your other fingers to provide support for your thumbs. Make sure your pressure is perpendicular to the body. The pressure will be more precise and directed, and the energy will come directly from your hara and into the receiver.

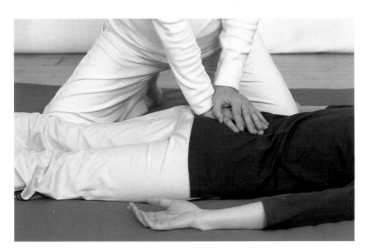

8 Sustain pressure and

breathe Place both hands on the sacrum and lean in. Stay in that position while you and your partner breathe in and out slowly a few times, and then gradually ease the pressure. Come back to position 1, with your hand on the sacrum. Notice if there has been a change in the feeling under your hand.

The Legs and Buttocks

As you work on the backs of the legs you will be accessing the rest of Bladder meridian, the longest meridian in the body. The buttocks are important in boosting energy to the reproductive system. There are some sensitive points in this area.

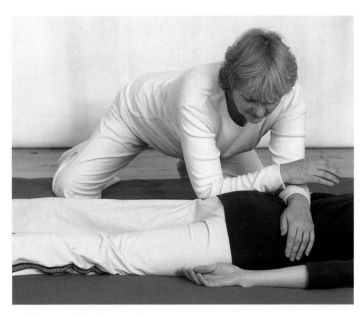

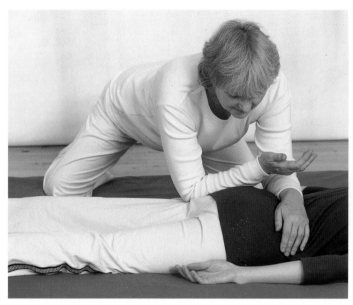

1 Forearm on buttocks Face your partner's body from the side with both knees on the ground but wide apart. Lean forwards so that you can comfortably work with your forearm on the buttocks. Start with your left forearm on the sacrum as the mother arm. Beginning at the side of the buttock nearest you, bending your elbow, place your right forearm gently on to the buttock, and roll your right arm away from you over the buttock and back.

2 Repeat the rolling motion Do this over the whole of the left buttock, altering your position if necessary in order to cover the whole area. Make sure that you are using the weight of your body as pressure, without putting too much pressure into the mother arm resting on the sacrum. Feel the energy coming from your hara, lowering your hara towards the ground for greater stability if necessary by adopting a wider kneeling position.

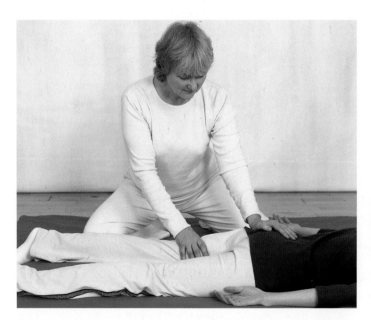

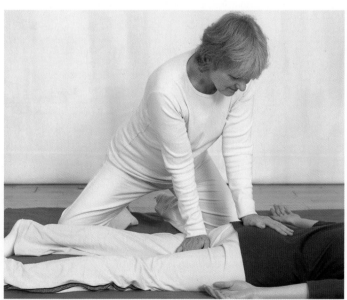

3 Sit up slightly and work your hand down the leg nearest you With the mother hand still on the sacrum, squeeze and knead down the leg to the ankle, using each squeeze to rock the leg gently and promote the movement of energy. If the knees are painful on the floor, place a small cushion under the calves.

4 Apply energy from your hara Come back up to the top of the leg and, keeping the left hand on the sacrum, palm down the back of the leg to the ankle. Use your body weight to apply energy, and feel it coming from your hara. Do not press on the back of the knee and go straight on to the lower leg.

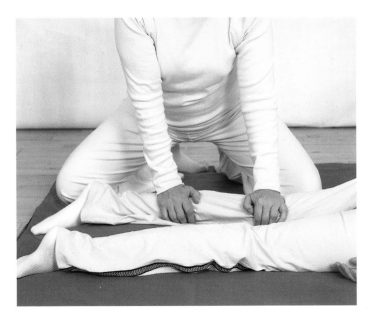

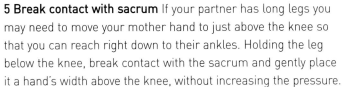

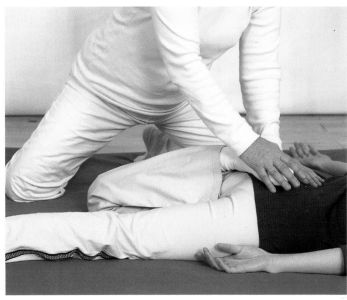

5 Break contact with sacrum If your partner has long legs you may need to move your mother hand to just above the knee so that you can reach right down to their ankles. Holding the leg below the knee, break contact with the sacrum and gently place it a hand's width above the knee, without increasing the pressure.

6 Stretch the foot Pick up the foot with one hand under the ankle, keeping your other hand on the sacrum. Stretch the foot to the buttock above this leg. You can push the top of the foot down so that the front of the ankle is opened, but be careful not to overstretch. Check with your partner for comfort.

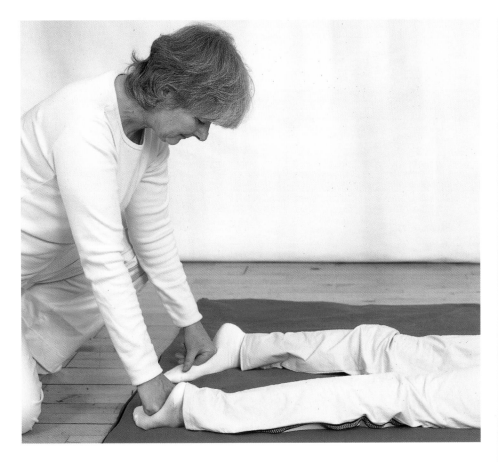

7 Pressure on soles and arches Come to the base of the feet and apply pressure to the soles and arches with your knuckles, without clenching your thumb into your hand. Lean in, putting your weight into your knuckles. To treat the other leg move to the other side and pick up the leg under the ankle and stretch it towards the buttock as in step 6. Change position so that you are at the top of the leg. Repeat steps 1–4 on the leg, using your other hand to work across the buttocks and down the leg. While you are moving, keep one hand as a mother hand connected to the body at all times.

Cushions

If you notice that your partner is not able to fully relax or that parts of the body do not make contact with the floor, this can show you where there are areas of stiffness and tension. When applying pressure use cushions to support any stiff or painful joints. For example, if someone has tight ankles or has had an ankle injury, you may notice that the shin is not touching the floor. Place a cushion under the shin so that as you apply pressure you will not put undue strain on the ankle joint. You can then safely let your weight drop on to the back of the leg. Similarly a cushion under the shin can protect a problem knee.

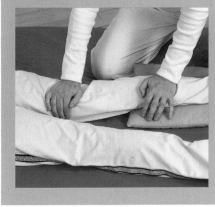

178

The Front and the Hara

Ask your partner to turn over on to their back, into the supine position. Make sure
they are comfortable, with the back and back of the legs in contact with the floor.
Place a cushion under the knees if the lower back is uncomfortable.

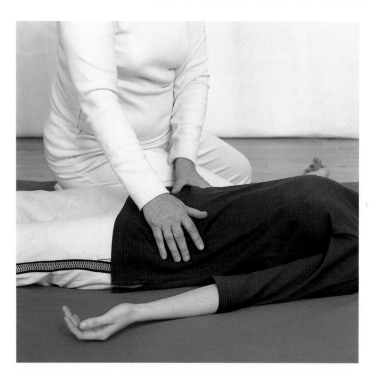

1 Hands on waist Sit in seiza next to your partner on the right
and place your hands either side of the waist, slightly to the front.
Keep the pressure gentle as this is a vulnerable area.

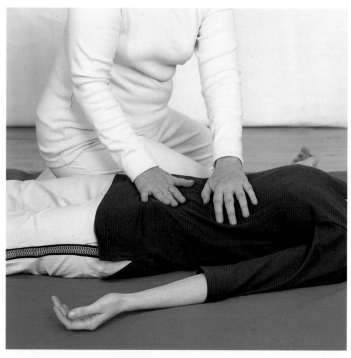

2 Feel the outline of the hara The ribs make the upper border,
and the hip bones create the lower border. The navel will be on
the waist level, slightly above the centre of the hara.

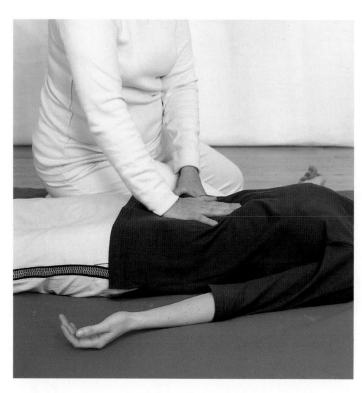

3 Slide your right hand gently to the centre of the hara
Do this with your palm resting just below the navel and your
fingers spread over it, but not reaching the base of the ribs.
Keep the left hand at the side of the waist as the mother hand.

Gentle pressure

Remember that this is a very vulnerable area of the body,
so pressure should be light to begin with. Check with your
partner if your pressure is comfortable. Tune in to their
energy. Observe any sensations under your hand. If
someone is ticklish make your contact firm and confident,
and if all fails, come back to the hara later in the session.

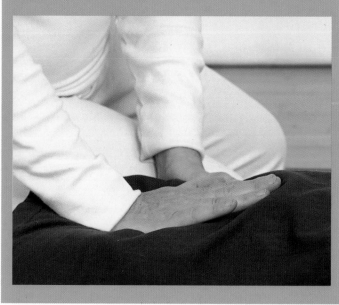

4 Create a wave-like motion Place your right hand on the hara with your fingers pointing towards the head, and the heel of your hand just above the pubic bone. Press the heel of your hand down with the out breath and release on the in breath, pushing the fingers down, making a wave-like motion from the heel of the hand to the fingertips. Keep the pressure soft and flowing, without any abrupt or jerky movements. Ask your partner to breathe in and out with your pressure, and keep the rhythm of the movement steady and flowing, following the breath.

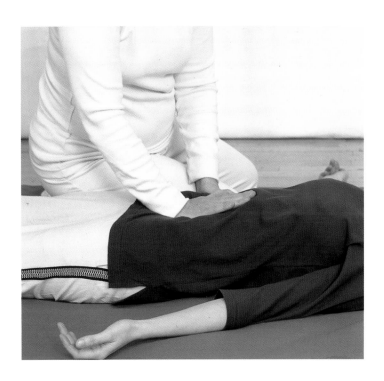

5 Stroke around the hara Do this with a light clockwise movement using both hands. This is a very relaxing movement that will focus the energy of your partner into the hara. Ask your partner to breathe slowly in and out, concentrating the breath into the hara and imagining it glowing with every in breath.

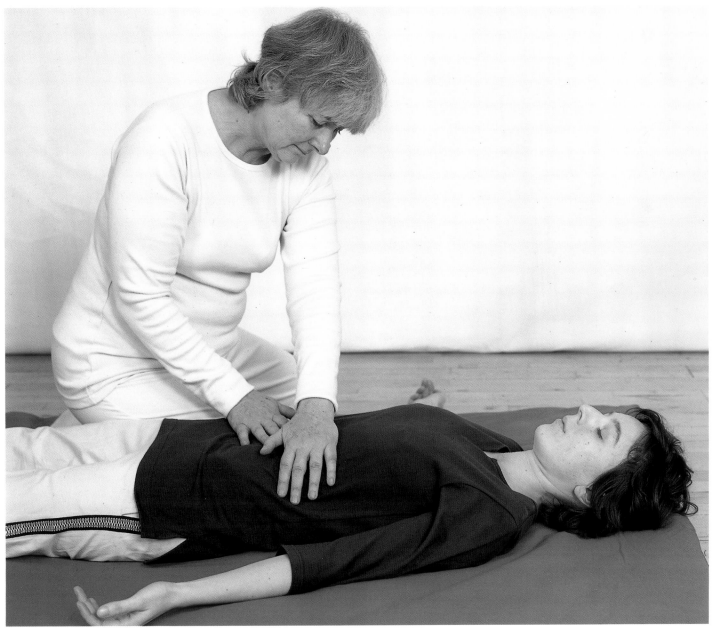

The Arms

There are six meridian pathways beginning and ending at the fingertips and flowing through the arms, some continuing into the shoulders and neck. This sequence stretching and palming the arms will help to increase chi flow into all these areas.

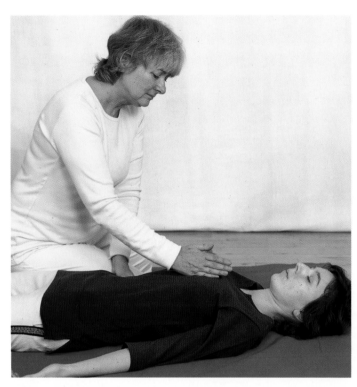

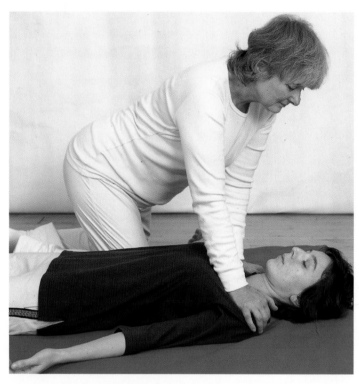

1 Work up the sternum Kneel comfortably on the right of your partner, the end of your knees about level with their elbow. Place your left hand on the side of the body as the mother hand. From the centre of the hara, using the little finger side of your right hand, work up the sternum to the left shoulder.

2 Stretch open the shoulders Change position to one knee forward and the other back. Bringing your hand on to the right shoulder, lean in with your body weight to stretch open the shoulders. Make a mental note of any tension or difference in the shoulders. Does one go down easier than the other?

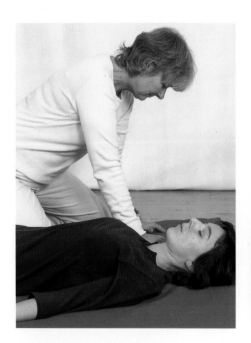

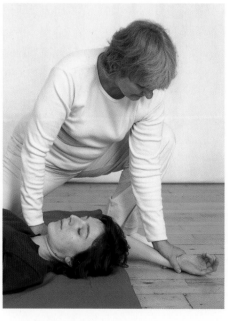

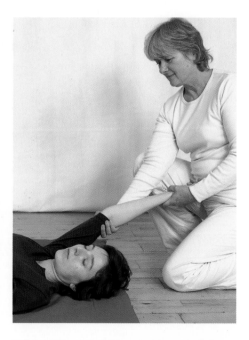

3 Palm down With the mother hand (now the right hand) on the right shoulder, bring the arm out at 90 degrees and palm down from the shoulder towards the hand.

4 Lift and stretch Lift the arm by the wrist and stretch it up over the head. Only stretch it up as far as it will move easily, without strain.

5 Arm off ground Move to the top of the head, lifting the arm up off the ground. Lean back and stretch the arm from the shoulder, supporting the elbow and wrist.

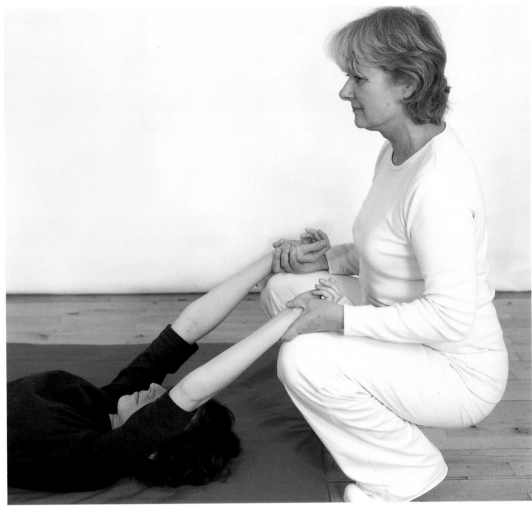

6 Stretch both arms Keeping hold of the right arm, lift the other above the head. In squatting position, lean back and stretch both arms. Be careful when stretching, holding the arms at the wrists with a soft hold. Never extend a stretch beyond your partner's natural extent, and be extra cautious on areas of the body that have previously been injured or are problematic.

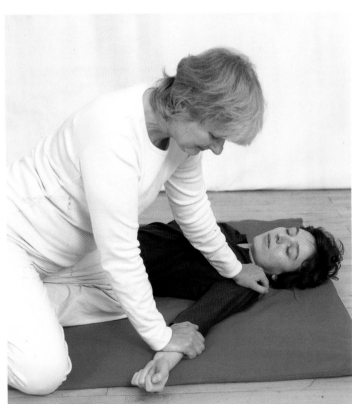

7 Palm down Let go of the right hand, move round so that the left arm is now at 90 degrees and palm down this arm.

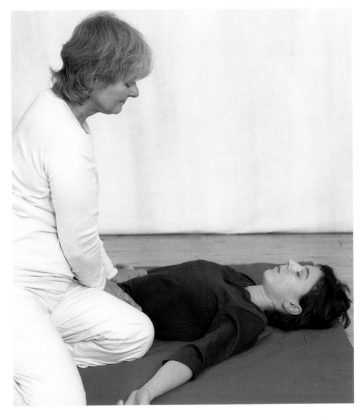

8 Rest gently Sit back in seiza at the hara and let your hand rest gently on the hara. Notice changes from the start of the exercise.

The Legs

As you work on the legs, notice any differences in the right and left sides: is one side easier to work than the other, or lighter and more flexible? The extent of the natural turn-out of the feet when lying down will be linked to the tension in the hip.

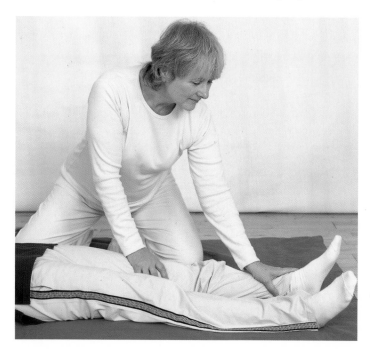

1 Palm down With your partner lying on their back, sit in seiza on the left side. Palm down the outside of the left leg, with your mother hand moving from the hara to above the knee if necessary.

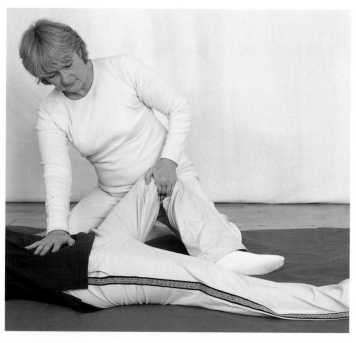

2 Pick up the leg With your mother hand on the hara, pick up the leg by placing your left hand under the knee and bringing it towards you. Move your hand to the front of the bent knee, and bring it back to vertical, then up towards your partner's head.

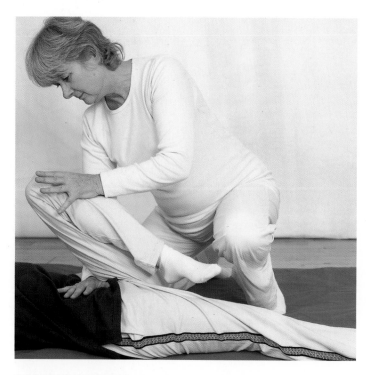

3 Rotate leg outwards As you bring up the leg, change your position to one knee up, and rotate the leg outwards to follow the natural movement of the hip joint. Keep your hand on the hara. Ask your partner to let you know if you are stretching too far. Notice any stiffness in the hip as you rotate.

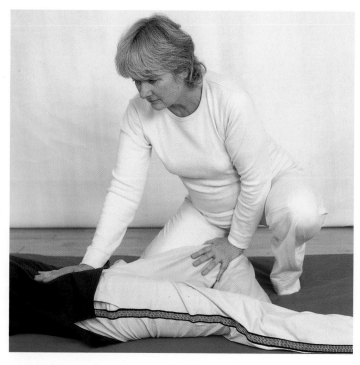

4 Stretch and support Bring the leg down and, still bent, let it drop out to the side. Place the instep against the opposite knee and stretch by applying gentle pressure to the left knee towards the floor. If the bent leg does not reach the floor, support the leg with your thigh wedged under your partner's thigh.

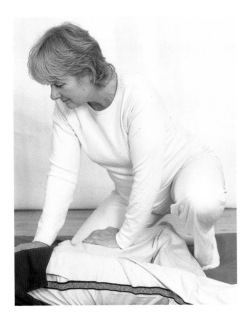

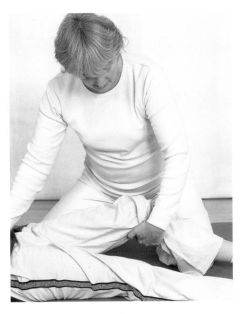

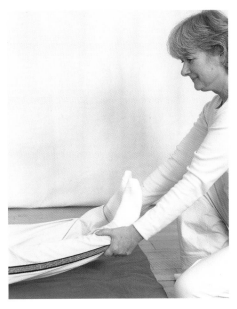

5 Palm up the leg With your hand still on the hara, palm up the inside of the leg, from above the ankle along the inside of the calf and thigh. Balance the pressure of your working hand with your mother hand. Remember to use perpendicular pressure and notice any areas of stiffness or emptiness.

6 Gently straighten the leg Supporting the leg under the knee, return it to its original position. When you lift or bend the legs and when you ease them back down again, always do so by supporting under the knee. Take extra care if your partner has knee problems.

7 Lift feet off the floor Move your position to below the feet, kneeling on one knee. Take both ankles in your hands and slowly lift them off the floor with your arms straight. Stretch both legs by using your body weight to lean backwards, opening up and stretching the legs from the abdomen.

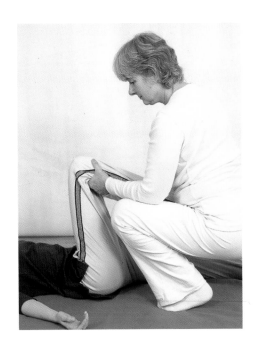

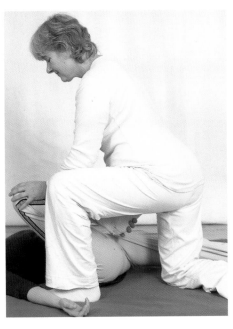

8 Transition Step to the other side of the body. Place your left hand beneath the knee and the right hand beneath the ankle of the right leg and lift the leg off the floor. As you step forward bend your partner's knee up, changing the position of your left hand to the front of the knee and the right hand to support the foot. Slide your lower leg forward so that you are in a position to rotate the leg. This should be a flowing movement.

9 Rotate the leg Note the two different kinds of leg rotations: in the first rotation your hand is on the hara so that you can monitor the ease of movement of the hip; while in the second you may be able to make a bigger range of movement, useful if your partner has heavy legs, or has difficulty in letting go. Repeat steps 4–6 on this leg, ensuring that you are not over-stretching or forcing. Come back to the hara on this side.

Positions for giving Shiatsu
Many practitioners find it comfortable to sit with the legs wide apart and both knees on the floor. You will have to maintain this posture for some time, so it is important that you do not tense or strain your own spine. The knees can be brought up or down so that you can move around easily, stretch over the body, and sink your weight properly into your hara when necessary.

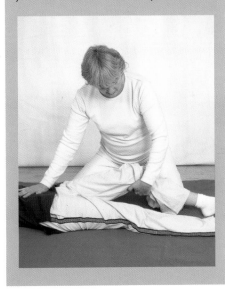

The Neck and Shoulders

The neck and shoulders are often an area of tension and discomfort. This short sequence can be done as a stand-alone treatment or incorporated into the basic treatment. Releasing tension in the neck and shoulders can increase blood flow to the head and improve alertness.

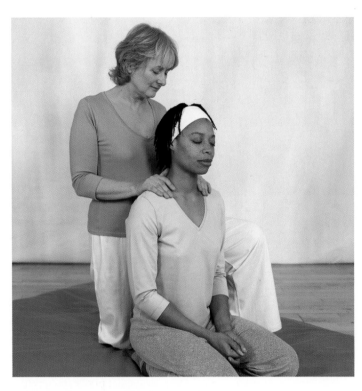

1 Tune in to your partner's energy With your partner sitting in seiza (or cross legged if this is more comfortable) kneel behind your partner, placing your hands on the shoulders.

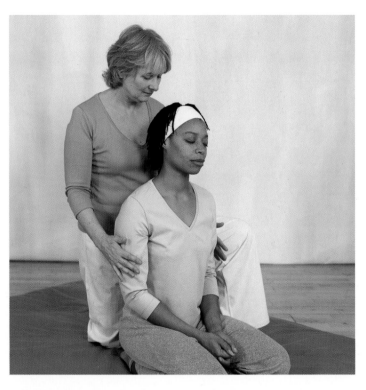

2 Palm across the shoulders and down the arms Use a hugging hand to work down the arms to the elbows. Repeat two or three times to loosen the arms and shoulders.

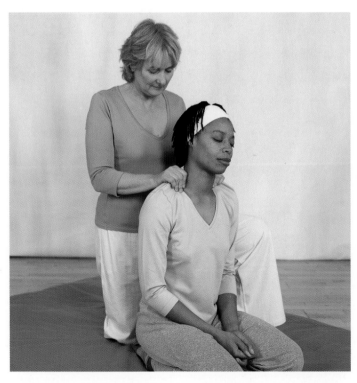

3 Squeeze the shoulders Do this by holding the trapezius muscles that run along the top of the shoulders and into the back of the neck. Try shaking, rocking, and kneading with the squeeze.

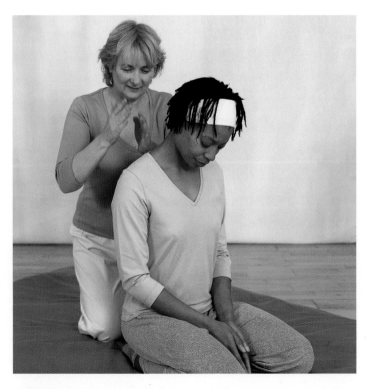

4 Light taps With your hands straight but relaxed and the sides of your hands towards your partner, cover the shoulder and upper back area with rapid, light taps.

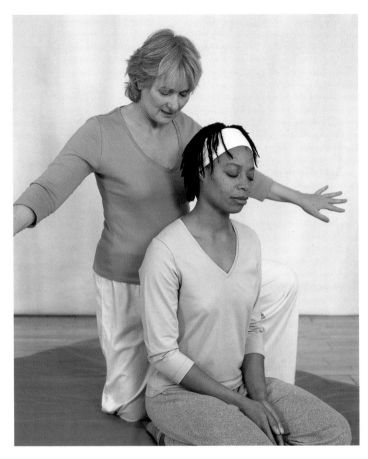

5 Brush hands out In one great sweeping motion, sweep your hands from the top of the shoulders, brushing them out.

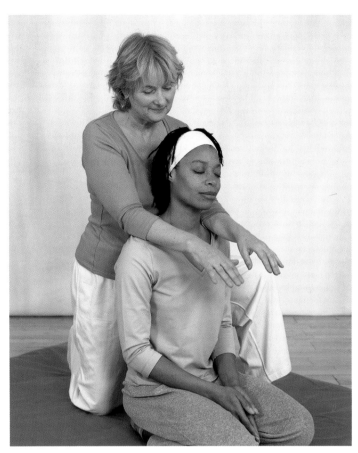

6 Pressure down Balance your forearms on the shoulders of your partner, next to the neck, and gently put pressure down.

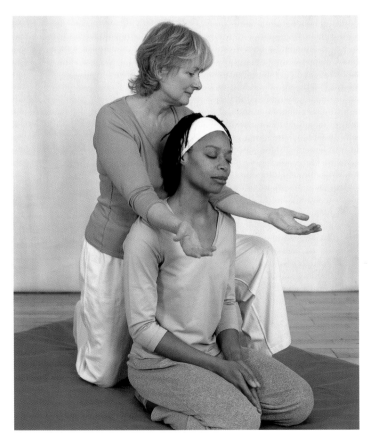

7 Rolling on shoulders and turning palms Roll your forearms along the tops of your partner's shoulders, turning the palms of your hands upwards.

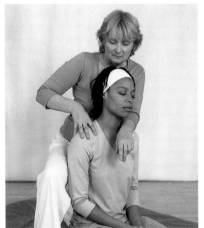

8 Press with thumb Leaving one of your arms on your partner's shoulder, press along the top of the shoulder with your thumb. Repeat on other shoulder.

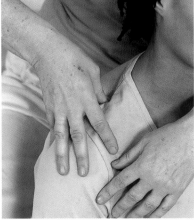

9 Focus on pressure point Work in to the pressure point GB 21, situated on the top of the trapezius muscle midway between the base of the neck and the end of the shoulder. This is a good point for releasing tension in the shoulder. Do not work on this point during pregnancy.

▷

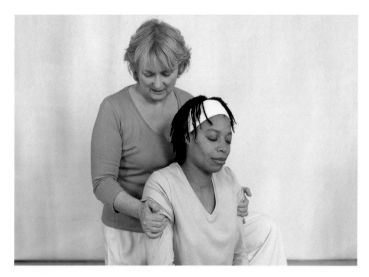

10 Shoulders in shrug Holding the top of the arms, lift up the shoulders into a shrug to see if the shoulders are relaxed.

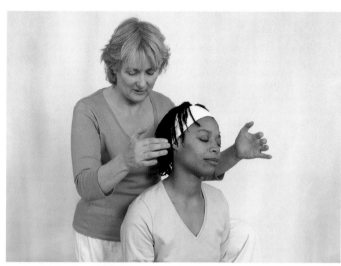

11 Release the shoulders Having done this, the shoulders should return to their natural position. Repeat a few times.

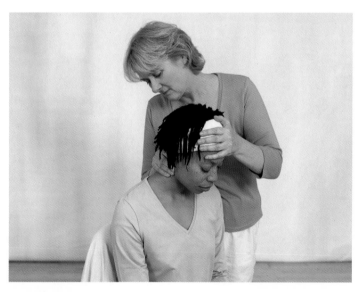

12 Drop head Holding the front of the head, let it drop forward. Squeeze down the back of the neck either side of the spine.

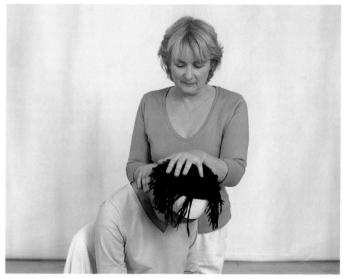

13 Hold stretch Let the head drop forwards gently, taking care not to overstretch. Hold the stretch for a few seconds.

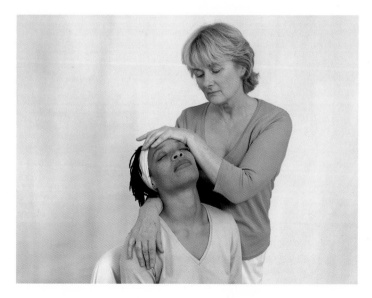

14 Drop head back Do this holding the forehead with one hand and with your other forearm behind the neck for support.

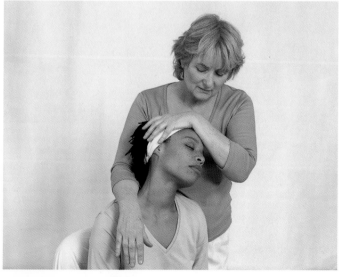

15 Head towards you Holding the side of the head, bend it to the side towards you, with your arm on the opposite shoulder.

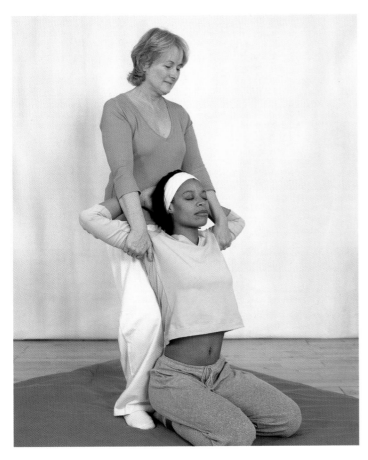

16 Stretch arms Stand with your knees against your partner and ask them to clasp their hands behind their head. Reaching under the arms, stretch up and back.

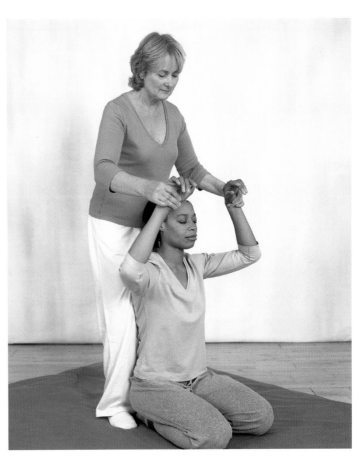

17 Hold arms Taking your partner's arms up by the wrists, hold them gently above the head, checking they are relaxed.

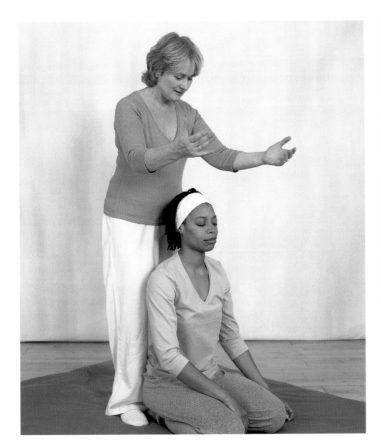

18 Let arms drop Release your hold and let your partner's arms drop naturally back into place, falling on to the lap.

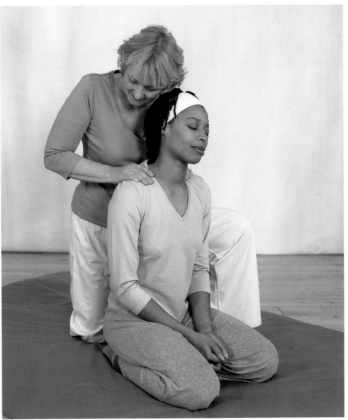

19 Tune in Kneel down again, place your palms back on your partner's shoulders and tune in. Notice any changes.

The Hands

The hands are worked in a similar way to that described in the Do-in section.
There are many important meridian points on both hands and feet. Include this
sequence into the basic routine when working on the arms.

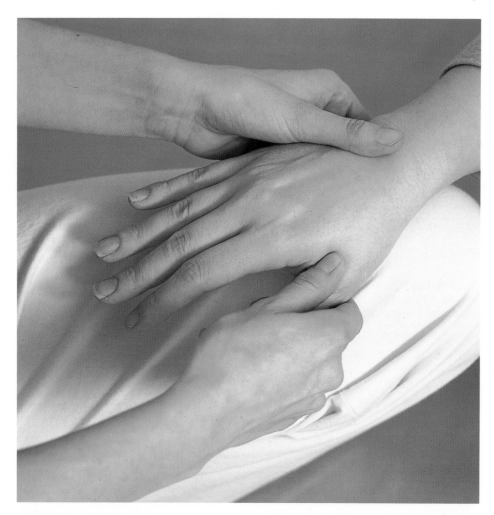

1 Rotate and flick Holding your partner's hand, rotate the thumb and fingers both
ways, and then flick them one by one.

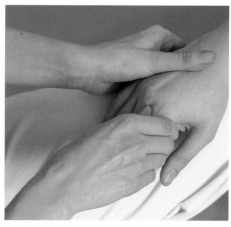

2 Massage fingers Massage thumbs
and fingers, squeezing along each.

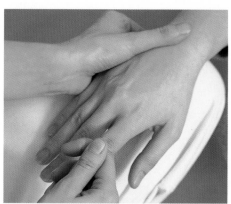

3 Stretch Holding the wrist, gently pull
each finger and the thumb.

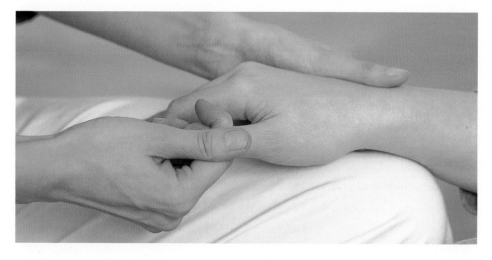

4 Find the point LI 4 This pressure point is located in the depression where the two
bones of the thumb and index finger meet. Press in with your thumb towards the
bone of the index finger and hold. This point is good for constipation or diarrhoea
and is known as "the great eliminator". Do not use in pregnancy.

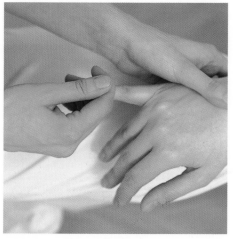

5 Squeeze fingertips Squeeze the sides
at the base of the fingernails – this
stimulates the finishing points of the
arm meridians.

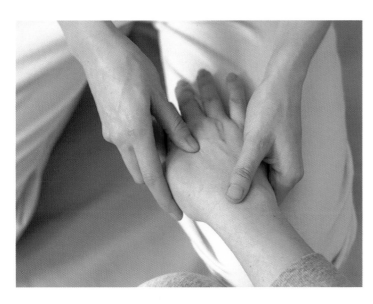

6 Fingers to wrist Holding with one hand, work with your thumb between the metacarpals from the fingers to the wrist.

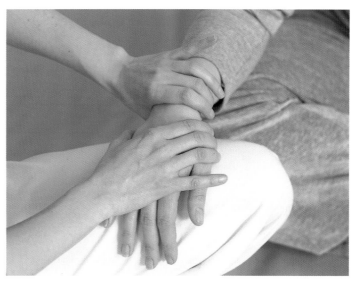

7 Encircle wrist and twist Rotate the wrists by encircling the upper and lower wrist and gently twisting to either side.

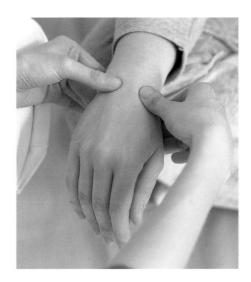

8 Shake hand Holding wrists between the thumb and forefingers, shake the hand up and down to relax the wrist.

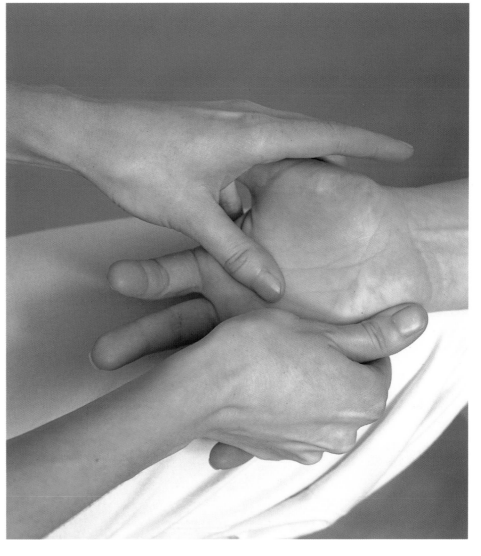

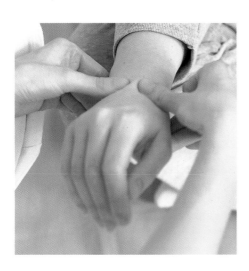

9 Work the wrists Use your thumbs to work the wrists, easing between the bones of the wrist on the front and back.

10 Open the palm With your partner's palm up, open up the palm by slotting your little fingers between the thumb and forefinger and the little finger and fourth finger. Stretch open the palm and use your thumbs to massage into the palm. Find HP 8 in the centre of the palm – fold the fingers down and it is where the middle finger touches the palm – and massage with your thumb. Repeat the full sequence on the other hand.

The Feet

There are many key points in the feet meridians, which you can include when giving a complete treatment. Finishing a treatment with the feet is a nice way to ground the energy. Shiatsu on the feet should be given through clean, preferably cotton socks.

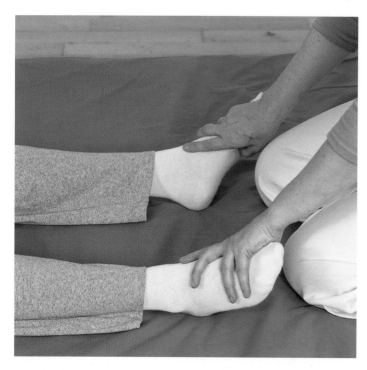

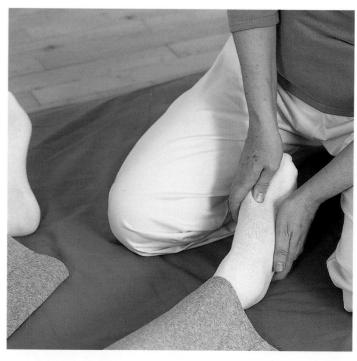

1 Bubbling spring Find KD 1 on the sole of the feet where the pad of the big toe and the ball of the foot make a "V", about a third of the way from the middle toe to the heel (see page 206). This "Bubbling Spring" point is a revitalizing point.

2 Open up foot Working on the top of the foot, use the side of your thumb and the heel of the other hand to work into the top of the foot from the middle to the edges, squeezing and pressing towards the outside edge.

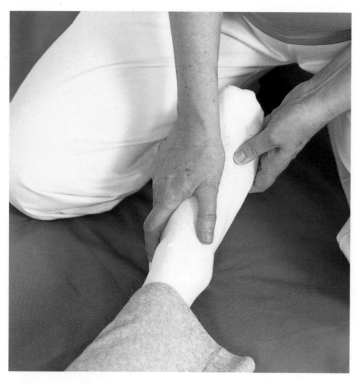

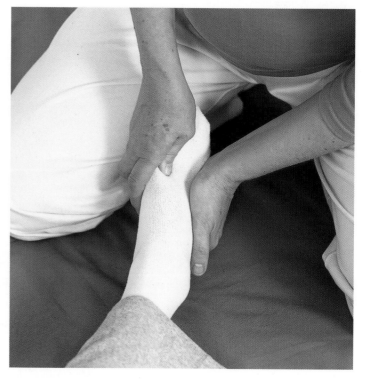

3 Open up sole of foot Squeeze the feet between your palms, grasping the sides of the feet and opening up the sole of the foot like a book. Work from the toes towards the heel a couple of times.

4 Work into the bones Work in between the metatarsals (the bones of the foot which become the toes) with your thumb. Be aware that there are some painful points here.

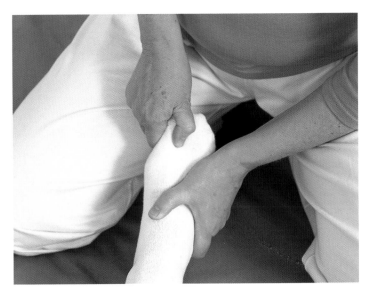

5 Unblock Liver energy Find LV 3, between the big toe and the second toe, two finger-widths below the webbing.

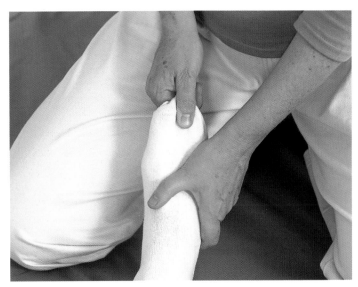

6 Massage, rotate and flick Do this to each toe to stimulate the meridians. Pinch between each of the toes.

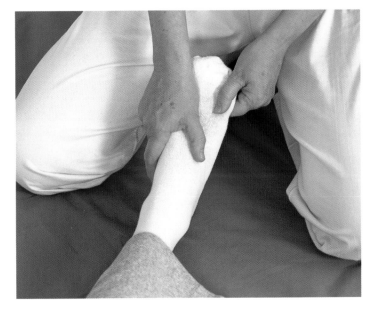

7 Hold and pull Holding the foot with the other hand, hold each toe, gently pulling to straighten it.

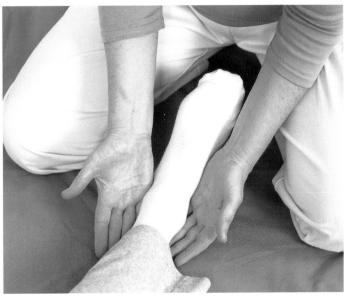

8 Rub around the ankle Do this with the sides of your hands, moving your hands firmly over the whole area.

9 Achilles tendon With fingers and thumb, squeeze down either side of the Achilles tendon. Find KD 3 on the inside of the ankle between the Achilles tendon and the tip of the ankle bone. This point is good for lower back pain.

Repeat the whole exercise on the other foot.

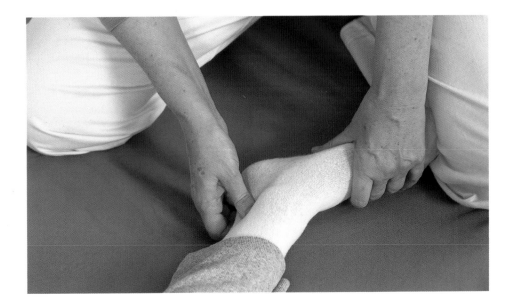

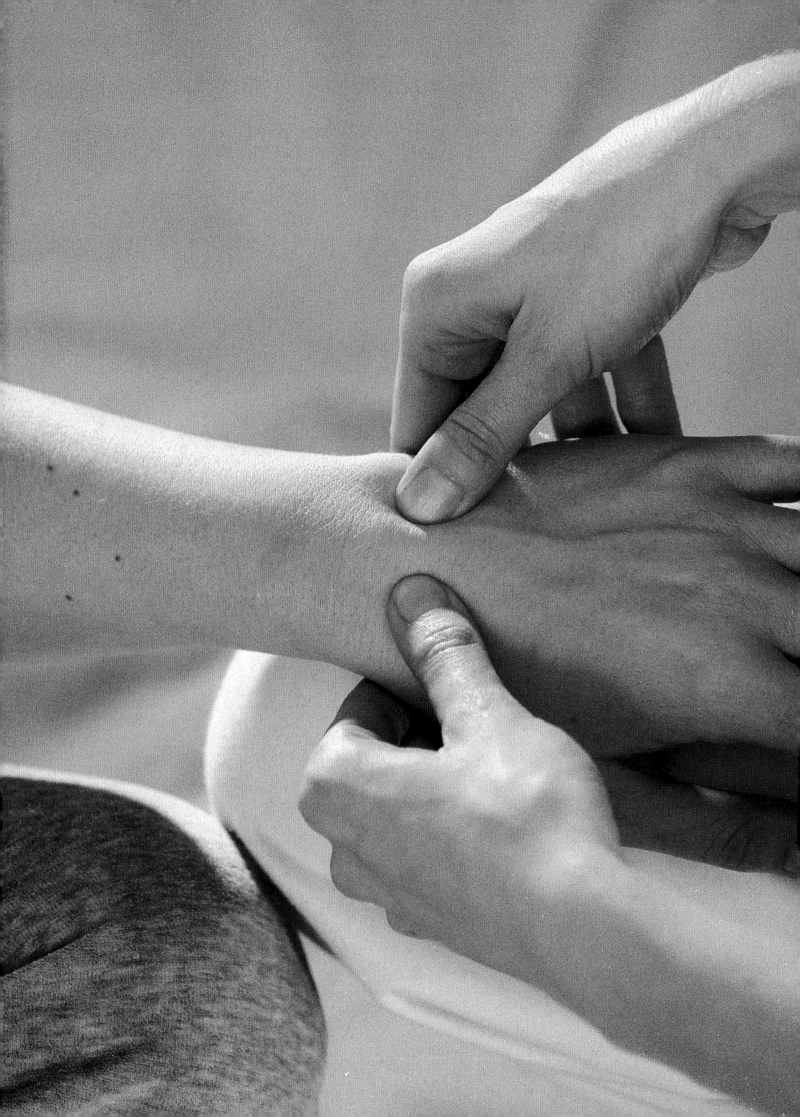

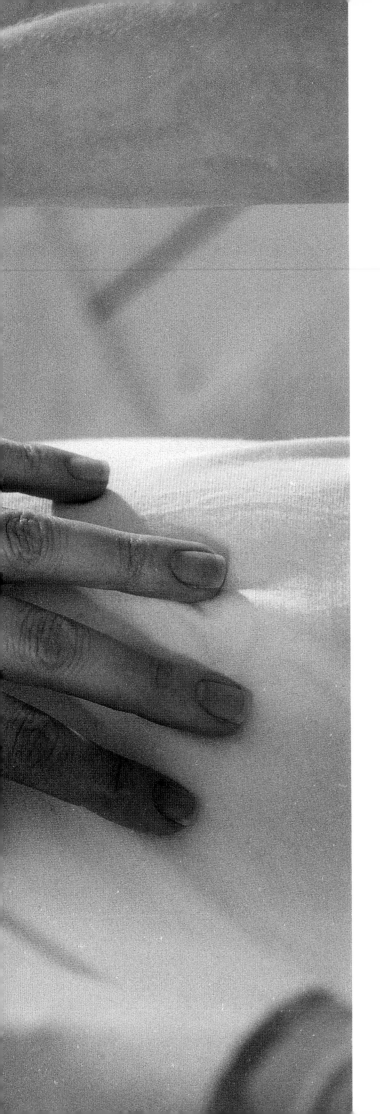

The Elements and Meridians

Here we look at the general nature of the five elements – Earth, Metal, Water, Wood and Fire (which breaks down into Primary Fire and Secondary Fire). Exploring the connection between the characteristics of each element and its associated pair of meridians, a series of Shiatsu sequences are then introduced, designed to work on each of the meridian pathways.

Although the meridians have, in most cases, the same name as a major organ in the body, their function does not necessarily correspond to the Western view of that organ. The Traditional Chinese Medicine practitioner takes a much wider view of the organ functions, ranging from emotional and psychological influences to the colour and sounds associated with the organ.

The Shiatsu treatments shown here can be used to rebalance the element in question, or used as part of a more general Shiatsu workout.

Working the Meridians

Each of the five elements has two meridians that control specific functions and body parts. In Shiatsu you can work these meridians to improve the general healthy function of the body, or to treat problems related to an element or a meridian. For simplicity, this section shows how to treat the parts of these meridians on the leg or the arm, clearly showing the first and last points of the meridian and some landmark points along each one.

PREPARATION

Before you start a treatment, do some preparation work (see preceding chapters), especially massaging and bringing energy to your hands. Also reread the contraindications section on page 171 and check that the receiver does not have any conditions that would make treatment inadvisable. Always listen to your partner's feedback. If they say that something is painful, slow down or stop what you are doing. And finally if someone has a serious complaint do not treat them. Shiatsu is not a medical treatment and should never be used as such. If you are in doubt about someone's condition refer them either to another practitioner or to a doctor.

GENERAL POSITIONS FOR MERIDIAN WORK

When treating your partner, always put the leg or arm in the position that will give you the easiest way of treating the meridian. Keep a steady rhythm going as you move along the meridian finding the landmark points. You may have to change your position slightly when you find the end points on the hands or feet.

Let the mother hand rest on the body while palming or working the points with the other hand. This hand keeps a constant pressure and gives a sense of security to the receiver, leaving the other hand free to move from point to point along the meridian. The pictures shown throughout this chapter will give you an indication of where the mother hand should be, but you can sometimes adapt the position if it is uncomfortable or hard to reach. Remember to relax, using your body weight and perpendicular pressure as you go into the meridian.

RESPONSIVENESS

As you work on your partner, go in slowly until you feel a resistance and then wait. Be aware of how the area under your hand or thumb feels. Sometimes the resistance will melt and you will be able to go further. Never force pressure on your partner: take your time and don't rush. Check with your partner if the pressure feels all right: if there is pain use less pressure or go in more slowly, or move on to a different part of the body and return to the tender part later.

As you practise you may be able to get a sense of how different areas or points on the meridian feel. Sometimes under-energized or over-energized points can be felt as a softness or stiffness, a fullness or emptiness.

INTEGRATING MERIDIAN WORK

Having practised working the individual meridians, then use the basic framework (see pages 168–91) and slot one or two meridian sequences into it. For example, while

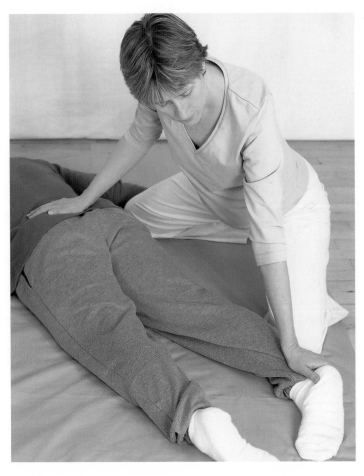

Left Use a wide seiza stance and apply pressure through your own body weight, originating from your hara.

Palming and thumbing the meridians

Palm the meridian to get a feel for where it is and the quality of the energy you are feeling (below). Then work down the points with your thumb, finding the beginning point, gradually moving along the meridian and then finding the landmark points. Keep your thumb straight when treating points, supporting it by making a fist with the fingers (below).

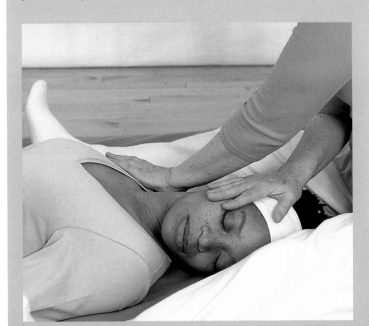

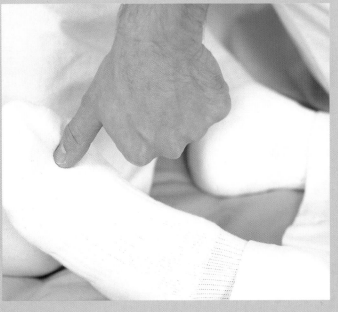

treating the legs in supine put the leg into position for Spleen meridian and work this meridian (see pages 198–9). Work all the meridian and points on one leg and then work the other side, using the transition in the basic framework outline. If you are treating two meridians on the leg, for example, treat both meridians on one leg first before moving around the body to start work on the other leg.

Use your powers of observation to see how the body is responding. Sense what is going on under your hand or thumb and ask your partner for feedback. Using observation and feedback are ways of improving and developing your intuition – a combination of knowledge, observation and an ability to "listen" (hearing sounds, but also sensing, feeling and responding to the subtle signals you pick up).

MERIDIANS AND ASSOCIATED PROBLEMS

Remember the first touch in the basic framework outline and use the time while your hand is resting on the sacrum to scan the body looking for areas of tension or lack of energy. Which meridians pass through these areas? If your partner reports an area of tension or a particular pain, match the area to a meridian or point.

Usually in a treatment the practitioner will treat only two or three meridians appropriate to that person's condition. Start to think about which meridians would help with specific problems when reading the section describing the characteristics of each of the five elements. For someone with digestive problems, for example, the best meridians to work could be Spleen and Stomach; for someone with a cough you could work on Lung meridian. In the next section there is a more detailed account of diagnostic skills and how to choose which meridians to work on (see pages 228–35).

Right A model showing some of the key pressure points in Traditional Chinese Medicine on the human torso.

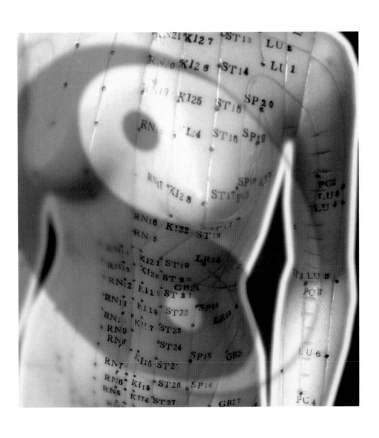

Earth

Earth represents solidity, nurturing and support, and is dependable and constant. It is associated with fertility, the cycles of nature and the reproduction of life. It provides us with food and gives us the ground beneath our feet, providing a home that grows and renews itself to support our existence. Earth's associated meridian pair is Spleen and Stomach: Spleen is the yin meridian and Stomach is the yang meridian.

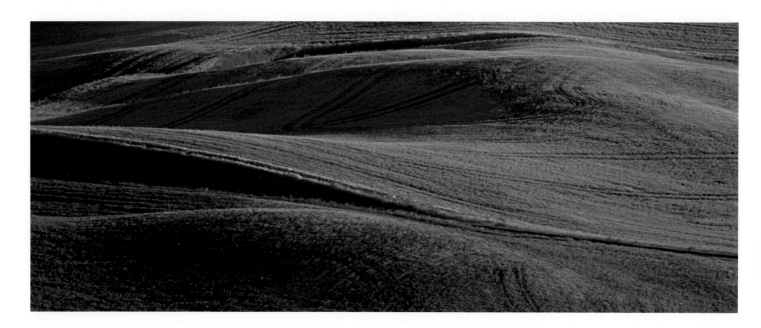

This element creates energy for digestion and governs the flesh. Earth's influence is felt throughout the front of the body, bringing energy and tone to the front muscles, especially the abdominal muscles.

When Earth is in balance a person is grounded, centred, and has the capacity to be still. The individual is then in a position to provide comfort because they feel secure and supported. The digestion is good and the appetite is stable.

Anxiety, worry and over-thinking damage Earth, knotting the energy and causing blockages in flow. Imbalance in Earth can result in digestive problems, diarrhoea, eating disorders, weight problems and menstrual problems. Someone out of balance in Earth will feel insecure, jealous or may have a victim mentality.

The most active time of day for Earth energy is 7–11a.m. This is the best time to digest food. If you hate getting up in the morning you may be out of balance in Earth. The time of year relating to Earth is late summer, and ill-health around this time could be a result of disharmony in this element. The taste attraction for Earth is sweet, especially the slow releasing, balanced

Above and below Mother Earth provides plentifully for us, bringing us nourishment, and providing stability and fertility.

sweetness of grains and root vegetables. The intense, fast-release sweetness of refined sugar will damage Earth. A craving for sweets and sugary food and drink shows a disharmony in the Stomach and Spleen meridians, indicating Earth element problems.

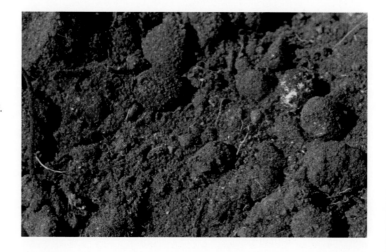

Pathway of the Stomach Meridian

Stomach meridian runs down the front of the body either side of the mouth,
through the breast and either side of the stomach. Indigestion, nausea and vomiting
can be helped by treating Stomach meridian, as well as eating disorders.

The Stomach meridian starts under the eye and runs past the side of the mouth, down the neck, crosses the collarbone and passes through the nipple. It then turns inwards at the belly and runs two finger-widths either side of the midline, branching out to the outside of the

thigh. It follows the outside border of the thigh and proceeds down the outside edge of the tibia (the shin bone). It then passes on to the front of the foot and finishes at the inside corner of the toenail of the second toe, where it meets the big toe.

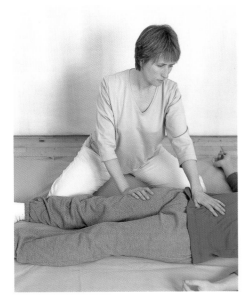

1 Turn leg inwards With your mother hand on the hara, place your lower knee against the lower leg, your hand on the thigh, and turn the leg inwards.

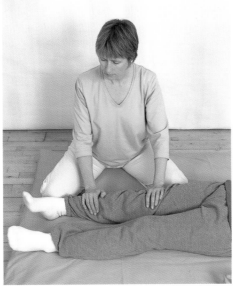

2 Palm down Keeping your hand on the hara, palm down the leg from the thigh to the ankle, changing the position of your mother hand to just above the knee.

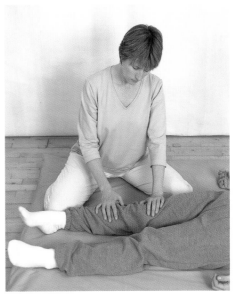

3 Thumb down Thumb down the meridian, moving the mother hand to just above the knee for the lower leg. Shift your position downwards as you go.

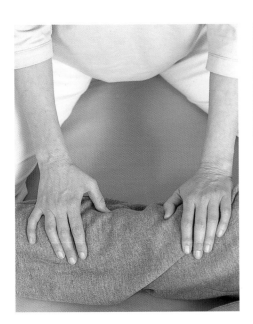

4 Find the point ST 36 This is situated three finger-widths below the knee on the outside of the leg. This is a good point for knee problems and tired legs.

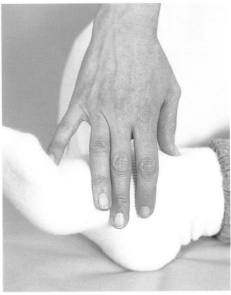

5 Find the point ST 41 This is on the front of the foot at the ankle crease between the two tendons. Use this point to help indigestion and nausea.

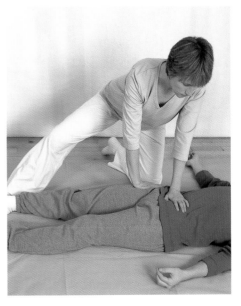

6 Foot against foot As an alternative position, you can use your foot against your partner's foot to turn the leg inward into Stomach position.

Pathway of the Spleen Meridian

Spleen helps in the digestive process by transforming food into energy and transporting this "food chi" and other fluids around the body. Treating it can help tiredness and digestive problems, such as diarrhoea and irritable bowel syndrome.

The Spleen meridian starts at the inside edge of the big toe, at the base of the toe nail. It passes along the centre of the top of the foot, and up in front of the ankle bone. As it runs up the leg, it remains along the inside edge of the tibia bone to the front, on the fleshy part. The meridian then runs along the inside edge of the thigh muscle, passing through the centre of the groin. It then pursues a course up through the front of the belly, a hand's width either side of the body's midline. It branches outwards at the ribs, continuing around the outside edge of the breast as far as the second rib, turning down to finish just below the armpit.

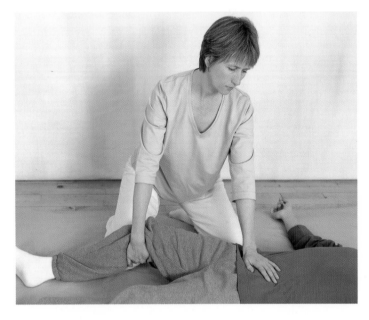

1 Face the hara Sit in seiza on the right side of your partner with your left hand on the hara. Turn to face the hara, keeping your hand on the hara as a mother hand.

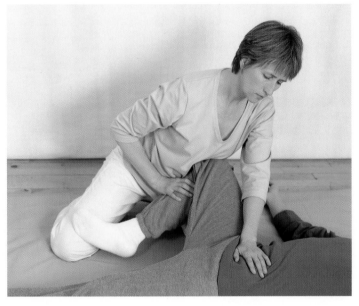

2 Leg towards you Bring up the right leg with your right hand under the knee, sliding it towards you. Change your hand to the front of the bent knee and press the leg up and sideways.

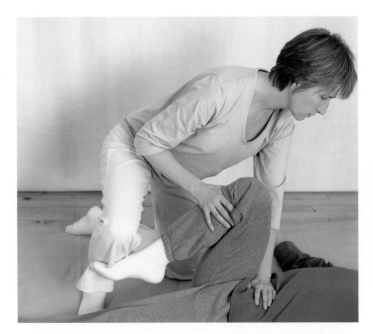

3 Rotate leg As you bring up the leg, change your position to one knee up, the other down and rotate the leg in a wide rotation. Feel for stiffness and check that it is comfortable.

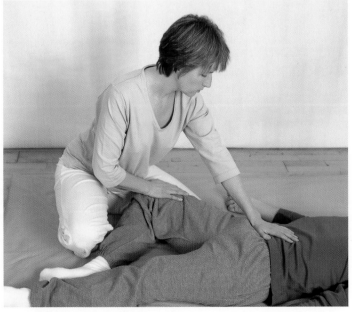

4 Lower leg down Lower the leg gently back down to the floor, with the knee bent and the heel lying just above the other ankle. Keep your hand on the hara.

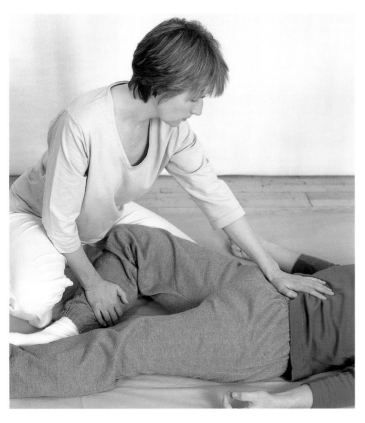

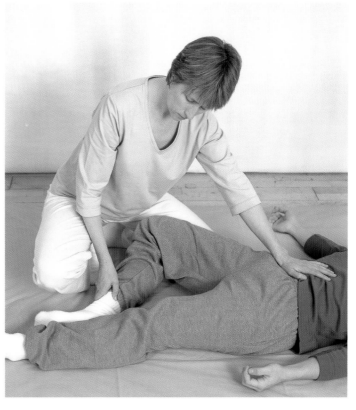

5 Palm inside leg Palm up the leg on the Spleen meridian pathway, up the inside of the leg, towards the front. Use your body weight, shifting your position when necessary.

6 Thumb pressure Use your thumb to press up the meridian. Keep your mother hand on the hara as you go, and once again move as necessary. Feel for kyo and jitsu as you work.

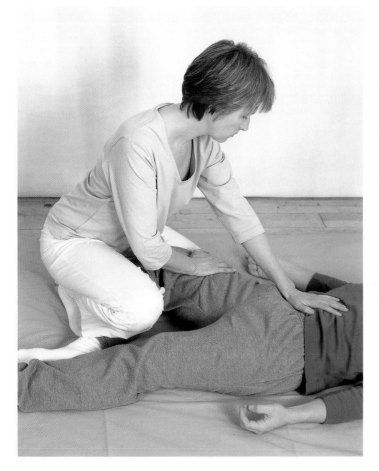

7 Turn to face the head When working on the thigh you can turn to face the head, swivelling slightly to be in position.

Spleen meridian points

Two important points on Spleen meridian are SP 6 and SP 9. SP 6 influences the digestive system, hormonal disorders and immune disorders. SP 9 is used to treat urinary diseases, abdominal and back pain and female reproductive system disorders.

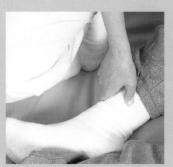

SP 6

Find this point by placing your first three fingers above the ankle bone on the inside of the leg. This point is helpful for menstrual pain and is also good for diarrhoea. Do not use during pregnancy.

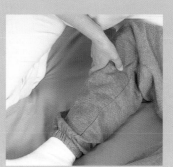

SP 9

This point is at the top of the shin bone on the inside leg in the fleshy part. It can help with knee problems, especially if the knee is swollen or is recovering from injury or surgery.

Metal

Metal is the densest of the elements, often aligned with rock and minerals. It is the force of gravity, the power of magnetism, the minerals within the earth – the rocks, the gems of the earth, the concentration of finely tuned particles. Metal is associated with strength, force, structure and boundaries. Metal's meridian pair is Lung and Large Intestine: Lung is the yin meridian and Large Intestine is the yang meridian.

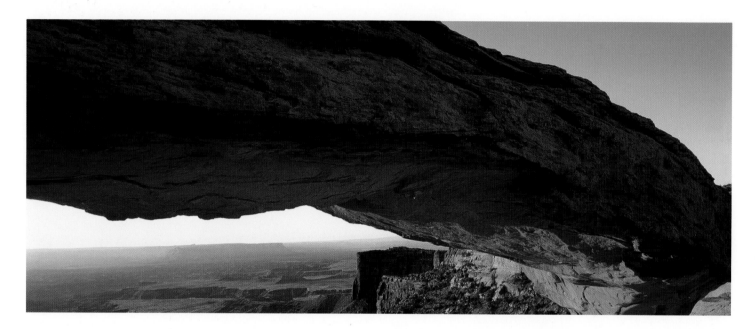

Metal governs the intake of chi and breath, inspiration and expiration. Chi from the air is transformed into what is called "true chi" and spreads throughout the body. The first of the Metal meridians, Lung sends "defensive chi" around the body, making the first line of defence against what the Chinese call "external pathogens" and what we know as infectious diseases, particularly colds and flu. If the Lung energy is weak there can be a susceptibility to diseases such as colds and coughs. Excess grief damages Lung. The second meridian, the Large Intestine, eliminates the waste products of the body.

Metal is to do with communication, boundaries, and taking in and letting go. The skin is the tissue associated with Metal. The skin makes the boundary of our bodies but it is not rigid. It is a permeable, living, breathing organ. The Lungs and Large Intestine act as boundaries which control the passage of substances in and out of the body.

People with a healthy Lung and Large Intestine function are open with a positive attitude. Good communicators, they have an ability to let go when needed but maintain boundaries when necessary. They will have healthy eliminations, a strong voice and be resistant to disease.

Above Rocks are symbolic of the Metal element in the environment (see also below), forming a cold, solid structure.

People with an imbalance in Metal can be either rigid and unable to let go or the opposite, having no boundaries. They will have a susceptibility to excessive colds and coughs and respiratory disease. Skin problems and constipation can be a sign of Metal imbalance. The taste attraction for Metal is pungent or spicy, but excess spicy food can cause Large Intestine problems. The season when Metal is most active is autumn.

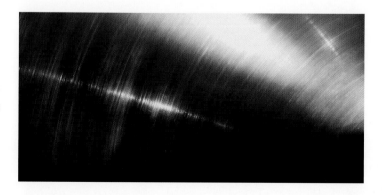

Pathway of the Lung Meridian

Lung is associated with the taking in of breath, transforming it into "true chi" and spreading it throughout the body. Lung is the first line of defence to fight off "external pathogens", which cause diseases such as colds, fevers and flu.

The Lung meridian starts between the first and second ribs, just under the middle of the collarbone, the small bone that links the shoulder to the breastbone. It then travels up crossing the collarbone and across the front of the shoulder, towards the arm. It follows a path down the outside edge of the biceps muscle in the upper arm, through the elbow and towards the wrist. It passes through the wrist, into the hand, and then progresses up the side of the thumb, ending on the outer edge at the corner of the thumbnail.

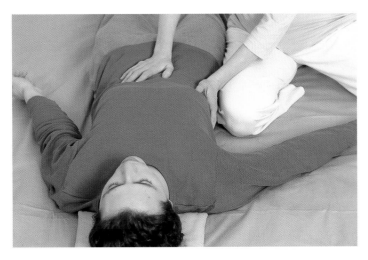

1 Arm straight, palm up Sit in seiza with your hand placed gently on the hara. Bring your partner's arm to an angle of 45 degrees from the body. Lay the arm straight with the palm up.

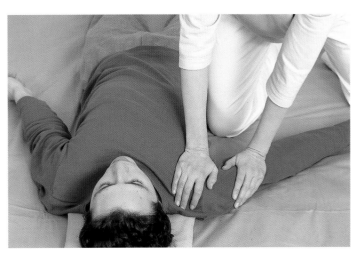

2 Palm down to the thumb Come into wide leg seiza and move up so that you can stretch towards the shoulders. Palm down Lung meridian all the way down to the thumb.

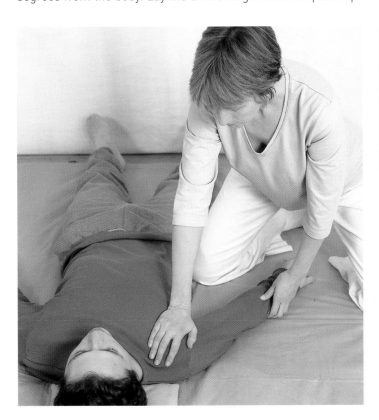

3 Thumb down Lung meridian To do this, change your position so that you are kneeling astride the hand.

Lung meridian points
Two points on Lung meridian are LU 1 and LU 5. Both can be used for respiratory problems, especially for chronic coughs, and prevention of colds and the flu.

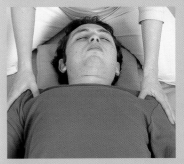

LU 1
Find this point between the first and second ribs, below the middle of the collarbone. This is best accessed from above the head. This is a good point for coughs and chest pain.

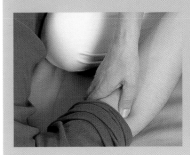

LU 5
This point can be found when you make a fist. It is in the elbow crease at the outside edge of the tendon. LU 5 is good for chronic coughs, arm and elbow pain.

Pathway of the Large Intestine Meridian

The Large Intestine eliminates the waste products of the body. It is like the internal skin, allowing waste products and toxins to pass out of the body. Skin problems, such as acne, and constipation can reflect problems in Large Intestine.

The Large Intestine meridian starts at the corner of the nail of the index finger at the side closest to the thumb. It then travels up the arm, passing through the elbow at the end of the elbow crease on the outside and across the shoulder. It then pursues a course up the side of the neck, crossing the large muscle at the side of the neck towards the nose. The meridian ends at the outside corner of the nostril. Remember that the point LI 4 is contraindicated in pregnancy (see page 171 for more information on contraindications).

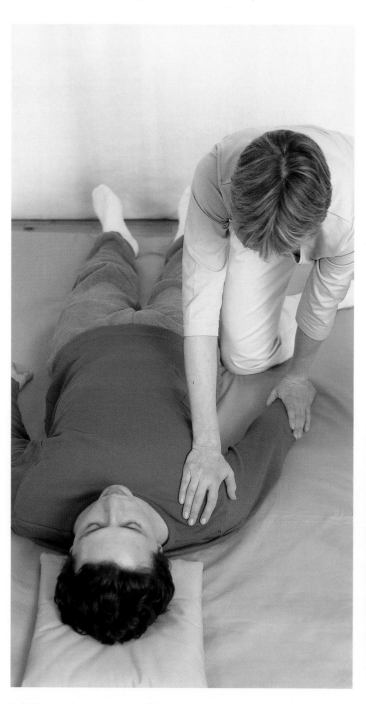

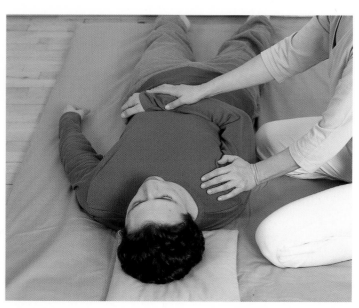

2 Bend arm Bend the arm at right angles and put it across the body so that Large Intestine meridian is at the top of the upper arm. Palm up towards the shoulder.

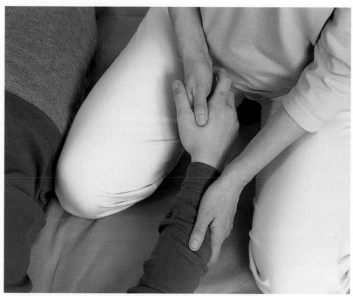

1 Palm up from wrist to elbow Place the arm palm down on the floor alongside the torso. Palm up the meridian from the wrist to the elbow. Move the mother hand to the shoulder. Then use your body weight, coming from the hara, to apply pressure to the shoulder.

3 Thumb up the meridian To work the meridian with your thumb, bring the arm out to the side and adopt a wide seiza position. Thumb up the meridian – you can hold LI 4 point with your mother hand as you work up the rest of the meridian.

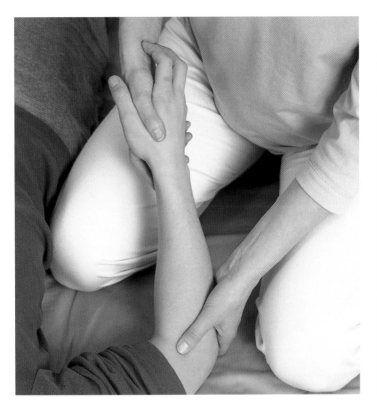

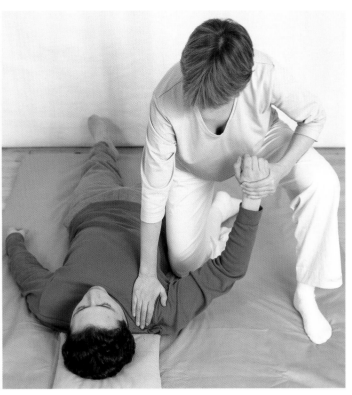

4 Move into point LI 11 Bend the elbow slightly as you go into the point LI 11. This point is on the outside edge of the elbow crease and useful in the prevention of colds, flu, shoulder and arm problems. Hold LI 4 with the other hand.

5 Rotate the arm To make a transition to the other side, lift the arm by the wrist and with mother hand on the shoulder step forward and rotate the arm. Use your mother hand on the shoulder to gauge the ease or stiffness in this joint.

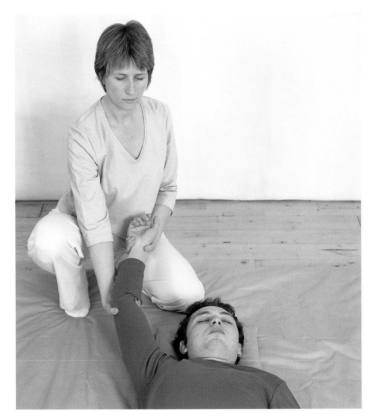

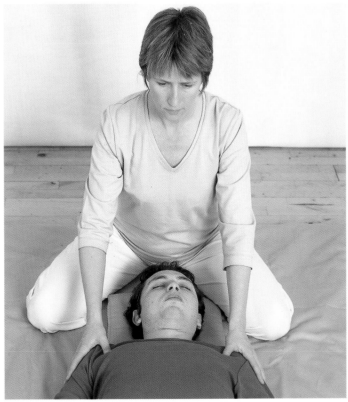

6 Face feet, lean back and stretch arm Step up to the top of the receiver's head, keeping hold of the arm, and turn to face the feet. Lean back and stretch this arm, holding it with one hand under the wrist and the other hand under the elbow.

7 Press into the LU 1 points Reposition yourself in wide seiza above the head and press into the LU 1 points, just below the middle of the collarbones. Move to the other side and work the other arm.

Water

The fluid nature of water means that it can flow into and out of any container, be it a vast ocean or a tiny pool. It is infinitely yielding yet infinitely powerful, ever changing and often dangerous. In nature, without a supply of water, nothing can sprout and grow, flower and blossom and finally be harvested. Water is the ultimate yin: quiet, cold, the resting time of winter. Water's associated meridian pair is Kidney (yin) and Bladder (yang).

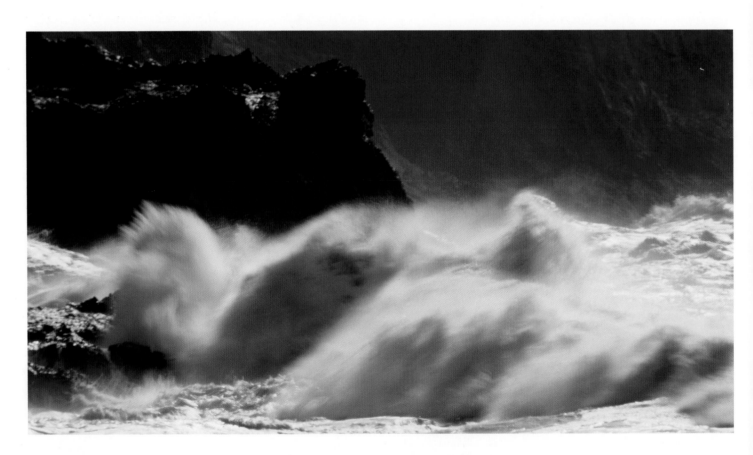

The potential of Water is called the jing or essence. It governs reproduction, fertility and sexual energy. Weakness here can lead to impotence, infertility and reproductive problems. The jing can also be likened to our genes – the constitution we inherit from our ancestors – giving us our vital energy. Water houses the will and give us the impetus to move. The teeth and bones are the related tissue. Weakness in Water can show up as bone disease, lower back pain and sore knees. It controls the water in the body – fluid retention, problems with urination and water metabolism may show imbalance in this element. The sense organ of Water is the ears and hearing.

The emotion associated with water is courage, enabling us to move forward and find new challenges. The converse emotion, fear, is felt if this element is weak. Chronic tiredness can be another symptom of this, as well as a grey complexion, and a dryness in the skin and hair.

Above and below Water can be highly dynamic and powerful, even destructive. It can also have a waiting, silent, still quality that can be described as "stored potential".

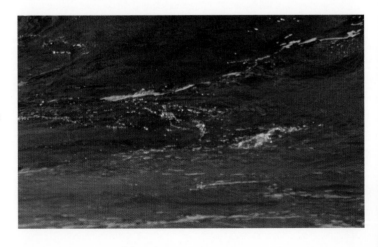

Pathway of the Kidney Meridian

The Kidney stores the jing — our genetic inheritance or constitution. Jing governs
the cycles of life: birth, puberty, reproduction, maturity and death. We are born with
a finite amount of jing and this affects our health, fertility and longevity.

The Kidney meridian starts on the sole of the foot, appearing through the arch on to the inside of the foot. Before it runs up the inside of the leg, there is a small loop, with a number of important points, just above the ankle. The meridian continues up under the main muscles in the front of the thigh and through the groin. It travels up the middle of the front torso, one finger-width either side of the midline until it reaches the ribs, where it branches out (three finger-widths from the midline) and finishes under the inner end of the collarbone.

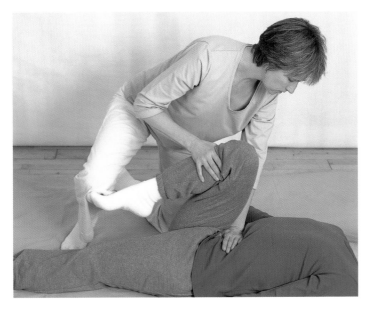

1 Rotate leg With your hand on the hara bring up the leg and rotate, feeling the relative ease or stiffness in the hip joint. Rotate twice to help the joint loosen up.

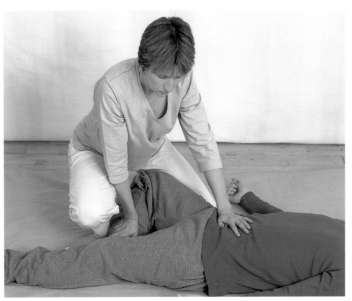

2 Instep against thigh With your hand on the hara let the leg drop out with the instep against the inner thigh of the other leg. Palm up the meridian from the foot to the knee.

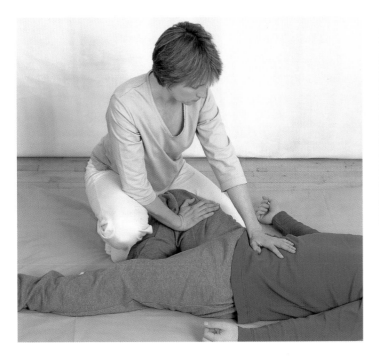

3 Palm up meridian Turn towards your partner's head and continue along the Kidney meridian in the inner thigh, using your mother hand to gauge the depth of pressure.

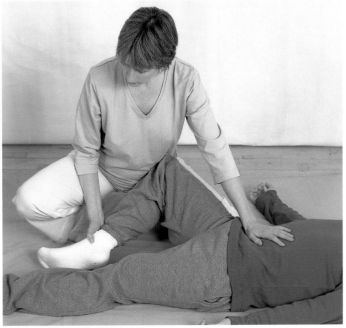

4 Thumb up leg Come back to the ankle and starting at KD 3, thumb up the lower leg. KD 3 is between the inside ankle bone and the Achilles tendon. It helps to strengthen the kidneys.

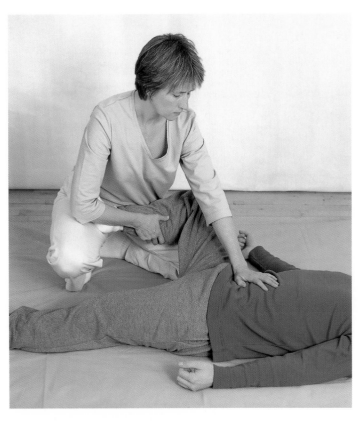

5 Thumb up towards knee Thumb up the meridian towards the knee, and up into the inner thigh, keeping your thumb straight and applying perpendicular pressure.

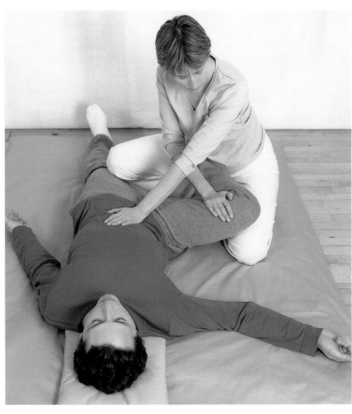

6 Drop leg out You can stretch and open the Kidney meridian by letting the leg drop out so that the knee rests on your thigh. Apply pressure with your palm on the inner thigh.

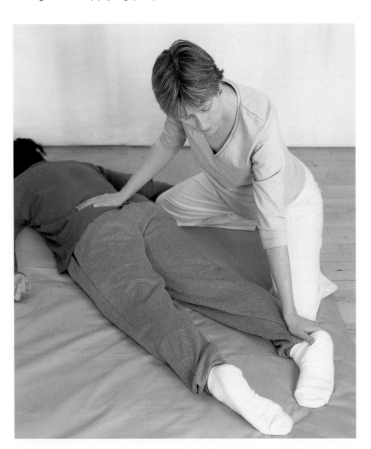

7 Alternative position Lie your partner on their front, turning the feet slightly inwards. Find the point KD 3 on the inside of the ankle between the heel and the ankle bone. Palm up meridian on inside of calf and inside of thigh.

Kidney meridian points

Kidney points can balance the water metabolism and ease problems of the lower back. The first and last points on the Kidney meridian are KD 1 and KD 27. Holding these points will help to stimulate the flow of chi along the whole meridian.

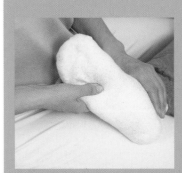

KD 1
This pressure point is on the sole of the foot where the pad of the big toe and the ball of the foot make a "V". This point, known as "Bubbling Spring", is a revitalizing point.

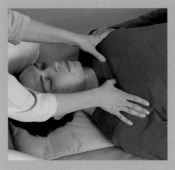

KD 27
This point is nestled in the hollow just below the collarbone at its inner end. This is a good point for coughs and asthma.

Pathway of the Bladder Meridian

Bladder meridian is the longest meridian in the body, starting at the bridge of the nose and ending at the little toe. Treat Bladder meridian on the back to deeply relax your partner by calming the central nervous system and balancing all the organ functions.

The Bladder meridian starts either side of the bridge of the nose, passes over the head and runs down either side of the spine, dividing at the top of the back into two distinct lines on each side, that run two finger-widths from the centre of the spine, and four finger-widths from the centre of the spine. Between BL13 (between the shoulder blades)

and BL28 (the base of the spine) there are 12 yu points, which directly influence the 12 organ functions. The meridian continues down the back of the legs, rejoining into two single lines at the knee, and ending at the outside edge of the little toenail. The part of the Bladder meridian on the back is covered in the basic framework on page 175.

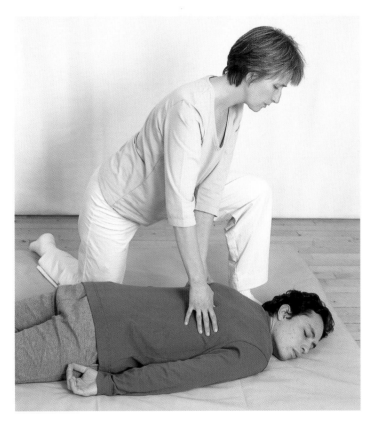

1 Thumb down Thumb down two finger-widths either side of the mid-line, moving down little by little.

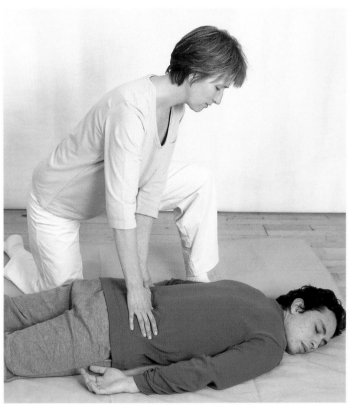

2 BL 23 When you reach the waist, find BL 23, which is in line with the space between the second and third vertebrae. This point is good for treating the kidneys and lower back.

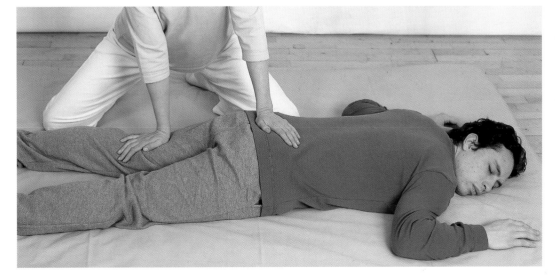

3 Palm down meridian
Repositioning yourself in a wide seiza position next to your partner's lower back and legs, let your mother hand rest on the sacrum. Palm down the Bladder meridian on the leg with your other hand, using your body weight to apply pressure. Avoid pressing directly on to the back of the knee.

▷

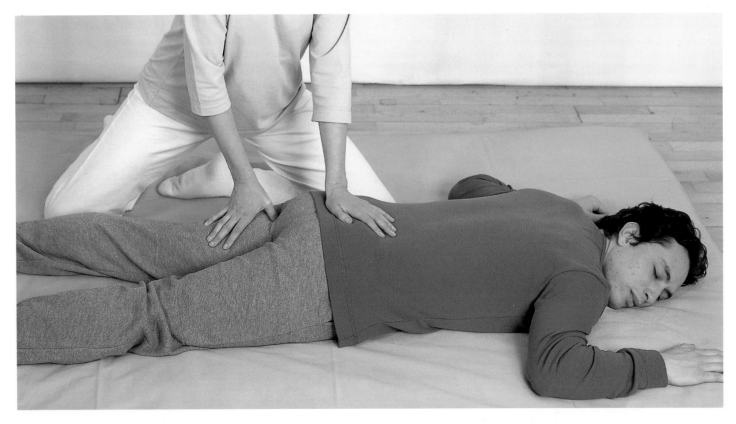

4 Thumb down With the thumb perpendicular to the body, thumb your way down the back of the legs to the knee.

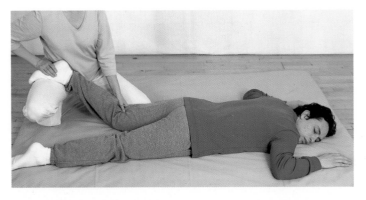

5 Work into the back of the knee Do this by lifting the ankle to bend the knee. BL 40 is in the centre of the crease at the back of the knee – a point good for lower back ache.

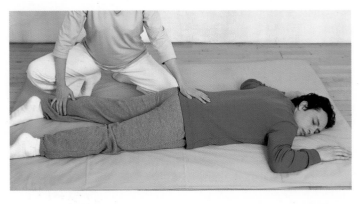

6 Thumb down Continue thumbing down to the ankle. Find BL 57 on the calf muscle halfway between the back of the knee and the heel, another point for lower back ache.

Bladder meridian points

Two important Bladder pressure points on the foot are BL 60 and BL 67. Both points at the opposite end of the meridian from the head, they can be used to treat headaches. They can also be used when working on the foot to improve the flow of chi within the Bladder channel. They can be used with the foot massage as part of the basic framework outline.

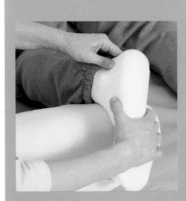

Bladder 60
This point is between the Achilles tendon and the tip of the ankle bone on the outside of the ankle. This is a good point for headache and pain in the neck and occiput. It can also be used for chronic back pain and pain in general.

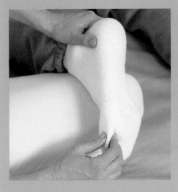

Bladder 67
Locate this point on the outside corner of the base of the little toenail. This can be used for frontal headaches and eye strain. Also used in the last month of pregnancy to turn a breech baby (with caution).

Wood

The energy of the Wood element moves upwards like the growth of a tree. A tree is flexible and can bend in the wind. Flexibility gives us the ability to adapt to circumstances while always growing upwards, towards the light. The function of the Wood element is to make plans and decisions. It harmonizes us and makes all the organs run smoothly. The meridians associated with Wood are the Liver (yin) and Gall Bladder (yang).

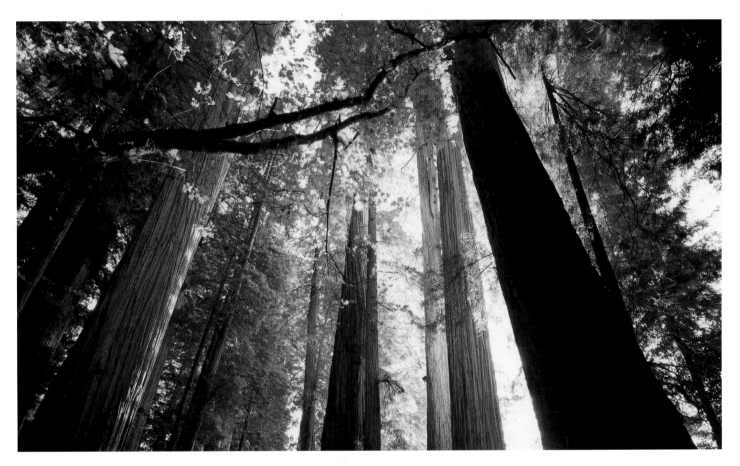

The season for Wood is spring, a time for new growth. If you feel low or hyperactive in spring, you may be suffering from a Wood imbalance. The tissue associated with Wood is the sinews: the nails, tendons and ligaments. Tendons and ligaments cross the joints, holding them together and making smooth, subtle movements possible.

Wood's function is organization and planning. It brings creativity and the intellectual skills required for making things happen. Anger can damage Wood. Repressed anger can lead to a feeling of stuckness and depression. People with Wood problems can be angry and controlling, unable to delegate and prone to workaholism. At the other extreme, they can be stuck, unable to move or make decisions. Look for joint problems, bloating (stuck digestion), headaches (energy stuck in the head), eye problems and brittle nails.

Above and below The function of Wood is organization, planning and creativity, good for bringing a new project to fruition.

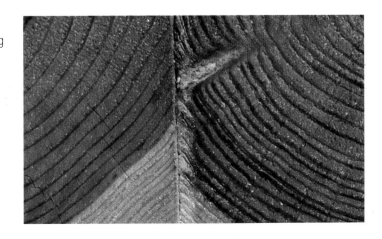

Pathway of the Liver Meridian

Liver governs the smooth flow of chi in the body, ensuring that all the organ
functions are operating in harmony with each other, giving flexibility when needed.
Liver is good for treating headaches, joint problems and premenstrual tension.

The Liver meridian starts at the outside edge of the big toe, at the corner of the toenail. It then passes in front of the ankle bone and pursues a course up the inside of the leg. At the thigh it runs parallel to and above the stringy muscles on the inside of the thigh (the adductors), passing through the groin and continuing up through the belly, across the hara, and finishing under the nipple between the sixth and seventh ribs.

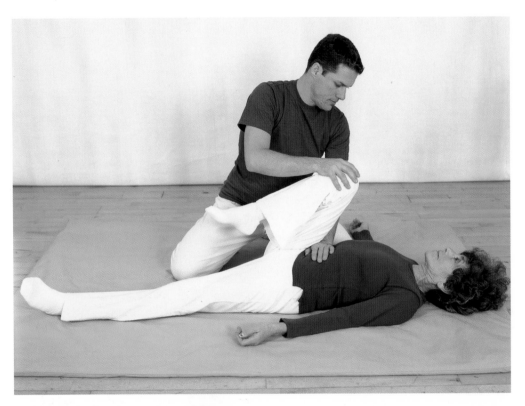

1 Knee up and rotate Sit in a wide seiza position facing your partner, placing your hand on the hara as a mother hand. Pick the leg up from the back of the knee gently and bring the knee up to the body. As you bring the leg up, move your hand to the front of the leg and rotate the leg outwards. Notice any stiffness or restriction as your rotate.

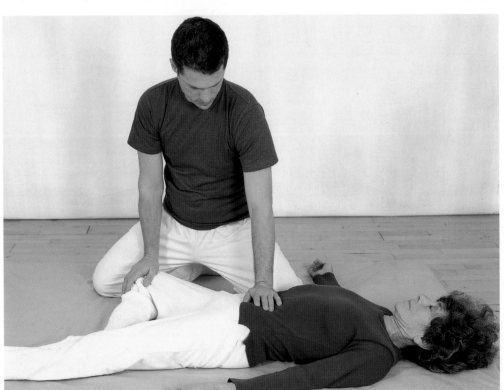

2 Drop knee to side Coming into wide seiza, allow your partner's knee to drop to the side, with the sole of the foot against the inside of the other thigh. If necessary, balance the outstretched knee on your leg for extra support. With your mother hand still on the hara, apply pressure gently downwards to open up Liver meridian and to stretch the thigh. Ask your partner to let you know if they feel any pain or discomfort.

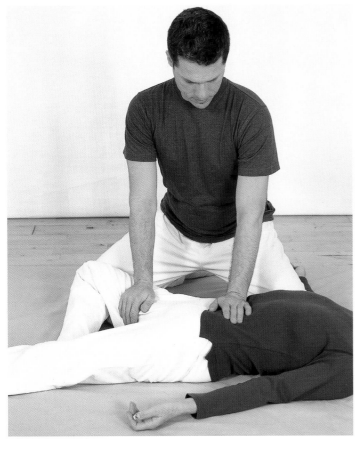

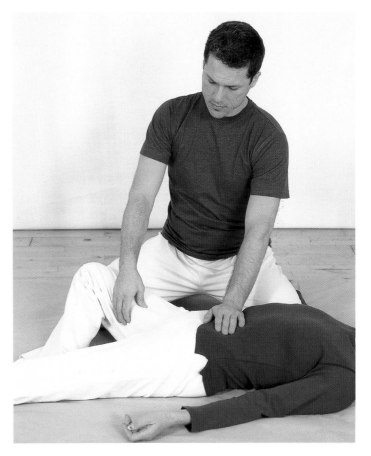

3 Palm up Move up the meridian, up the lower leg and inner thigh, keeping your mother hand on the hara.

4 Thumb up slowly Thumb your way up the meridian taking care to go in slowly and with perpendicular pressure.

Liver meridian points

Four main landmark points on the Liver meridian are LV 3, LV 8, LV 13 and LV 14. LV 3, LV 13 and LV 14 are very good general points for unblocking Liver chi stagnation. Symptoms of stagnation include bloating, digestive problems, depression, moodiness, premenstrual tension and irregular periods. As well as moving stagnation, each of these points will have a specific action.

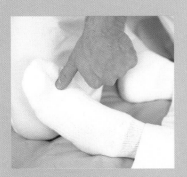

LV 3
This point is two finger-widths below the webbing between the big toe and the second toe. An important point and often painful, it is used for migraine headaches and can also be used for calming frustration.

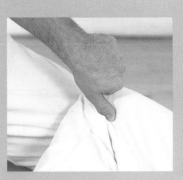

LV 8
To locate this point, bend the knee and it is found at the end of the knee crease on the inside leg. Very often painful, this is a useful point for knee problems.

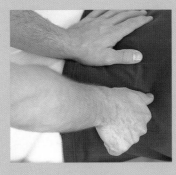

LV 13
This point is at the free end of the eleventh floating rib. It is a good point for treating digestive problems that result in diarrhoea.

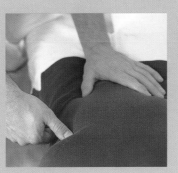

LV 14
Find this point between the sixth and seventh ribs directly below the nipple. Good for treating digestive problems that result in nausea and vomiting.

Pathway of the Gall Bladder Meridian

Gall Bladder is important in the process of decision-making and can become out of balance in people with high-level jobs. Its position on the head, neck and shoulders makes it ideal for treating headaches and shoulder tension caused by stress.

The Gall Bladder meridian starts at the outside corner of the eye and circles around the back of the ear and the side of the head, making three concentric arcs. It runs down the back of the neck, crosses the shoulder and runs in front of the ball and socket joint of the shoulder to the side of the body under the armpit. It then zigzags towards the front ribs and back to the hip, continuing down the side of the leg and ending at the outside edge of the fourth toe at the nail. Remember that the point GB 21 is contraindicated during pregnancy.

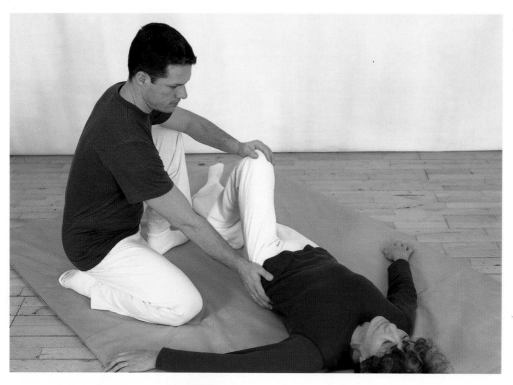

1 Lift leg from under knee
Sit with one knee up and one down and bring the leg into position to treat Gall Bladder by lifting the leg from under the knee. Bend up the leg and place your partner's foot next to the other knee. Bring your hand on to the front of the knee to support it as your mother hand rests on the hip.

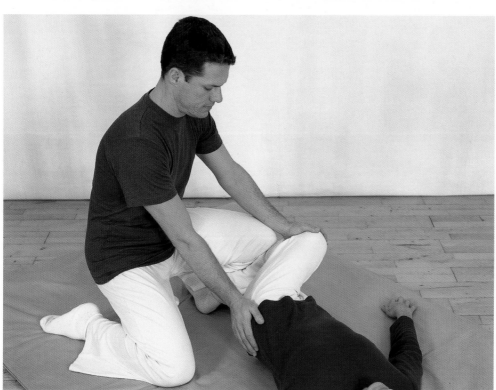

2 Stretch the meridian Adjust your hand so that the palm is on the outside of the knee, forming a base from which pressure can be applied. Gently push the leg down towards the floor over the other leg, which remains on the floor. Keep your mother hand on the hip throughout, applying pressure to prevent the hip from rising off the floor. Ask your partner to tell you if you are over stretching or causing discomfort.

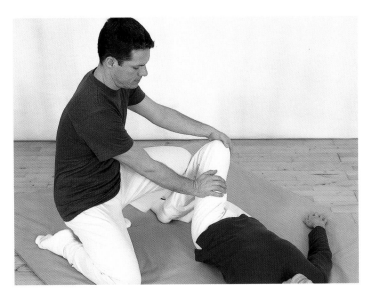

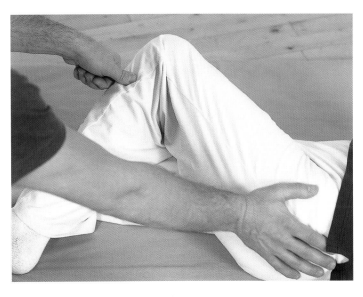

3 Support the calf with your knee and put your foot against your partner's foot to anchor it. Palm down the meridian.

4 Thumb down the meridian with the mother hand on the hip, moving it on to the knee as you move down the leg.

Gall Bladder meridian points

As it travels through most of the major joints, the Gall Bladder meridian is good for joint problems, particularly the knee and hip joints. There are seven important landmark points on the Gall Bladder meridian: GB 1 and GB 44 (the first and last points) and GB 20, GB 21, GB 31, GB 34 and GB 40.

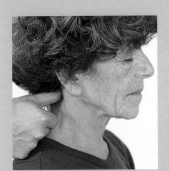

GB 20
This point is under the base of the skull, halfway between the mid-line and the lower edge of the skull. Press the thumb up towards the forehead for the correct angle. Good for neck tension and headaches.

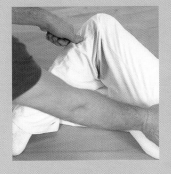

GB 34
This point is in a hollow under and in front of the small head of the fibula below the knee (the bone on the outside of the leg). A general point for joint problems and for treating the knee.

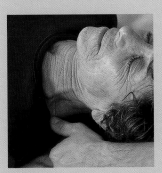

GB 21
This point is located midway along the shoulder on the highest point. It is nearly always painful and is good for a stiff, painful or frozen shoulder. Not to be used during pregnancy.

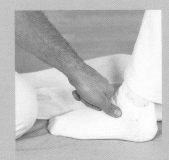

GB 40
In the hollow in front of and underneath the external ankle bone. This point can be used to treat ankle problems and is good for freeing stuck Liver energy and for helping decision-making.

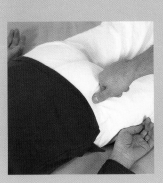

GB 31
Find this point one-third of the distance between the hip and the bottom of the sacrum in the hollow. This is a useful point for treating hip problems and sciatica.

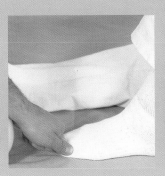

GB 44
Located at the outside edge of the fourth toe just at the corner of the toenail. Effective for headaches around the eyes as well as for red, sore eyes.

Primary Fire

The Fire element embodies consciousness or spirit, the spark of life. Fire gives warmth and is active. While it can blaze with energy, it can also be calming: through the beat of the heart Fire creates a constant and stable rhythm in the body. It governs the emotions and how we interpret our environment through them. The blood vessels and the circulation are controlled by Primary Fire, and the associated meridian pair is Heart (yin) and Small Intestine (yang).

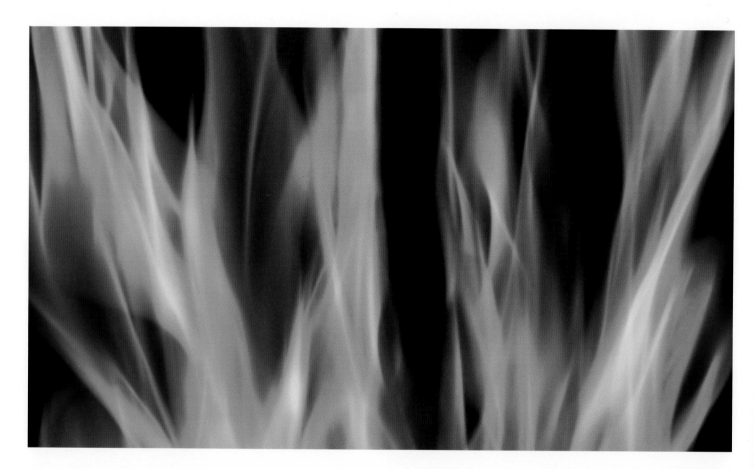

The emotions related to Fire are love and joy. Long-term stress can damage the heart and create hysteria. The emotions can become chaotic and erratic. A person with strong Fire energy may laugh a lot – and is likely to be a comedian. The functions of Fire are communication and awareness, and the Fire inside us will let us know how we are affected by the external world. Conditions caused by Fire imbalances include heart disease, poor circulation and difficulty in assimilating nutrients through the small intestine. The season associated with Fire is the summer, and if you feel hot and bothered at this time of year, it may indicate that you have too much Fire energy. The taste is bitter. The colour of Fire is red – someone with a red face may be showing an imbalance in Fire.

Above and below Fire provides the emotions of love and joy, although too much Fire can lead to over-excitement or hysteria.

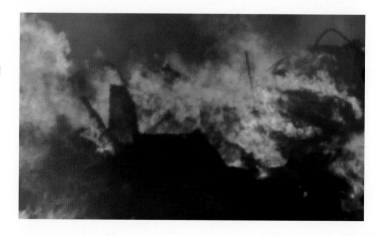

Pathway of the Heart Meridian

The Heart houses the shen which can be translated as "spirit" or "consciousness".
The shen must be rooted and stable and needs a calm heart. Imbalances in shen
can show up as insomnia, disturbing dreams and, in extreme cases, mental illness.

The Heart meridian starts under the armpit, within the hollow that forms when you hold your arm right up. With the arm by the side and the palm towards the front it travels down the inside of the arm, along the inside edge of the biceps muscle. It passes through the elbow and along the inside of the wrist towards the palm. Passing along the little finger side, it ends at the little finger on the side nearest the ring finger at the base of the nail.

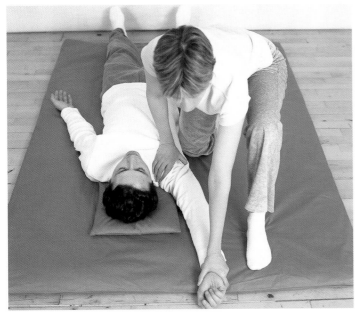

1 Open up the Heart meridian Hold the arm loosely by the wrist and step forward, lifting the arm vertical and then bringing it up over the head, pushing to stretch the arm.

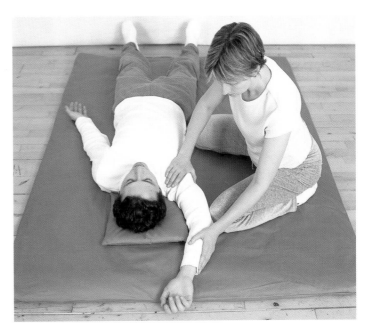

2 Place the arm in position for Heart meridian Release the wrist and bend the arm slightly, allowing it to lie comfortably above the head.

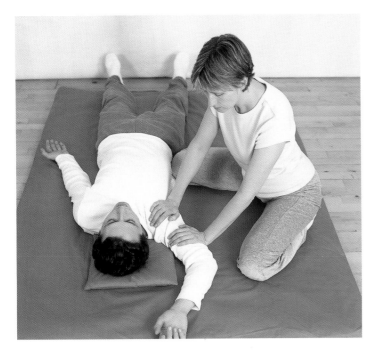

3 Palm up Work up the meridian from the armpit on the outside of the arm towards the little finger. Keep your mother hand on the shoulder.

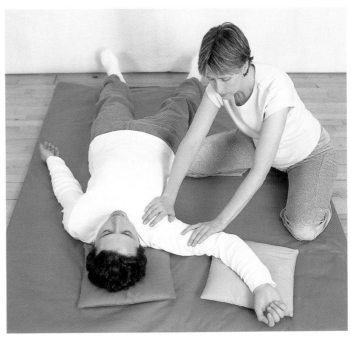

4 Variation If your partner's arm is uncomfortable pointing straight up you can put the arm slightly more out to the side and rest it on a cushion.

▷

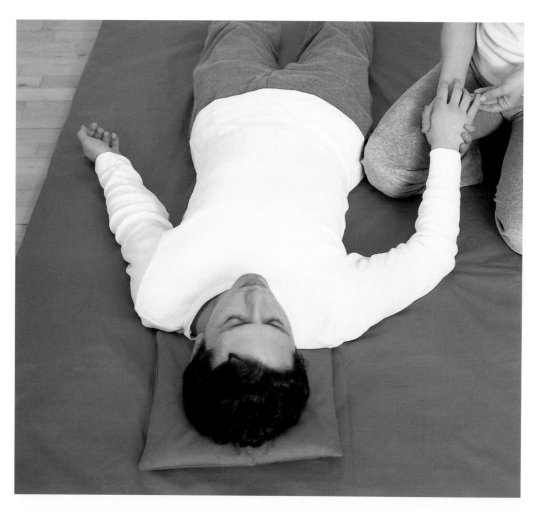

5 Working the hand When working the points in the hand (see HT 7 and HT 9 below) sit back in seiza by your partner's side and bring the arm down to rest it on your thigh. Turn the hand palm side up to work along the edge of the palm and turn it palm side down to work on the little finger – the end of the meridian.

Heart meridian points

There are four landmark points on the Heart meridian: HT 1, HT 3, HT 7 and HT 9. The two hand points can be treated when working on the hands. Caution should be taken when treating someone with a serious cardiovascular condition and beginners should avoid this altogether. If in doubt refer them to a more experienced practitioner.

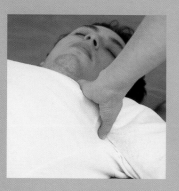

HT 1
This point is located in the deepest part of the armpit at the centre. It can be used for treating insomnia.

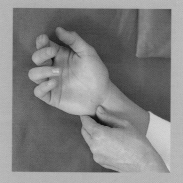

HT 7
Located in the crease on the side of the wrist nearest the little finger, this point calms anxiety and worry caused by stress, and helps with insomnia.

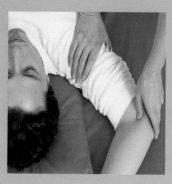

HT 3
This point is located at the end of the elbow crease at the little finger side of the arm. It calms the mind and can be used for elbow problems.

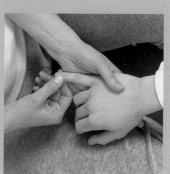

HT 9
This point is at the end of the little finger at the inside corner of the fingernail. This is a revival point in cases of heart attack.

Pathway of the Small Intestine Meridian

The function of the small intestine is to assimilate nourishment. It receives food
from the spleen and separates the pure from the impure. The pure is assimilated
and the impure is sent to the large intestine for elimination.

The Small Intestine meridian starts at the outside edge of the little finger, runs along the back of the arm and passes through the space between the ulna and the humerus on the little finger side. It then travels along the back of the arm towards the back of the shoulder. After this, it does a zigzag on the scapula and moves up the neck behind the big muscle at the side of the neck, ending just in front of the ear.

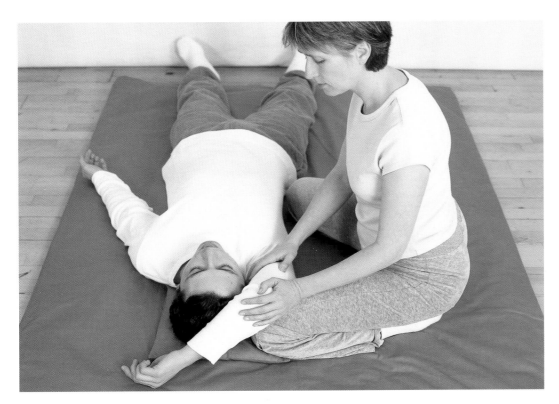

1 Expose Small Intestine meridian Bring your partner's arm up over the head so that the elbow is pointing up and the side of the arm is uppermost. This position will expose the Small Intestine meridian. You can support the arm on your thigh so that it can relax. Hold the upper arm with your hand.

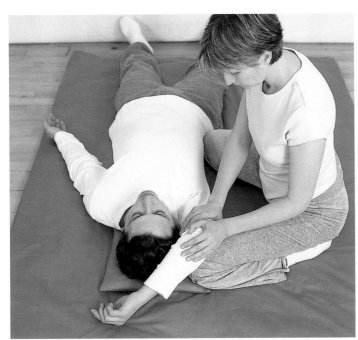

2 Work from wrist to armpit Palm down the Small Intestine meridian from wrist to armpit. Have your mother hand on the elbow when working from the elbow towards the shoulder.

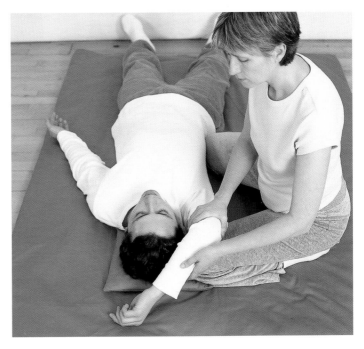

3 Thumb down Work down the meridian from the wrist towards the elbow. When you reach the elbow, change your mother hand to the elbow and continue towards the shoulder. ▷

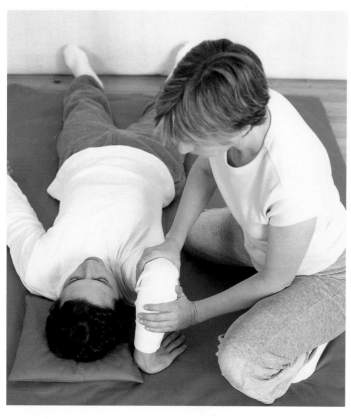

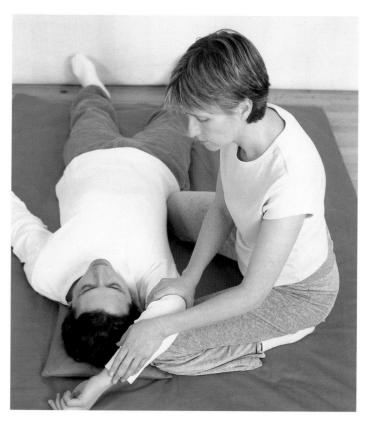

4 Variation This alternative position for working the Small Intestine meridian involves pointing the elbow up and placing the palm of the hand on the ground next to the head with the fingers pointing towards the shoulder.

4b Variation Palm the meridian from wrist to shoulder. This is a good position for opening up the Small Intestine meridian but is better used on people who are more flexible in the shoulder.

Small Intestine meridian points

The Small Intestine meridian is important for treating shoulder problems as the meridian crosses the shoulder blade. Shock is also very often treated by working Small Intestine meridian (the body's inability to assimilate). Four important landmark points on the Small Intestine meridian are SI 1, SI 8, SI 11 and SI 19.

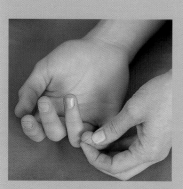

SI 1
This point is found on the end of the little finger at the outside corner of the fingernail. It is good for treating a stiff neck.

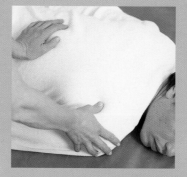

SI 11
Located in the middle of the shoulder blade in the depression, this point is always a painful point and very good for shoulder pain.

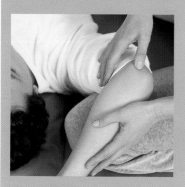

SI 8
This point is located at the back of the elbow in the hollow between the two bones on the little finger side. It can be used for elbow and neck pain and helps to calm the mind.

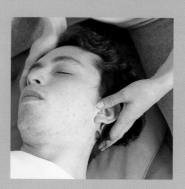

SI 19
This point is found in the hollow in front of the middle of the ear formed when opening the mouth. Use it to treat deafness and tinnitus.

Secondary Fire

Secondary Fire shares the same characteristics as Primary Fire. The meridians associated with Secondary Fire are Heart Protector (yin) and Triple Heater (yang), functions with no Western equivalent but which could be described as Circulation and Protection. Heart Protector protects the heart, and Triple Heater governs the peripheral circulation. Together they are responsible for a healthy and balanced emotional state.

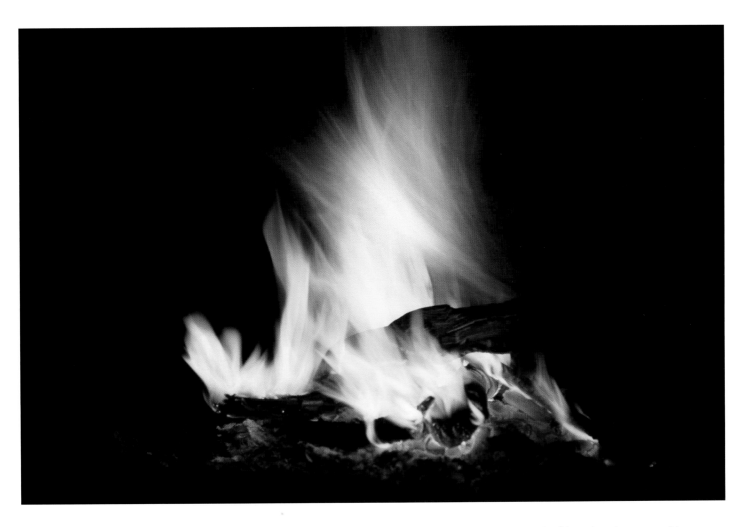

The Heart Protector acts as a buffer for the heart and protects it from physical and emotional trauma. The Heart Protector is often seen as the relationship meridian – emotional trauma will deeply affect the Heart Protector. When relationships go wrong, we can become very protective of our heart, bringing energy into the Heart Protector. It also governs the circulation, and conditions such as varicose veins and high blood pressure can show up as an imbalance in this function.

The Triple Heater governs what are known as the "three burning spaces" in the body: the upper, middle and lower burners. The Triple Heater keeps them in

Above The Triple Heater keeps the "three burning spaces" in balance and acts as the body's thermostat.

balance. Each space corresponds to certain internal organs: the upper heater is the heart and lungs, the middle heater is the stomach and spleen and the lower heater is the kidney, bladder, liver, and small and large intestines.

Symptoms associated with the Triple Heater function can be feeling the cold and difficulty in adapting to the environment. Those suffering from low Triple Heater energy may have a low immune system function, and it can also lead to other auto-immune problems such as allergies.

Pathway of the Heart Protector Meridian

Heart Protector supports the heart, protecting it from both physical and emotional pressure. It is associated with the pericardium, the outer layer of tissue which surrounds the heart. It can help open the chest and ease emotional problems.

The Heart Protector meridian starts at the side of the breast, adjacent to the armpit. It runs up above the armpit and then travels down the centre of the inside of the arm, passing through the elbow and wrist between the Heart and Lung meridians. It ends on the front of the middle finger, at the very tip.

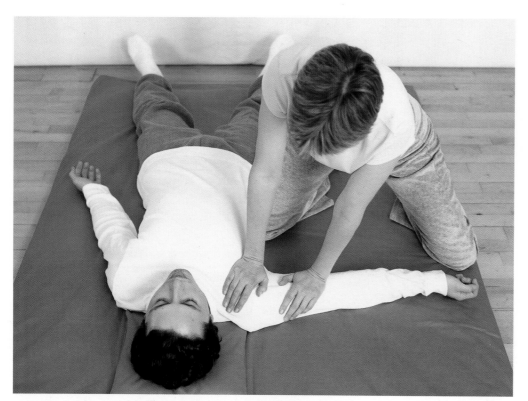

1 Palming Start in seiza position next to your partner. Turn your body slightly towards the head and pick up the arm lightly by the wrist. Lift and place it back on the floor so that it is at right angles to the body. Keep the palm facing upwards, and place your mother hand gently on the shoulder. Use your other hand to palm all the way down the Heart Protector meridian, from the shoulder down the middle of the arm to the middle finger.

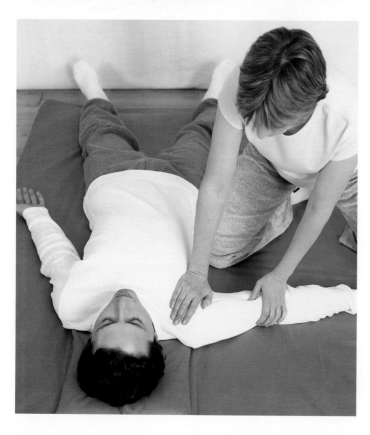

2 Thumb down to elbow Keep your mother hand on the shoulder, and thumb the Heart Protector meridian from the shoulder to the elbow.

Heart Protector

The function of the Heart Protector does not have an equivalent in Western medicine, the nearest being the pericardium, the protective tissue which surrounds the heart. In Chinese medicine the Heart was described as the Emperor or supreme controller overseeing the spiritual health of his subjects. The Heart Protector was the ambassador who guarded the functions of the supreme controller and shielded the spirit from danger, so that internal peace and harmony was restored.

In some early texts the Heart was seen as sacred and so was rarely treated. Heart can be treated through the Heart Protector meridian, especially in cases of emotional trauma. Heart Protector particularly governs the circulation of the body and can be used effectively to treat mild cases of high blood pressure.

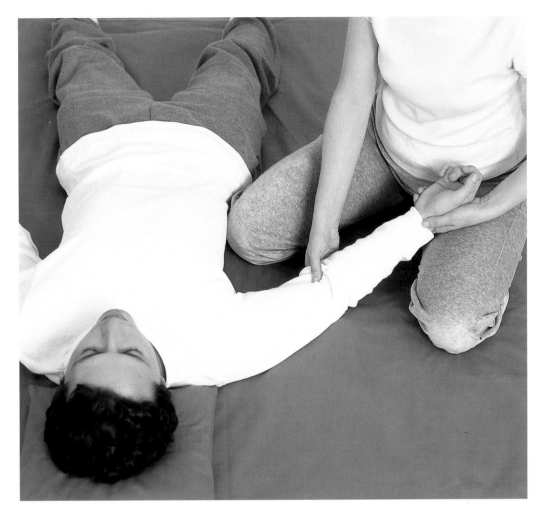

3 Thumb down from elbow to finger When you reach the elbow, bend it slightly as you go in with your thumb. This will allow you to go in deeper. Continue down the lower arm until you reach the hand, finishing at the tip of the middle finger. Ask your partner to keep the arm relaxed.

Heart Protector meridian points

You can treat the Heart Protector meridian in cases of some cardiovascular conditions, such as high blood pressure and mild angina, rather than working directly on Heart meridian. Four main landmark points on Heart Protector meridian are HP 3, HP 6, HP 8 and HP 9. All these, except for HP 9, will help to release anxiety.

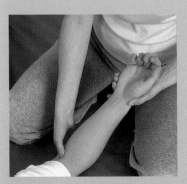

HP 3
This point is located on the elbow crease on the inside of the tendon you feel when bending the arm. This point can be used to calm the mind in cases of anxiety and to treat nausea and vomiting.

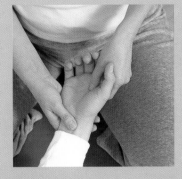

HP 8
Find this point in the centre of the palm – fold the fingers down and it is where the middle finger touches the palm. This point calms the mind and is good for exam nerves.

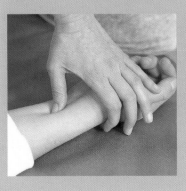

HP 6
This point is located three finger-widths below the wrist crease in between the two tendons. A very useful point for nausea and travel sickness. Calms the mind and relieves chest pain.

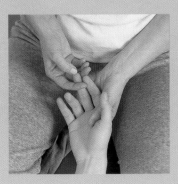

HP 9
This point is at the tip of the middle finger. It is the last point on the meridian and is a revival point.

Pathway of the Triple Heater Meridian

Triple Heater governs the "three burning spaces" roughly equivalent to the chest cavity, the solar plexus area and the lower abdomen. It ensures that these areas maintain their correct temperatures and that the organs are working harmoniously.

The Triple Heater meridian starts at the fourth, or ring, finger at the base of the nail on the outside edge, nearest to the little finger. It then runs along the back of the arm and passes through the elbow joint on the thumb side of the arm. It then travels along the back of the shoulder, up the back of the neck, behind and around the ear and finishes at the very outside corner of the eyebrow.

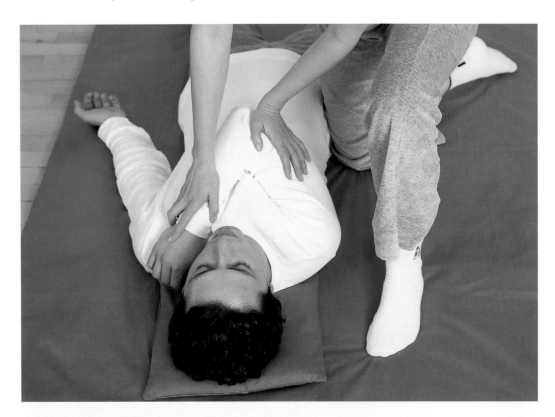

1 Stretch arm Bring the arm across the body so that Triple Heater meridian will be exposed on the top of the arm. With one hand just above the elbow and the other hand on the wrist you can stretch the arm towards the opposite shoulder to open up the back of the shoulder and open up Triple Heater on the upper arm. Check with your partner – sometimes women can find this stretch uncomfortable.

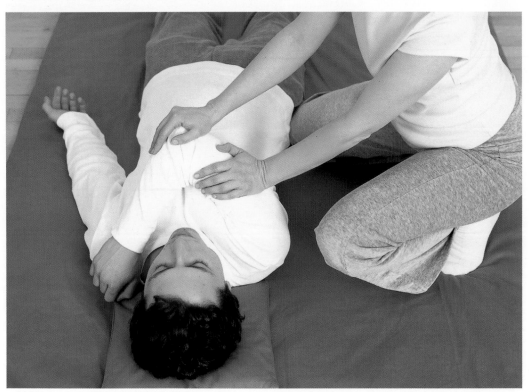

2 Palm up Placing your top hand down on to the elbow to become the mother hand, palm your way up from the wrist to the elbow and then, changing hands, from the elbow to the shoulder. Make sure that your pressure is perpendicular to the arm and not pushing the arm on to the chest, which can be uncomfortable and constrict the breathing.

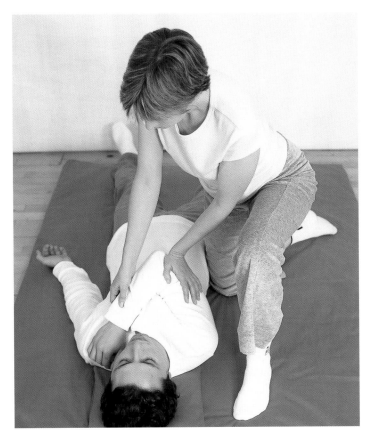

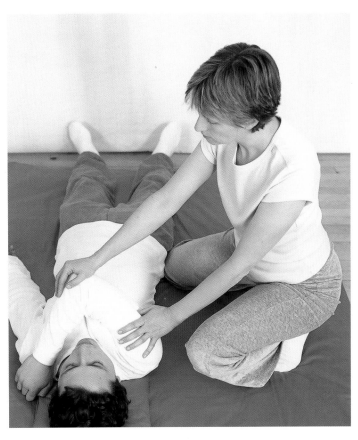

3 Thumb down Returning your mother hand to the upper arm, just above the elbow, thumb down the forearm. Once again make sure that your partner can breathe freely.

4 Thumb upper arm Swap your mother hand, so that your mother hand now rests on the elbow. You can now thumb the upper arm with the other hand.

Triple Heater meridian points

The main landmark points on Triple Heater meridian are TH 4, TH 10, TH 15 and TH 23. Triple Heater is like the thermostat of the body, so fevers or excessive cold will affect its functioning. It governs peripheral circulation, and cold hands or feet reflect a problem in Triple Heater.

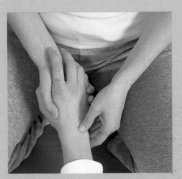

TH 4
This point is located in the back of the wrist joint in a depression in line with the fourth finger. This point is good for headaches and shoulder pain.

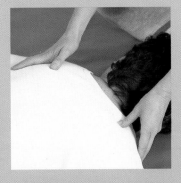

TH 15
This point is one thumb width below GB 21 (see page 213). Use it for shoulder and neck pain and stiffness.

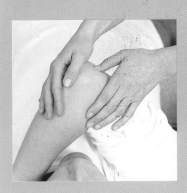

TH 10
Bend the elbow and this point is in the depression one thumb-width above the point of the elbow. This point is good for tennis elbow, elbow pain and stiffness in general.

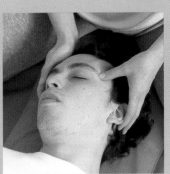

TH 23
This point is in the hollow at the outside tip of the eyebrow. It is good for eye problems and headaches.

The Conception Vessel

Considered as an "extraordinary" meridian, the Conception Vessel is not usually treated like the other meridians. There are important points on this meridian, called Bo points, which can be used to treat and diagnose the energy of other meridians.

The Conception Vessel, running down the centre of the body, governs all the yin channels and is a reservoir of energy for these channels. It influences all stages of conception and pregnancy and the female reproductive system. It can be used to strengthen the yin energy of the body. There are points called Bo points on the Conception Vessel which relate to individual meridians and these points can be used to treat and diagnose their corresponding meridian, especially its emotional and spiritual aspects. The Conception Vessel starts at CV1, a point on the perineum between the anus and the genital organs. It continues up through the front of the body on the mid-line and ends just under the lower lip. CV 1 and CV 8 in the umbilicus are contraindicated points.

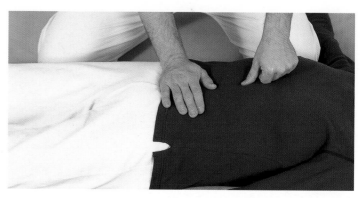

2 Hold CV 12, located midway between the navel and the lower end of the sternum, good for stomach problems.

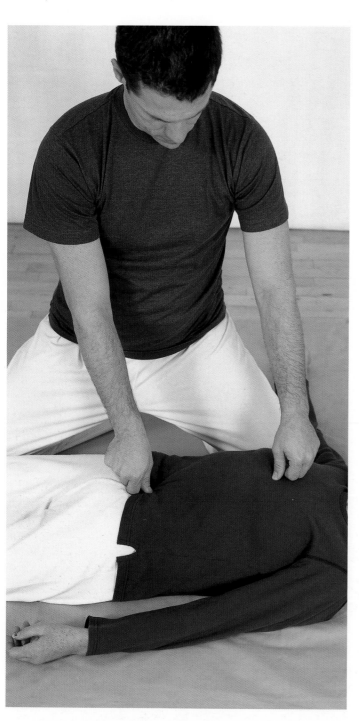

1 Hold the points CV 6 and CV 17 and feel the energy between these points, connecting the Heart and the hara.

Conception Vessel points

All the yin channels are governed by the Conception Vessel, which acts like a reservoir of energy for these pathways. CV 6 and CV 17, mentioned earlier, are important points on the Conception Vessel meridian, linking the whole system.

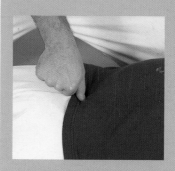

CV 6
This point is two finger-widths below the navel. It is known as "Sea of chi", and is an important point because it builds up chi. It can be used for physical and mental exhaustion and depression.

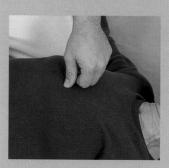

CV 17
Located in between the nipples on the mid-line, this point is important in relation to the Heart Protector (called a Bo point) and has a beneficial effect on the chest, easing pain and tightness in the chest.

The Governing Vessel

Running along the spine, the Governing Vessel plays a similar role to the Conception Vessel, for the yang meridians instead of the yin. It can be used for strengthening the spine and nervous system.

The Governing Vessel governs all the yang meridians. It is a reservoir of energy for these meridians and can be used to strengthen all the yang energy in the body. It influences the spine, the brain and the kidney.

Imbalances in the Governing Vessel will affect the spine and the nervous system on a deep level. Conditions such as epilepsy and serious spinal degeneration may result. Governing Vessel can have a beneficial effect on the spirit and mind. GV 20 is an especially good point for lifting the spirits.

The Governing Vessel starts at a point between the anus and the base of the coccyx. It follows the mid-line of the spine, continuing over the head, and finishes at a point under the top lip on the gum.

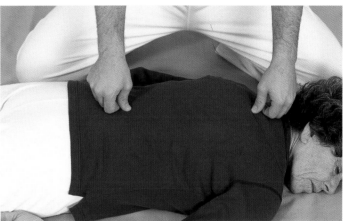

2 Find and hold GV 4, which is between the second and third lumbar vertebrae. This is an important point for stimulating Kidney energy and for easing any lower back problems.

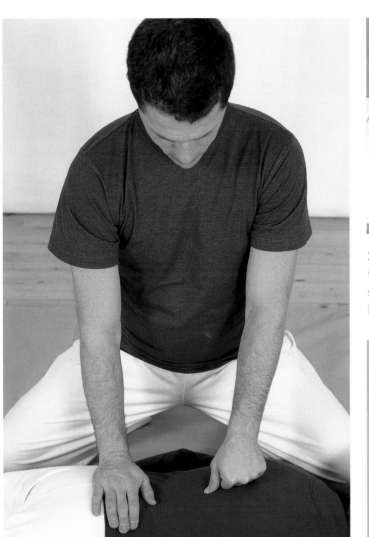

1 You can work on Governing Vessel meridian by finding individual points down the spine. Notice where there is a kyo area in the back and hold there.

Governing Vessel points

Two other points of interest on the Governing Vessel are GV 16 and GV 20.

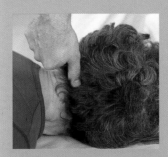

GV 16
Find this point in the hollow on the mid-line just below the base of the skull. This point clears the mind and stimulates the brain.

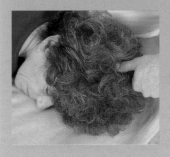

GV 20
Located on an imaginary line between the tips of the ears, and on the mid-line, this point has a strong lifting action. It can lift depression and is used for haemor-rhoids.

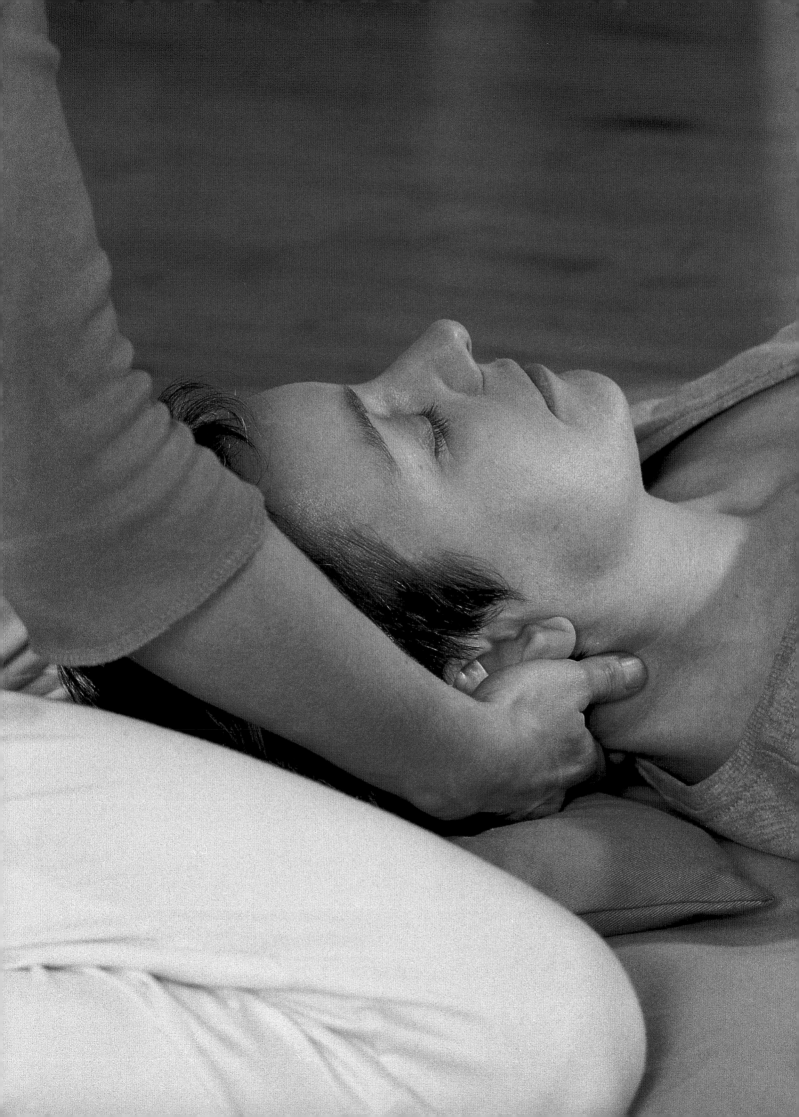

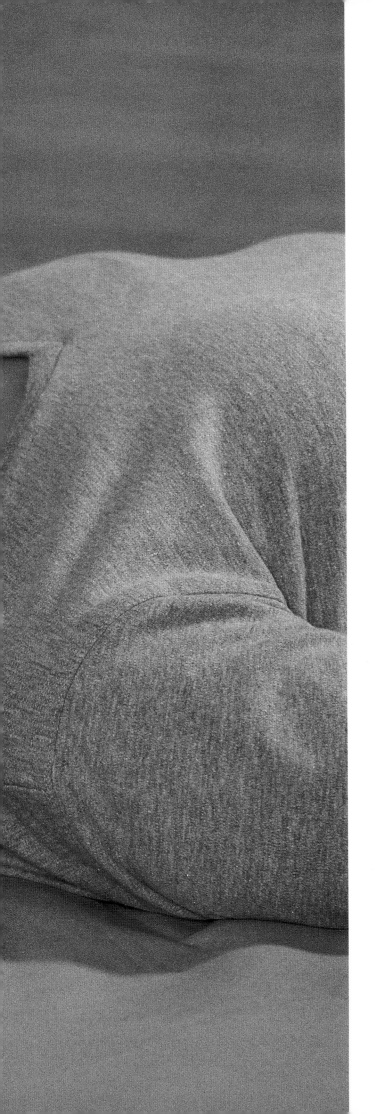

A Full Treatment

Usually a treatment takes an hour from start to finish, with the actual hands-on part lasting about 35–40 minutes. This gives you time to take a case history and make a diagnosis at the beginning, perform the full treatment, and have some time left at the end for your partner to recover and for you to advise them on further action to take.

In this section we look at how to put everything together. The first part is the art of diagnosis – how to assess your partner so that you can devise the best possible treatment to address his or her particular condition. There are four methods of diagnosis: looking, listening and smelling, questioning, and touching. After that we follow a full treatment, showing how to put a session together and decide on any recommendations.

Diagnosis

Evaluation and advice play a central role in Shiatsu. The first stage is to gather information about the receiver so that an assessment can be made in relation to any energy or elemental imbalances. A treatment appropriate to the condition can then be decided upon. Shiatsu diagnosis is not a medical evaluation and, if you suspect that your partner has a medical condition, you should advise him or her to seek medical advice.

To develop good diagnostic skills in Shiatsu you have to observe carefully and develop your intuition. Intuition is really just a finely developed form of observation.

In traditional Eastern medicine there are four methods used to assess a client's condition: looking, listening and smelling, questioning, and touching.

LOOKING

This includes observing areas such as style of dress, hygiene, presentation, skin tone, posture and energy patterns. Immediately your partner comes into sight you will unconsciously begin to assess his or her condition. Is your partner fidgety, upright and tense, or lazy, hunched and slow to react?

Influenced by our cultural and social conditioning we will make judgements based on gender, age, appearance, style of dress, and so on. Many people present themselves to reflect their inner countenance, by dressing in bright colours, for example. We naturally make intuitive assessments of our partner's health based on our observation. We may say "you're looking well" or "you look a bit off colour". In Shiatsu we seek to formalize these assessments by looking for particular markers, such as face colour, hair, posture, and so on.

KYO AND JITSU

These terms are both used to describe the presence or absence of chi in the meridians and in areas of the body. An overall impression can be gained about the relative kyo or jitsu condition of a person: do they appear to be full of energy or do they look weak and tired?

In a more kyo condition, the person is slumped, the belly is sagging or the shoulders are rounded. There is a lack of vitality, tiredness and shallow breathing. Kyo people can be thin and frail or obese and sluggish.

In a more jitsu condition, a person has a high level of tension. They can have hyperactive, jerky movements and a more stiff posture, possibly with chest thrust out and the shoulders held back.

Below and below opposite Look at your partner's posture from all sides, standing and walking. Look for energy imbalances.

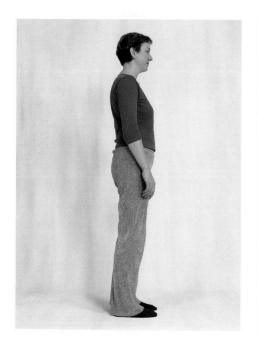
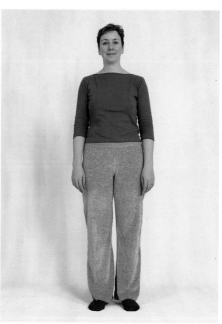
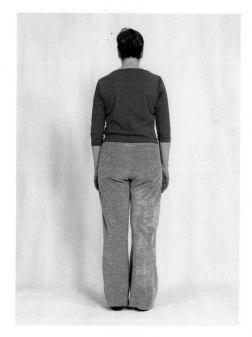

POSTURE

Bad postural habits develop over many years and can be a response to an internal condition, an emotional problem or some kind of trauma. We tend to want to protect weakness and veer away from pain. For example, if someone has a painful ankle they usually put more weight on the other foot to protect the bad ankle and walk with a limp. After a while this can become a habitual way of walking and, even when the pain has receded, the habit may remain. The body may adapt to this change and, as the body compensates, this could result in other postural habits developing.

Looking at the posture will give you clues as to areas of weakness, pain and tension in the body and the emotional state of your partner. Observe the posture from the front, the back and sides, and walking if you can. Take note of the following questions:

- What do you notice first?
- Is one shoulder higher than the other?
- Is one arm longer than the other?
- Are the shoulders rounded or tense?
- When walking is there a part of the body that doesn't move, such as the shoulders or hips?
- Does one arm move more than the other?
- Is there a trace of a limp?
- Is the head thrust forward, or leaning?
- Is the body stooping or hunched?

If you see any of the above conditions, for example rounded shoulders, this can be an area you can address in your treatment. Look at your partner's posture again after the treatment and see if it has changed. In your recommendations, you may want to suggest that your partner improves their posture, giving pointers to the areas to be addressed.

Posture exercise

Get together with a partner and watch them walking towards and away from you

- See if you can copy their walk
- How does it feel to walk like them?
- Can you sense an imbalance?
- Can you locate an area that needs attention?
- Are there areas of tension you notice or feelings you have walking in this way?
- Does your partner recognize the posture when you copy them, and notice the postural habits?
- Can you make any suggestions to improve this posture?

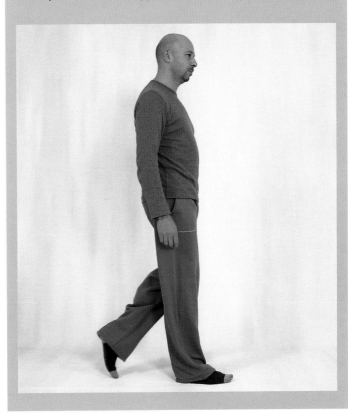

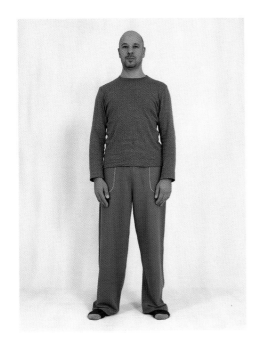

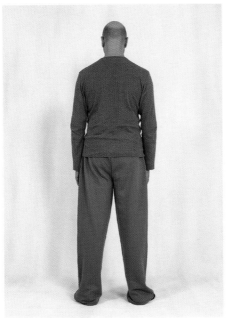

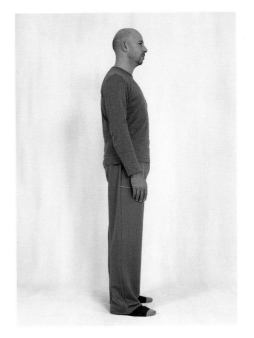

Facial Diagnosis

The face is a reflection of a person's health. The condition of the skin and the vitality in the eyes show the energy levels of the five elements, and the colour or hue of the face shows the element that is out of balance. Each part of the face is related to a specific body organ, set of functions and element. A fullness or an emptiness in any of these areas demonstrates that there is an imbalance within that meridian.

The face can be divided into different areas, each relating to one of the organ functions. Skin blemishes or discoloration in one of these areas may show some imbalance or build-up of toxins in that organ. For example the tip of the nose represents Heart and under the eyes represents Kidney. A redness in the end of the nose can indicate circulation problems, and dark bags under the eyes may show that Kidney is under stress.

In Shiatsu, a person's constitution – their reproductive health, longevity and resistance to disease – tends to show up in the face. Strong, prominent eyebrows show power and vitality, especially in Liver, Kidney and Triple Heater. A healthy head of hair is believed to indicate good sexual energy, again relating to the Kidney energy.

The size of the ears is linked to the health of Kidney, a meridian that governs vital essence, reproductive health and longevity. A good exercise to gauge the strength of the ears is to take firm hold of both ears and gently pull and rotate them to see how rooted they are. If they move easily then Kidney (and the constitution) may be weak. Large earlobes, as well as being considered a sign of longevity, are thought to indicate wisdom.

Look also for colour or hue of the face, which will often show the element that is out of balance. For example, someone who is red-faced may have problems in the Fire element and this could indicate cardiovascular problems, such as high blood pressure. A very pale-faced person may have Lung problems.

The shape of the face

In Shiatsu, you should also look at the shape and structure of the face. If the shape of the face is rectangular or oval with high cheekbones and pale hair, the person is likely to have more of a Metal personality and could be creative or intuitive. A longer face that is more triangular indicates a Wood person who tends to be decisive and goal-oriented. A square-shaped face, with a square jaw and broad features, is probably an Earth personality – someone who is practical, stable and grounded. A Fire personality is likely to have a more pointed face and chin, maybe with red hair and freckles or a redder complexion, and therefore likely to be be enthusiastic and inspirational. A rounder, softer face, usually with dark hair, may be a Water personality who will be sociable, wise and more in touch with their emotions.

Many people will have a mixture of the five elements in the shape of the face, and there will not always be one prominent element.

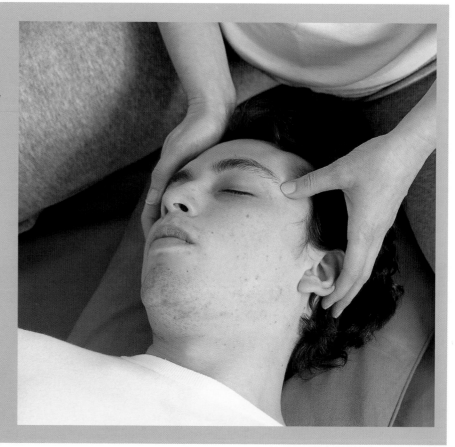

The Face Map

A person's constitution – including reproductive health, longevity and resistance to disease – will show up in the face. For example, redness on the end of the nose or upper cheeks can indicate cardiovascular problems relating to Heart.

This diagram shows the different areas of the face and how they relate to each element and the organs of the body. The face can be divided into different areas, each relating to one of the organ functions. Look at the diagram of the face: the colours show the areas of the face that are represented by each element. Look for skin blemishes, discoloration (particularly one of the colours relating to one of the five elements), puffiness or lines in any of these areas. This will show some imbalance or build-up of energy or toxins in that organ and element.

For example, dark patches under the eyes show conditions in Stomach, Liver and Kidney. If they are bluish, Kidney may be under stress; if the discoloration is more greenish, it could indicate a build-up of toxins in the liver. Redness on the end of the nose or on the upper cheeks shows cardiovascular problems relating to Heart. Pallid, white or sunken cheeks can indicate a Lung weakness. A swollen lower lip could show a sluggish or weak large intestine. Prominence of the V-shaped forehead wrinkles indicates Gall Bladder conditions.

Gall Bladder
Look for excessive lines or discoloration, maybe greenish, in this area on the forehead. Above the eyebrows you may see small V-shaped wrinkles.

Kidney
Under the eyes, dark blue circles show stress in Kidney, or bluish puffiness may show water retention. Puffiness or discoloration on the chin can be kidney related.

Lung
The lower cheeks will reflect a Lung condition. Look for grey or pallid cheeks, sometimes pitted, spotty or sunken.

Key to the meridians
- Gall Bladder
- Large and Small Intestine
- Stomach
- Triple Heater
- Heart
- Bladder
- Spleen
- Liver
- Lung
- Kidney

Large and Small Intestine
A swollen lower lip or blemishes here indicate problems in the small or large intestines. For Large Intestine you may also see deep lines at the side of the mouth.

Spleen
The area above the mouth indicates Spleen conditions. Look for a yellowish discoloration, puffiness or blemishes.

Bladder
Two strong lines on the forehead will indicate some stress in Bladder. Sometimes you will see puffiness, pitting or discoloration on the lower chin.

Triple Heater
Very little hair at the end of the eyebrows or the eyebrows being short can indicate an imbalance in Triple Heater.

Stomach
A deep central line between the eyebrows, a yellowish colour directly under the eyes or yellowish, sunken or pitted skin at the side of cheeks indicate problems.

Heart
Look for redness or broken veins along the bridge of the nose and top of cheeks. The tip of the nose may additionally be red and swollen. (Heart Protector doesn't have a specific area of the face, but will be the same as Heart and sometimes shows up as a red complexion.)

Liver
A greenish puffiness at the upper corner of the mouth or under the eyes shows stagnation in the Liver. Two deep frown lines between the eyebrows can indicate excess anger affecting Liver.

Listening and Smelling

The sound of the voice and a person's body odour give you a clue to the element that is out of balance. Look at the table below to see the correspondences of voice and smell with each element. Diagnosis by listening means assessing the sound and tone of the voice to see if it has a particular characteristic. Body smell can be related to different organs within the five element system, as shown in the correspondences table.

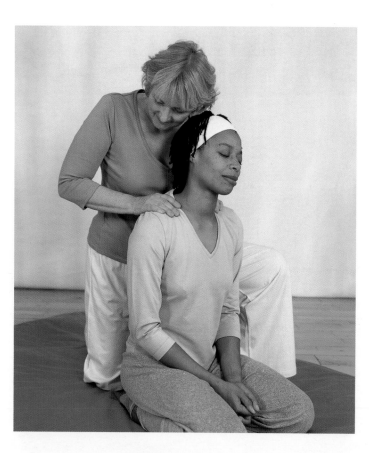

SENSITIVE EVALUATION

Listening is not just hearing what your partner has to say, but also the way in which it is said. A listening assessment can begin during the first phone call or initial contact by noting the tone of voice. Sometimes it helps to listen with your eyes closed and hear it as if you were listening to music. You are looking for a predominance of a tone of voice which may not necessarily be in harmony with what they are saying. A weeping, weak or breathy voice relates to the Metal element. A laughing, hearty voice can indicate a Fire personality, and those who laugh for no reason may have a Fire imbalance. Those with an Earth personality will exhibit a sing-song or lilting voice.

The smell is more difficult to assess in Shiatsu as the receiver remains clothed, although in some cases you may be able to pick up a distinctive odour. Acupuncturists smell the area just below the back of the neck by lifting the back of the collar. This area is less likely to be washed regularly as it is difficult to reach.

Left Listening and smelling can be performed while in the process of massaging the neck and shoulders – this will put your partner at their ease.

Five Element organs, seasons and senses

	WOOD	FIRE	EARTH	METAL	WATER
YIN ORGAN	Liver	Heart	Spleen	Lung	Kidney
YANG ORGAN	Gall Bladder	Small Intestine	Stomach	Large Intestine	Bladder
SEASON	Spring	Summer	Late Summer	Autumn	Winter
CLIMATE	Wind	Heat	Damp	Dryness	Cold
COLOUR	Green	Red	Yellow	White	Blue/Black
TASTE	Sour	Bitter	Sweet	Pungent	Salty
SMELL	**Rancid**	**Scorched**	**Fragrant**	**Rotting**	**Putrid**
ORIFICE	Eyes	Tongue	Mouth	Nose	Ears
TISSUE	Tendons	Blood Vessels	Flesh	Skin	Bones
EMOTION	Anger	Over-excitement	Pensiveness	Grief	Fear
VOICE	**Shouting**	**Laughing**	**Singing**	**Weeping**	**Groaning**

Questioning

An important part of a Shiatsu treatment is asking your partner questions. The aim of the questioning is to locate the disharmonies that are causing your partner's symptoms so that you can plan a treatment that will help to correct the imbalance. There is a simple questionnaire (see case-history form on p235) designed to elicit "the signs and symptoms" as well as asking about a person's general health, lifestyle and emotional condition.

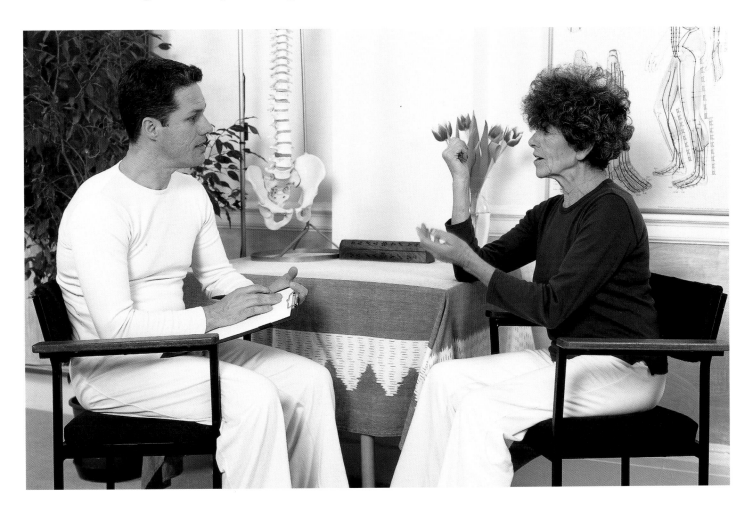

Above Set aside five or ten minutes at the beginning of each session to talk to your partner and understand any health issues.

ASSESSING THE SYMPTOMS

When you ask your partner why he or she is seeking a Shiatsu treatment, they will give you an indication of the organ functions that are out of harmony and tell you the health issues they would like addressed. Further questioning may uncover other conditions or symptoms (see box on page 234). All these findings should be carefully noted in a case-history form (see pages 234-5).

TAKING A CASE HISTORY

You need to ask questions that will enable you to assess your partner's condition and decide on what kind of treatment to give. Already you may have made some diagnostic assessments relating to their posture, tone of voice or facial characteristics; as you ask questions you can be checking how the answers match up to these initial assessments. It is also important to explain what you are going to do, answer any questions your partner has, reassure them about the treatment and help them to feel relaxed and secure. People often find it hard to talk openly about their problems, so you should always accept what they say without criticizing or judging.

One of the first questions will be about their current conditions. Do they have any symptoms? This question will often be an indicator of the kind of treatment that is expected. For example, if someone is coming to you because they have stiff shoulders, they will expect you to treat their shoulders, and hope to feel better afterwards. As a practitioner you need to address the symptoms that concern your partner, although there may be other areas you want to work on as well.

Asking about emotional states can be difficult. Ask questions such as "Do you suffer from depression or anxiety?" or "Do you find yourself frequently frustrated and irritable?". What you are looking for in their answers is a predominance or an absence of an emotion. It is normal to feel emotional in response to situations, but if someone is always angry or upset, for example, then this shows an imbalance.

SYMPTOM ASSESSMENT CLUES

- Medical history may show a pattern of disharmony in one element. For example, someone who has suffered a bereavement may then frequently suffer from colds and coughs, indicating the Metal element.
- Medication can mask symptoms or produce side effects which can confuse the diagnosis.
- Digestive system problems show a condition in the Earth element. Loose bowels show Spleen deficiency, constipation is linked to Large Intestine. Appetite and eating problems are related to Stomach.
- Diet and taste attraction will give clues as to out-of-balance organs. Someone with a sweet tooth may have other symptoms in Earth, such as loose bowels.
- Excessive drinking of coffee and tea can affect Kidney as caffeine stimulates the production of adrenalin. Alcohol may also affect Liver.
- Menstrual problems and PMS can be signs that Liver is not doing its job of moving chi. Lack of periods can be caused by a deficiency in Spleen.
- Back problems, particularly in the lower back, show Kidney and Bladder imbalances.
- Night-time urination also relates to Kidney and Bladder.
- Breathing difficulties, coughing or frequent colds indicate that the Metal element is out of harmony.
- Headaches, eye problems and stiff joints are all symptoms indicating a Wood imbalance.
- Insomnia or disturbed dreams show Heart imbalance, as do circulation problems such as varicose veins.
- A site of pain may give you an indication of the meridian involved. Note the meridian that passes through or is dominant in this area.
- Energy levels at different times of day will indicate meridian imbalances. For example, if someone is always tired in the morning it indicates a Spleen imbalance.

Finally, you should write down your postural observations, the hara diagnosis and the treatment. Write down any extra changes or symptoms that you noticed. For example, you may have felt that the left shoulder was stiffer than the right, and you could come back to this next time.

In reaching a diagnosis you will be working from your hara diagnosis (see pages 236–7). The case history will help you to confirm your diagnosis or to see deeper underlying patterns. When assessing the case history, look for three or more symptoms or indications in a meridian. You can also use your diagnosis as a basis for any recommendations to your client on self-massage, exercise, diet or lifestyle.

THE CASE-HISTORY FORM

As a professional practitioner you will always need to keep accurate records of your clients' treatments and case notes, so get into the habit as soon as you start treatments of filling in a case-history form such as the one shown opposite. The form should be fully completed at the end of a treatment, although most of it will have been filled in before treatment has started.

When a client returns to you for a further session, you should refer back to the case-history form, to see at-a-glance the symptoms they had when they first came and then, over a period of time, whether or not their condition is improving. The case-history form will also show any significant changes in your diagnosis over successive treatments as well as the overall effectiveness of your treatment.

PREPARING YOUR PARTNER

A Shiatsu treatment will often result in an immediate improvement, but it is also quite normal to feel some adverse reactions. Let your partner know this before you start the treatment, in case they have a sudden reaction during or immediately after the treatment. You can then reiterate this after the treatment (see page 244).

Below Asking questions and listening well to your partner's problems play a central role in Shiatsu diagnosis.

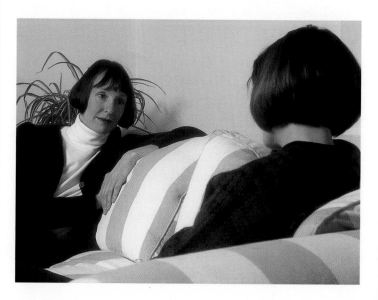

CASE HISTORY

Name:
Address:
Tel. no.:
Occupation:

Reasons for seeking a Shiatsu treatment:

Current symptoms:

Medical history:
(include surgery / major illnesses + when)

Medication currently taking:

Digestive system:
Bowels:
Appetite:

Diet:
Taste attraction:
Coffee / tea / alcohol:

Reproductive system:
Menstruation / PMT:
Back problems:
Chronic / acute where / when:
Urinary system:
Frequency / night:

Respiratory system:
Breathing/coughs:
Smoker:
Headaches / eye problems:
Joints:

Sleep:
Insomnia / dreams:
Circulation:

Energy levels:
Best time of day:
Worst time of day:
Dominant emotion:

Postural observations:

Pain – where / when:

Hara diagnosis (kyo and jitsu):

Treatment notes (treatment carried out / conclusions):

Below The overall treatment process will enable you to focus on individual health problems that need addressing. Often the diagnosis will simply support the symptoms your partner has specified, but sometimes the treatment uncovers other weak areas that need rebalancing – all these must be carefully recorded on the case-history form.

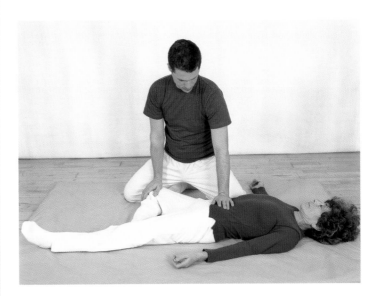

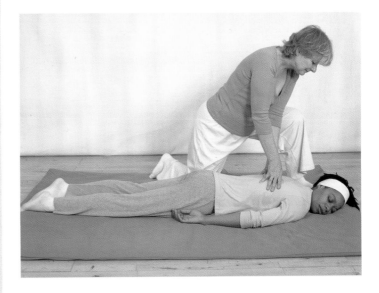

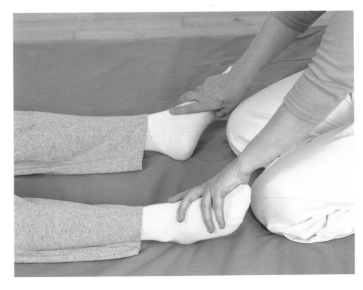

Touching

Touch is the most important diagnostic tool in Shiatsu. When palpating different areas of the body you are using touch to look for areas of kyo (empty) and jitsu (full). Diagnosis requires practice and an empty and receptive mind similar to that reached when meditating – detached, observant and focused. Try not to have any preconceived ideas about the result and remain open, calm and focused.

Hara Diagnosis

Each meridian has a corresponding diagnostic area in the hara. By palpating these areas we can assess for kyo and jitsu. The area with the most empty (kyo) energy state and the one with the most full (jitsu) are the two meridians chosen to work on.

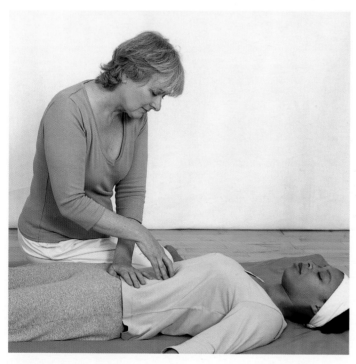

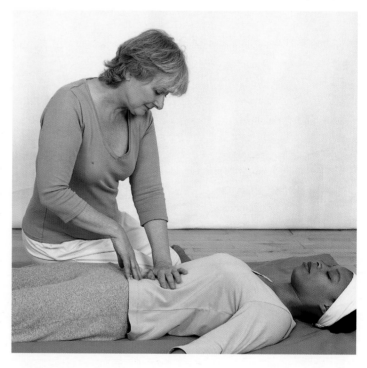

1 Palpate upper hara Leaving the mother hand on the lower hara, palpate the areas in the upper hara with the other (relaxed) hand, using the first three fingers. Follow the steps on the page opposite.

2 Palpate lower hara As you move through the steps, swap the mother hand and place it on the upper hara. Do not press directly into the navel but circle the fingers around it.

Preparing for hara diagnosis

Sit in seiza, close to your partner. Take deep breaths and assess your own state. Observe your partner's energy as you place your mother hand on the lower hara, and the other hand at the side of the belly. Ask yourself "which is the most jitsu area in the hara?" Use a light touch to assess each area, using the same order so that it becomes automatic. Use a cushion to practise.

Checking your diagnosis

When working the channels and points feel for relative kyo and jitsu. Sometimes you can use this to check your diagnosis. Does the meridian you have chosen from the hara diagnosis feel the most kyo meridian? There may be localised areas or points that are kyo or jitsu which relate to a particular condition but don't necessarily reflect the underlying cause and are not the most kyo meridian.

Step-by-step Palpations

The diagram below shows a suggested working sequence for hara diagnosis.
Each of the diagnostic areas in the hara is shown, starting with the Heart and
working gradually round to end with the Small Intestine.

With the mother hand on the lower hara, palpate the areas 1–9 in the upper hara, using the first three fingers and a relaxed hand. Change the mother hand to the upper hara and palpate areas 10–12. Using two hands, fingers pointing down at right angles to the body, work simultaneously on areas 13–14. Where there are two or three areas of the same meridian they should have the same energetic quality. Having moved around the hara quickly, no more than twice, ask the question "which is the most jitsu area?". If you don't know, take a guess and allow your intuition to guide you. Then go round the hara again holding the jitsu area with your mother hand and look for the kyo area, the place that creates a reaction in the jitsu – a softening, a feeling of connection, or some other change.

3 Liver is the pale green area further to the right just below the ribs, where the actual liver is. Continue to move to the right and palpate Liver area. Is it more kyo or more jitsu?

2 Gall Bladder is the purple area on the right below the ribs. Drop your fingers into the Gall Bladder. Is it more kyo or more jitsu than the previous area?

1 Heart is the soft red area at the base of the sternum. With a relaxed hand, using the first three fingers of one hand (the other is the mother hand on the lower abdomen), gently press down, feeling for kyo and jitsu.

4 Lung is the dark grey area further right towards the end of the ribs in the soft area at the waist. Move your relaxed hand to Lung area and again assess for relative kyo and jitsu.

5 Come back to the Heart area (1).

6 Stomach is the yellow area under the left ribs just over the stomach. Continue down the left side palpating the Stomach area.

7 Triple Heater is the pink oval further to the left under the ribs. Palpate Triple Heater area assessing for relative kyo and jitsu. By now you should have a most kyo and a most jitsu area.

8 Lung is the dark grey circle on the left, matching the right Lung area in step 4. Try to remember how it felt on the right side and compare. Return to these two areas again at the end, using two hands to compare.

9 Heart Protector is the deep red oval on the mid-line between the base of the sternum and the navel, just below the top Heart area. Gently palpate with three fingers, looking for relative kyo and jitsu.

10 Spleen is the mid-brown area around the navel. Move the mother hand to above the navel. Use the three fingers and your thumb around the navel. Avoid pressing into the navel directly.

11 Kidney is the blue horseshoe-shaped area below and around the sides of the navel. Palpate below the navel and then use two hands to feel the horseshoe sides.

12 Bladder is the pale blue outer horseshoe. Palpate just above the pubic bone and with two hands round the sides.

Key to the meridians

- Small Intestine
- Triple Heater
- Large Intestine
- Stomach
- Lung
- Heart
- Heart Protector
- Liver
- Spleen
- Kidney
- Gall Bladder
- Bladder

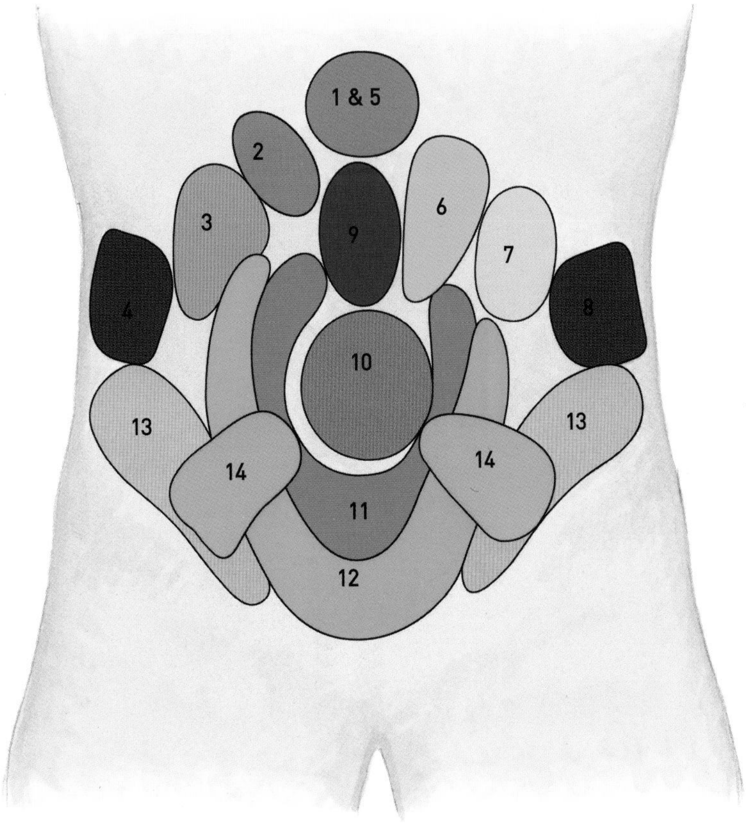

14 Small Intestine areas are the egg shapes superimposed over the Large Intestine, Bladder and Kidney. Palpate with two hands, comparing energetic quality and seeing if they have the same fullness or emptiness.

13 Large Intestine areas are pale grey flat ovals above each hip bone. Work with two hands.

Planning a Treatment

Having done all the background work setting up a Shiatsu treatment room and organizing loose cotton clothing (see page 170), you'll then need to come up with a treatment structure that suits you. The session should always include diagnosis using all the different methods, followed by the hands-on treatment (taking into account the contraindications listed on page 171) and some time afterwards for recovery.

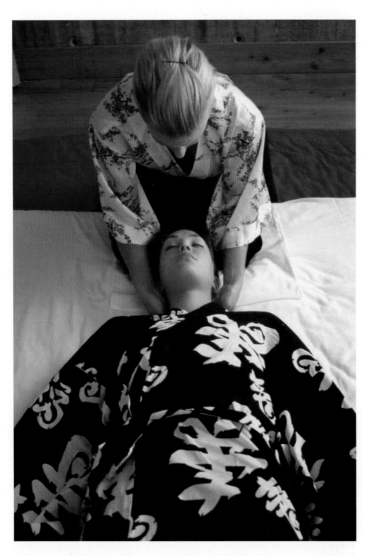

Above Both partners should wear comfortable, loose cotton clothing that covers as much as possible (Shiatsu treatments should not be carried out on exposed skin) and treatment should be on a firm, but soft, base such as a futon.

Right Always start every Shiatsu session with a hara diagnosis. Make a note of any full or empty areas, and return to the hara to feel for any changes as you progress. Having completed the diagnosis, Shiatsu practitioners generally work first on the kyo meridian: this helps to relax the jitsu and address the cause of the energy imbalance.

TREATMENT STRUCTURE

Start by following the basic framework outline in your treatments (see pages 168–91), starting with a hara diagnosis and slotting in the relevant meridians when you come to the arms or legs. As you become more experienced you can change the order of your treatment. You could start with a hara diagnosis, then work on the front of the body on the arms or legs, according to which meridians you have chosen. In some cases it is better to start working on the back after the hara diagnosis, especially if your receiver has not had Shiatsu before, as it is more relaxing.

Usually the actual hands-on treatment lasts about 35 to 40 minutes. This gives time at the beginning to take a case history and form a diagnosis and 5 minutes at the end for your partner to recover and for you to give them any recommendations you may have (see page 244). So altogether the treatment should take an hour from start to finish. When you are just beginning, it will almost certainly take longer, but with practice you should be able to hone down the treatment time to an hour.

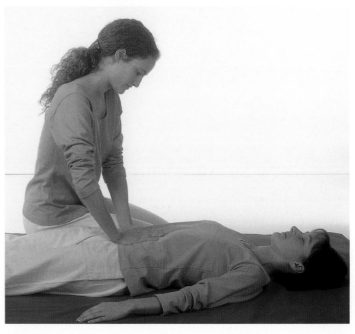

A Simple Treatment Sequence

Your treatment structure should always include work on the Bladder meridian, because of its relation to the spine and the nervous system. There are points on Bladder meridian either side of the spine that have a direct effect on each of the organ functions, known as yu points.

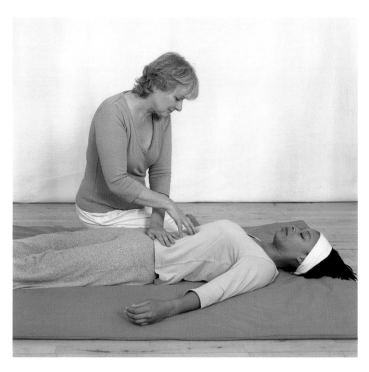

1 Hara diagnosis Sit in seiza position next to your partner's abdomen, placing your hand on the hara and tuning into your partner's energy. Do a hara diagnosis, moving quickly round the hara. Use the diagnosis as a focus for your treatment.

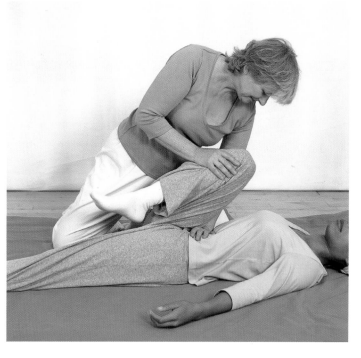

2 Leg rotation In this treatment we are using Spleen kyo, Lung jitsu as a diagnosis. Work the kyo meridian first – in this case Spleen. Start with leg rotation, keeping your hand on the hara and feeling for any stiffness in the hips.

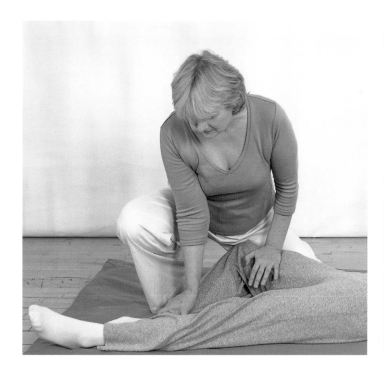

3 Palm the meridian Drop the leg down, lifting your own leg to kneel forward. Rest your partner's knee on your thigh for extra support if needed. Work the meridian with your palm and then your thumb, as shown on page 172.

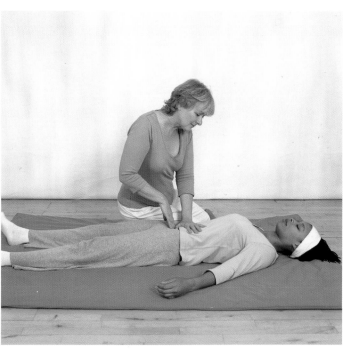

4 Reassess hara energy Return to a seiza position next to the hara as you draw back the leg and complete the Spleen meridian. Feel the difference in the energy in the hara: has it altered since you started the Shiatsu sequence?

▷

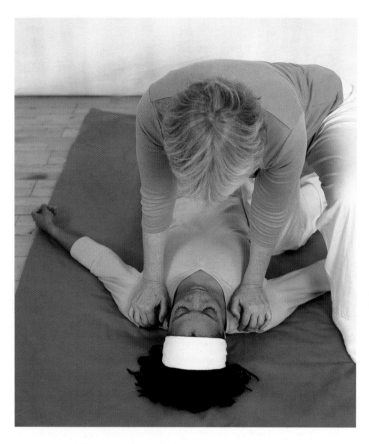

5 Open up the chest Move up to the shoulders by stepping up with one leg so that your foot is in line with your partner's shoulder. Place your hands on each shoulder and lean in with your body weight to open up the chest.

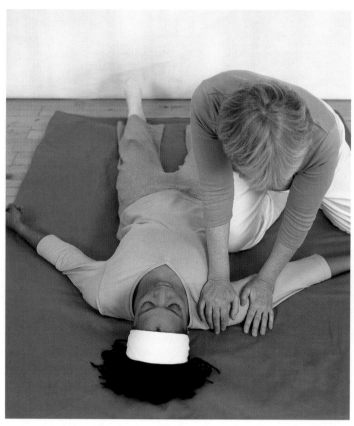

6 Thumb down Put the arm at 45 degrees – the position to treat the Lung meridian. With your mother hand firmly on the shoulder, palm and then thumb down the Lung meridian from the shoulder to the wrist.

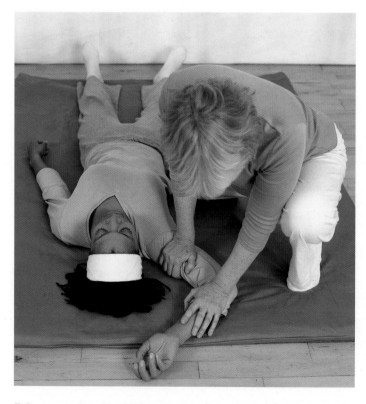

7 Open up the shoulder Holding the wrist, step up and bring the arm over the head. With your hand on the shoulder stretch the arm and open up the shoulder. Turn so that you are facing the feet in a position ready to work the head and neck.

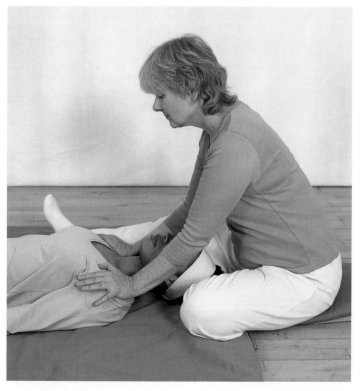

8 Pressure on shoulders Replace your partner's arms by their sides and move above the head. Adopt a relaxed seiza position with one leg straight for balance. Place your hands on the shoulders, pointing down the body, and apply pressure.

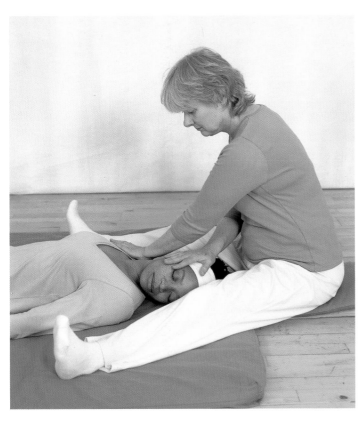

9 Rotate head Place one hand on the side of the head, the other on the shoulder and rotate the head, turning the chin towards the opposite shoulder. Open up the side of the neck by stretching the two hands away from each other.

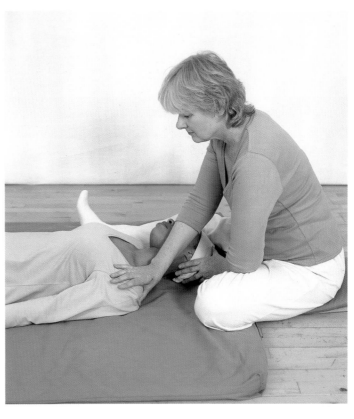

10 Head to the side Side bend the head by placing one hand on the side of the head and the other on the shoulder. Push the head sideways, away from the shoulder you are holding, to open up the neck. Repeat on the other side.

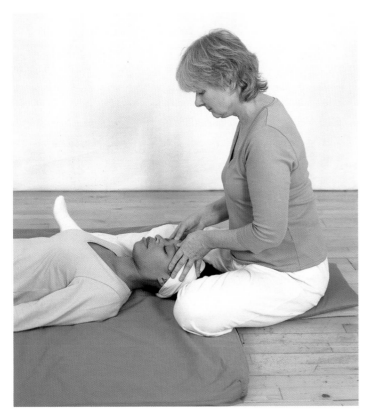

11 Thumb pressure Find the point BL 2, in the depression under the inner end of the eyebrow ridge. This point can be painful, so apply gentle but focused pressure with your thumbs making sure they are perpendicular to your partner's face.

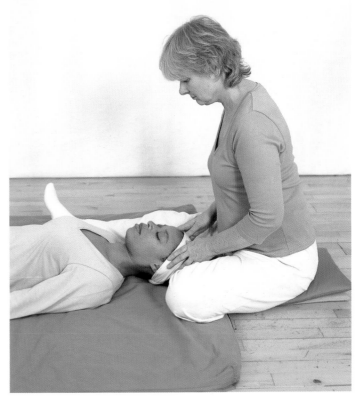

12 Thumbing up Continue in a straight line from BL 2, thumbing up Bladder meridian in the forehead and over and behind the head as far as you can reach. These last two techniques are good to release tension in the eyes and head.

▷

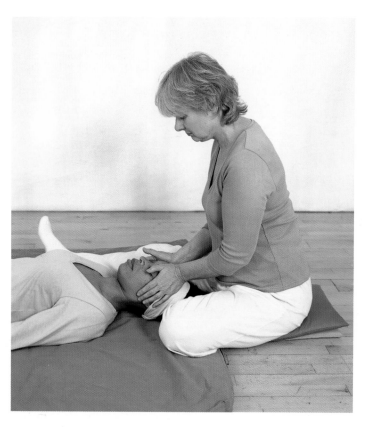

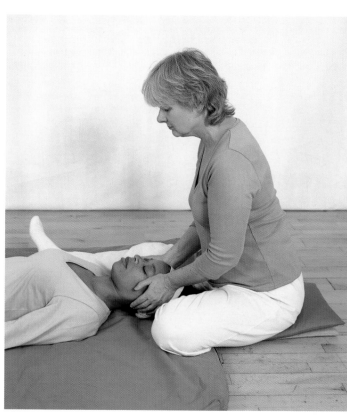

13 Palming head Palm around the top of the head with the heel of your hand. This covers the Gall Bladder meridian, which goes over the head several times. It is an important pathway for chi energy to circulate and activate the brain.

14 Rest head Bring your fingertips under the base of the skull and allow the head to rest in the palms of your hands. Come around to the other side and repeat the arm and leg sequence on the other side.

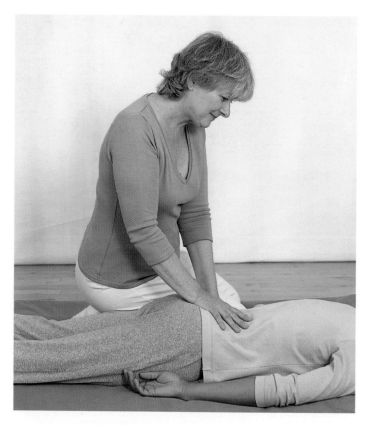

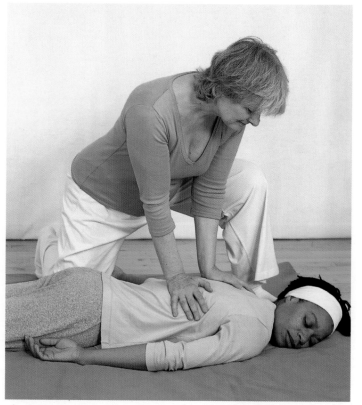

15 Assess energy flow Turn your partner over into prone position. Centre yourself by placing your hands on the sacrum. Tune in to the chi energy flow, feeling for any signs of fullness (jitsu) or emptiness (kyo).

16 Palm down Step up with one leg forward and palm down Bladder meridian in the back, starting one hand's width below the neck. Notice any over- or under-energized areas as you work down. Finish when you reach the sacrum.

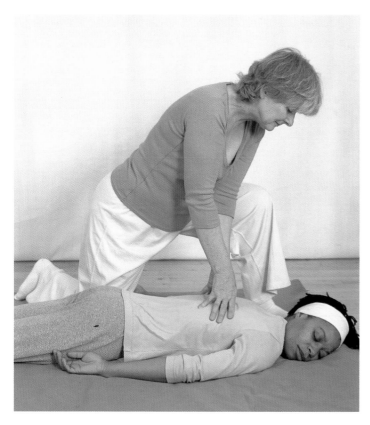

17 Thumb down Come back to the top and thumb down the Bladder meridian two finger-widths either side of the mid-line. Use perpendicular pressure leaning in with your weight. Notice kyo or jitsu points.

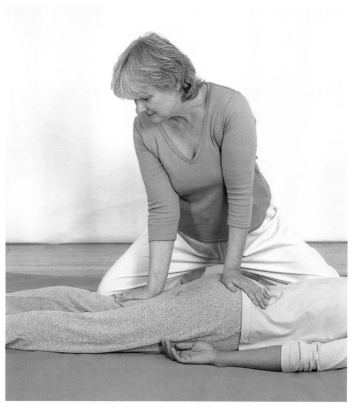

18 Palm down When you have completed Bladder in the back, turn to face the body and with mother hand on the sacrum and a wide seiza position, palm down the back of the leg. Shift your position down the leg as you work down.

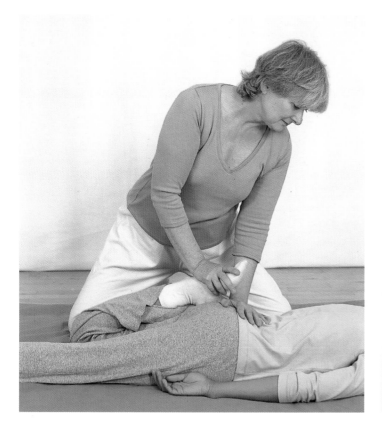

19 Stretch foot When you reach the ankle, pick up the leg under the ankle and stretch the foot to the buttock. Keep your hand on the sacrum and be careful not to over-stretch. Replace the leg and work down the other leg.

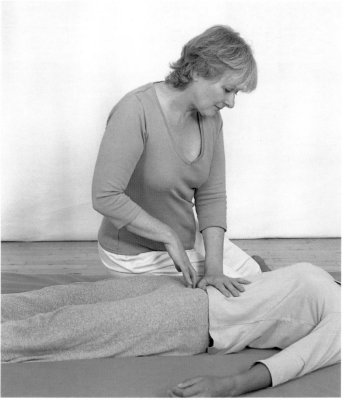

20 Hara assessment Turn your partner back over into supine position. Sit in seiza by the hara and check to see if there has been a change. Let your hand rest on the hara to finish, slowly breaking contact.

Finishing a Session

Having finished the physical Shiatsu treatment, first let your partner relax. Then remind them about how the treatment may affect them, alerting them to any ways that they may feel different, and offer yourself as a source of support if they are concerned by their physical or emotional reaction. Finally, complete the case history of their lifestyle patterns and the treatment that you carried out.

RELAXATION

After coming back to the hara to check whether it has changed, allow your partner to lie still for a few minutes to enjoy the feeling of deep relaxation and balance and allow the body to process any changes that have occurred. You may want to leave the room to allow your partner to be alone, and give yourself recovery time too.

TREATMENT REACTIONS

At the end of a treatment warn your partner that they should expect some changes over the following hours or days. Mostly they will feel better immediately, but it is quite common to feel tired, and you should advise them to have a rest if they do. Some people may have a headache or feel emotional, and this is also normal. Sometimes when the body's energy is changing it may be felt as discomfort. Encourage your partner to contact you for advice if conditions or problems develop.

Below Makka-ho exercises help to activate the meridians and are easy to do yourself at home – this one is a simple exercise to help the Spleen and Stomach meridians.

The effects of treatment

The immediate effect of Shiatsu treatment is individual, and partly depends on the length and depth of the treatment. A sense of well-being is common. The time taken for relief of symptoms depends on the nature of the condition. Because of the deep relaxation that usually occurs and the stimulus to the major body systems, your partner may experience "healing reactions": flu-like symptoms, aches, changes in bowel movements and urination, headaches or low energy may appear for around 24 hours. These are signs of elimination and show that healing is beginning.

If your partner suffers any serious adverse effects after treatment, he or she should seek medical help. If it is a more mild reaction, use the following guidelines:
• Take it easy and do not exert the body unnecessarily
• Avoid caffeine, alcohol and other drugs
• Take a lot of rest and go to bed earlier than usual
• Relax in a warm bath to sweat out some of the toxins
• Eat plenty of fresh fruit and vegetables, preferably raw
• Drink plenty of fresh water and hot water
• Avoid sugary and fatty foods

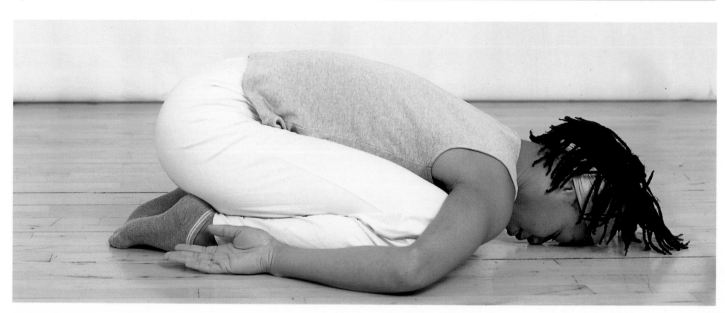

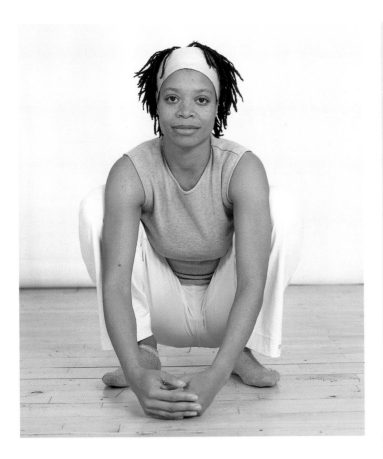

Above This makka-ho squatting exercise increases flexibility in the hips, knees and ankles. Be aware of your hara and let your weight drop into the feet from the belly.

RECOMMENDATIONS

Suggesting some simple recommendations will help your partner to continue the healing process. These may include activities, such as dancing, T'ai Chi or sports. You can teach them one or two of the makka-ho exercises described on pages 164–7 to help activate specific meridians. These are simple to do and can be applied to a particular condition. For example, if your partner has a problem with digestion or appetite you could recommend the Stomach/Spleen makka-ho exercise described on page 165. Or if your partner's emotions need bringing into balance, use the stretch on page 166 that works on the Heart and Small Intestine. If you want to give dietary advice, then keep it very simple or recommend a nutritionist. Look at the five elements correspondences table on pages 246–7 to see the taste attraction. If you have treated Spleen or Stomach, you could suggest substituting fruit or sweet vegetables for sugar. Restrict your advice to one or two recommendations that your partner can easily achieve; sooner choose something positive that can be added to a lifestyle, rather than something to give up. Don't be afraid to recommend other kinds of practitioners with more expertise in a particular area. Get to know some practitioners, such as counsellors, reflexologists, acupuncturists, homeopaths and herbalists, whom you feel confident to recommend.

Recommendations by element

An important part of every Shiatsu treatment is to give recommendations for suitable follow-up exercises to work on and lifestyle changes to be introduced. It can give your partner a real sense of empowerment to know that they can make changes to improve a condition. Make a point of giving simple recommendations that your partner can feasibly achieve.

EARTH – SPLEEN AND STOMACH MERIDIANS

- Dietary modification and measures for losing weight:
    Chewing each mouthful slowly (10 – 30 times)
    Eating a good breakfast
    Making meal times relaxed and stress free
- Grounding exercises such as T'ai Chi and Chi Kung
- Getting nourishment or pampering from sources other than food, such as music, receiving Shiatsu or other types of massage

FIRE – HEART AND SMALL INTESTINE, HEART PROTECTOR AND TRIPLE HEATER

- Meditation or relaxation tapes to calm the shen
- Skin brushing to improve the circulation
- Singing to encourage expression
- Counselling for emotional problems

METAL – LUNG AND LARGE INTESTINE

- Breathing exercises to encourage the taking in of chi
- Any vigorous exercise or a sport to encourage the intake of oxygen and to be more social
- Yoga to help with breathing
- Getting out of the house – going to a film, theatre or dancing – for a change of environment

WATER – KIDNEY AND BLADDER

Rest and moderation are important as Water people tend to overdo everything and become exhausted.

- Meditation is often difficult for a Water person to do, but they could try more active types of meditation, such as visualization or autogenic training
- Coffee over-stimulates the kidneys and cutting down or drinking decaffeinated coffee can help
- Alcohol and recreational drugs are particularly damaging

WOOD – LIVER AND GALL BLADDER

Wood people will often be workaholics and tend to be overly controlling.

- Encourage a good balance between work and play
- Creative pursuits such as pottery, writing, drawing etc.
- Non-competitive sport or outdoor activities, such as swimming, walking or gardening
- Dancing is excellent for encouraging flexibility, grace and self-expression

Five Elements Correspondences Table

	WOOD	FIRE
Yin organ	Liver	Heart Heart Protector
Yang organ	Gall Bladder	Small Intestine Triple Heater
Colour	Green	Red / Purple
Voice	Shouting	Laughing
Negative emotion	Anger Frustration	Excitement Hysteria
Positive emotion	Patience Humour	Calmness
Taste	Sour	Bitter
Smell	Rancid	Scorched
Sense	Sight	Speech
Orifice/body part	Eyes	Tongue
Season	Spring	Summer
Time of day	11 p.m. – 3 a.m.	11 p.m. – 3 a.m. 7 p.m. – 11 p.m.
Damaging climate	Wind	Heat
Body tissue	Tendons Ligaments	Blood vessels
Function	Organization Decisions	Consciousness Communication
Fluid secretion	Tears	Sweat
System	Joints	Circulation
Direction	East	South
Spirit	Life direction	Consciousness
Stage of development	Birth	Growth
Nurturing foods	Wheat Leafy green vegetables	Corn (sweetcorn) Beans

EARTH	METAL	WATER
Spleen	Lung	Kidney
Stomach	Large Intestine	Bladder
Yellow / Orange	White	Blue / Black
Singing Whining	Weeping	Groaning
Worry Victim	Grief Isolated	Fear Phobias
Compassion Grounded	Positive Open	Courage
Sweet	Pungent	Salty
Fragrant	Rotting	Putrid
Taste	Smell	Hearing
Mouth	Nose	Ears
Late summer	Autumn	Winter
7 a.m. – 11 a.m.	3 a.m. – 7 a.m.	3 p.m. – 7 p.m.
Damp	Dryness	Cold
Flesh	Skin Membranes	Bones Hair
Transformation Transportation	Exchange Elimination	Purification Regulation
Saliva	Mucus	Urine
Digestive	Respiratory Eliminatory	Nervous Reproductive
Centre	West	North
Intellect	Soul	Will
Transformation	Harvest	Hibernation
Rice Root vegetables	Lotus root Ginger	Millet Aduki beans

Further Reading

THAI MASSAGE

The Art of Traditional Thai Massage by Asokananda. Editions Duang Kamol, Bangkok, 1992.

Awakening of the Spine by V. Scaravelli. Harper Collins, 1991.

Baby Massage. A Practical Guide to Massage and Movement for Babies and Infants by Peter Walker. Piatkus, 1995.

How to Use Yoga (Practical Handbook series) by Mira Mehta. Lorenz Books, 2001.

Massage for Total Relaxation by Nitya Lacroix. Dorling Kindersley, 1991.

Qi Gong for Beginners by Stanley D. Wilson. Rudra Press, 1997.

Thai Massage by Ananda Apfelbaum. Avery Publishing, 2004.

The Muscle Book by Paul Blakey. Bibliotek Books, 1992.

Thai Traditional Massage for Advanced Practitioners by Asokananda. Editions Duang Kamol, Bangkok, 1997.

Total Body Massage by Nitya Lacroix, Francesca Rinaldi, Sharon Seager and Renée Tanner. Lorenz Books, 2004.

Yoga Mind, Body & Spirit by Donna Fahri. Newleaf, 2000.

The Yoga of Mindfulness by Asokananda. Editions Duang Kamol, Bangkok, 1993.

SHIATSU

Beyond Shiatsu: Ohashi's Bodywork Method by Wataru Ohashi and Ken Okano. Kodansha America, 2003.

The Book of Massage: The Complete Step-by-step Guide to Eastern and Western Techniques by Lucinda Lidell, Sara Thomas, Carola Beresford Cooke and Anthony Porter. Prentice Hall & IBD, 1986.

The Book of Shiatsu: Vitality and Health Through the Art of Touch by Paul Lundberg. Gaia Books Ltd, 2005.

Essentially Wai by Esther Wai Lin Lim. Minerva Press, 1999.

Healing with Shiatsu by Catherine Sutton. Newleaf, 1997.

Ocean of Streams: Zen Shiatsu – Meridians, Tsubos and Theoretical Impressions by Veet Allan. OMKI, 2006.

Shiatsu-doh: Improved Health and Enhanced Living Through the Japanese Healing Art by Kensen Saito. Cross Media, 2004.

Shiatsu Theory and Practice by Carola Beresford-Cooke. Churchill Livingstone, 2003.

Shiatzu: Japanese Finger Pressure for Energy, Sexual Vitality and Relief from Tension and Pain by Yukiko Irwin. Lippincott Williams & Wilkins, 1976.

A Study of Shiatsu by Cass Jackson and Janie Jackson. Caxton Editions, 2002.

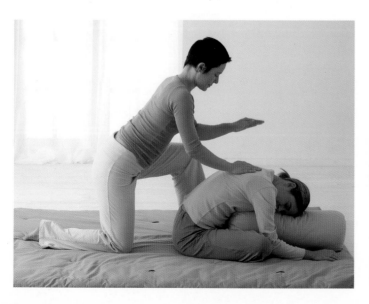

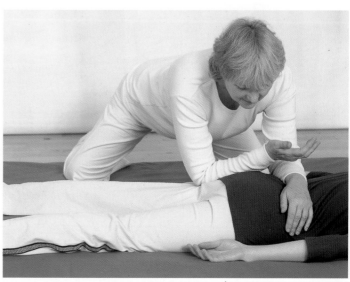

THAI MASSAGE

UK

Individual Thai massage treatment and training:
www.bodywisdom.org.uk

Thai massage equipment:
The Futon Shack
452 Hornsey Road
London
N19 4EE
Tel. +44 (0) 20 7561 0577
www.futonshack.com

Yoga equipment:
Yoga Mad
Tel. +44 (0) 1386 551930
www.yogamad.com

USA and Canada

Futons and related equipment:
Bodywork Central
5519 College Avenue
Oakland
CA 94618
Tel. 510 547 4313
www.bodyworkcentral.com

Training and treatment:
Lotus Palm School of Thai Massage
5870 Waverly Street
Montreal
Quebec H2T 2Y3
Canada
Tel. 514 270 5713
www.lotuspalm.com

Training and treatment:
Saul David Raye/White Lotus
Foundation Retreat Centre
Santa Barbara, California
www.thaiyoga.com

New Zealand

Thai massage training:
Sunshine Network Institute
www.asokananda.com

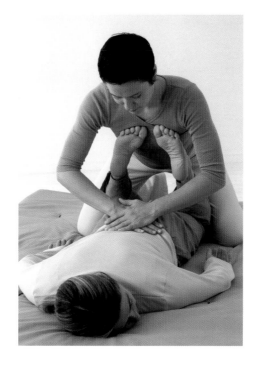

Australia

Futons and advice on equipment:
Fantasy Futon
Kings Street
Newtown
Sydney
NSW 2042
Tel. 02 9550 3939

Thailand

Thai massage courses:
Sunshine Network
www.infothai.com/thaiyogamassage

Sunshine School
Chiang Mai
www.sunshine-massage-school.com

The Foundation of Shivago Komarpa
Old Chiang Mai Medicine Hospital
Near Chiang Mai Cultural Centre
Wualai Road, Chiang Mai

Thai Traditional Medical School
Wat Pho
Bangkok

SHIATSU

The following organizations offer Shiatsu advice as well as training or treatment.

UK

The Shiatsu Society (UK)
Eastlands Court
St Peters Rd
Rugby CV21 3QP
Tel: +44 (0) 8451 304560
www.shiatsu.org

British School of Shiatsu-Do
Unit 3
Islington Studios
Thane Villas
London N7 7NV
Tel: +44 (0) 20 770 03355
www.shiatsu-do.co.uk

USA

AOBTA National Headquarters
1010 Haddonfield-Berlin Road
Suite 408
Voorhees
NJ 08043-3514
Tel: 856 782 1616
www.aobta.org

International School of
  Shiatsu
10 South Clinton Street
Doylestow
PA 18901
Tel: 215 340 9918
Email: info@shiatsubo.com
www.shiatsubo.com

Ohashi Institute
147 West 25th St
8th Floor
New York, NY 10001
Tel: 800 810 4190
Email: info@ohashiatsu.org
www.ohashi.com

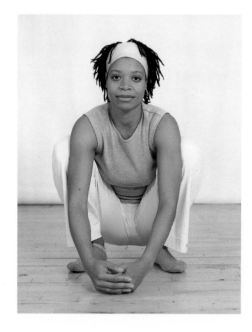

Canada

The Canadian Shiatsu Society of
    British Columbia (CSSBC)
www.Shiatsupractor.org
Shiatsu School of Canada Inc.
547 College Street
Toronto
Ontario, M6G 1A9
Tel: 416 323 1818
or toll-free: 1 800 263 1703
Email: info@shiatsucanada.com
www.shiatsucanada.com

Shiatsu Academy of Tokyo
320 Danforth Avenue
Suite 206, Toronto
Ontario M4K 1N8
Tel: 416 466 8780
Email: sait131@aol.com
www.kensensaito.com

Sourcepoint Shiatsu Therapy Centre
3261 Heather Street (at 16th Ave.)
Vancouver
British Columbia V5Z 3K4
Tel: 604 876 0042
Email: info@sourcepoint.bc.ca
www.sourcepoint.bc.ca

Australia

Shiatsu Academy
54 Brighton Road
Balaclava, Melbourne
Victoria 3183
Tel: 03 9525 7968

Shiatsu Therapy Association
    of Australia
c/o The Secretary
PO Box 91
Brunswick West
Victoria 305
Tel: 03 9380 9183 or 1300 138 250
www.staa.org.au

New Zealand

Tao Shiatsu Oceania
9 Hemington St
Waterview
Auckland
Tel: 09 828 3385
Mob: 025 989 726
Email: oceania@taoshiatsu.com
www.taoshiatsu.com

Japan

Japan Shiatsu College
2-15-6 Koishikawa
Bunkyo-ku Tokyo
Tel: 03 3813 7481
www.shiatsu.ac.jp

Europe

The European Shiatsu
    Federation
www.shiatsu-esf.org

Austria

Österreichischer Dachverband für
    Shiatsu
Postfach 109
A-1217 Wien
Tel/fax: +43 1 258 08 49
Email: info@shiatsu-verband.at
www.shiatsu-verband.at

Belgium

Belgische Shiatsu Federatie vzw
Gounden Leeuwplein 1
B-9000 Gent
Tel: +32 92 252 904
Email: info@shiatsu.be
www.shiatsu.be

Czech Republic

CAS Czech Shiatsu Association
Na Zderaze 5
120 00 Praha 2
Tel: +42 0603 156 708
Email: darja@shiatsu.cz

Greece

Hellenic Shiatsu Society
Zissimopoulou 16
115-24 Athens
Tel: +30 (0) 10 6980 168
Email: mcharl@tee.gr

Holland

Iokai Shiatsu Akademie
    Nederland
1E Jacob Van Campenstr. 40
BG Amsterdam
1072 Netherlands
Email: info@iokai-shiatsu.nl
www.iokai-shiatsu.nl

Ireland

Shiatsu Society of Ireland
P.O. Box 7683, Malahide, Co. Dublin
Tel: +353 1 845 3647
www.shiatsusocietyireland.com

Israel

Israeli Tao Shiatsu Center
Tzvika Calisar, Spinoza 5, Tel-Aviv
Tel: 03 524 9277
Email: Europe@taoshiatsu.com
www.taoshiatsu.co.il

Spain

Asociación de Profesionales de
    Shiatsu en España
C/ Atocha, 121-1°-izda
E-28012 Madrid
Tel/fax: +34 91 429 49 89
Email: Shiastu@terra.es
www.shiatsu-es.com

Sweden

Riksorganisationen för Shiatsu
Rusthållarvägen 6
S-18769 Täby
Tel: +46 8 766 40 05
Email: info@shiatsuriks.org
www.shiatsuriks.org

Switzerland

International School of Shiatsu
Hauptstrasse, Kiental / BE
CH 3723
Tel: +41 33 676 26 76
www.kientalerhof.ch

Acknowledgements

AUTHORS' ACKNOWLEDGEMENTS

Thai Massage (author Nicky Smith)

I would like to acknowledge and thank: Asokananda for his guidance, support and dedication to Thai massage; Pichet Boonthumme, Chaiyuth Priyasith, Claire McAlpine, Sean Doherty, John Stirk, and Silke Ziehl for their gifts of inspiration; my friends and family, for their love and support, especially my sister Fiona for her patience during the photo sessions; the models – Oriol, Spring, Nick and Dagma; and agoy.com for the beautiful yoga mats.

Many thanks also to Asokananda, for his helpfulness and for his permission to base the artworks on pages 23–5 on those featured in his book, *The Art of Traditional Thai Massage*.

Shiatsu (author Hilary Totah)

I would like to thank my editor Jennifer Mussett for encouraging me and, in difficult circumstances, helping me in the completion of this book. My heartfelt thanks go to all my teachers who have inspired me in this journey into the wondrous working of the human body and its energy patterns, especially to my first teachers Ray Ridolfi, Saul Goodman, Pauline Sasaki and Ohashi Sensei.

I would like to acknowledge my fellow teachers and students at the British School of Shiatsu-Do for the fund of knowledge that they have shared, which forms the basis of this book. Special thanks to Maura Bright for information on facial diagnosis and to Doe Warnes, Emerson Bastos, Kishaw Wheatle, Maya Babic, Cynthia Kee and Cesar Pinto for their patience and enthusiasm as the models. To Katy Bevan for organizing us all and first suggesting that I do this book.

I am deeply grateful to all my teachers, colleagues, students and clients who have shared this Shiatsu path with me – for all the healing, friendship, inspiration and support.

My special thanks to my two children Layla and Talal who have loved and supported me unconditionally and without whose father, Edward Totah, I would never have started on this road.

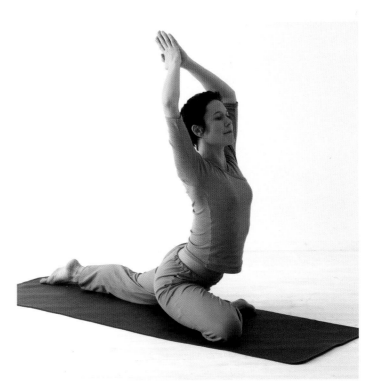

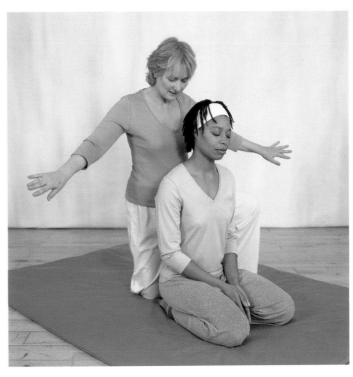

PHOTOGRAPHIC ACKNOWLEDGEMENTS

The publishers would like to thank the following for permission to reproduce their images (l=left, r=right, t=top, b=bottom, m=middle):

Page 6bl: Asokananda; page 18b: Corbis; page 19tl: Archivo Iconografico, S.A./Corbis; page 19br: Macduff Everton/Corbis; page 33br: Macduff Everton/Corbis; page 133 Charles Pertwee/Alamy Images; page 195m Image source/Alamy; page 238 image100/Alamy; page 136, page 137 Mary Evans Picture Library; page 173tr Robert Harding Picture Library. All other photographs © Anness Publishing Ltd

Index

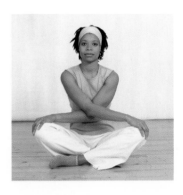

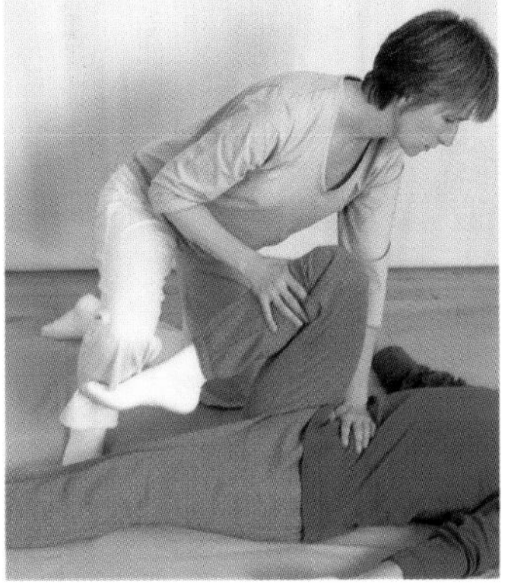

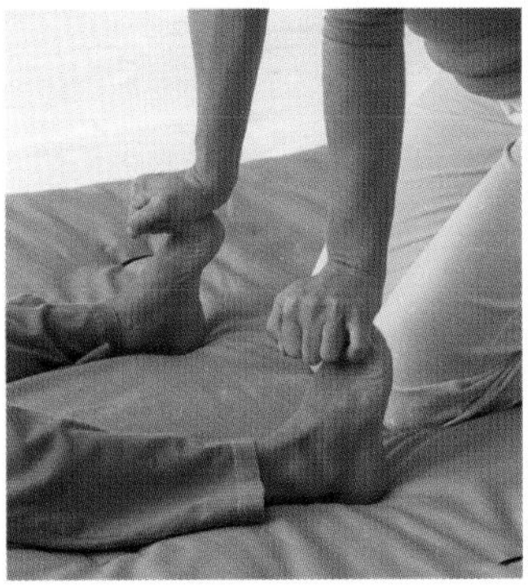

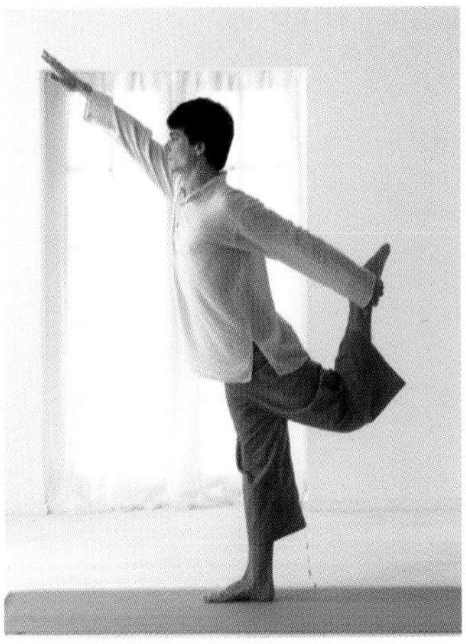

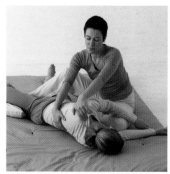

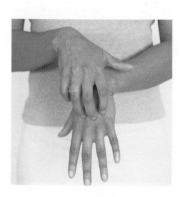

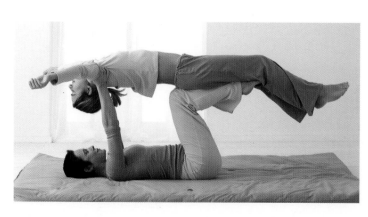

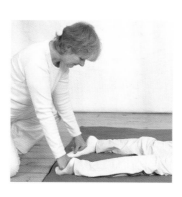

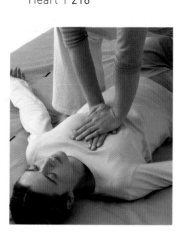

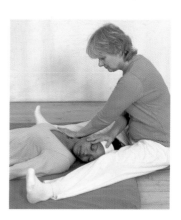

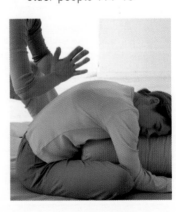

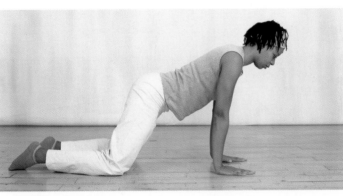

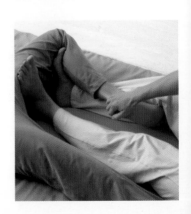

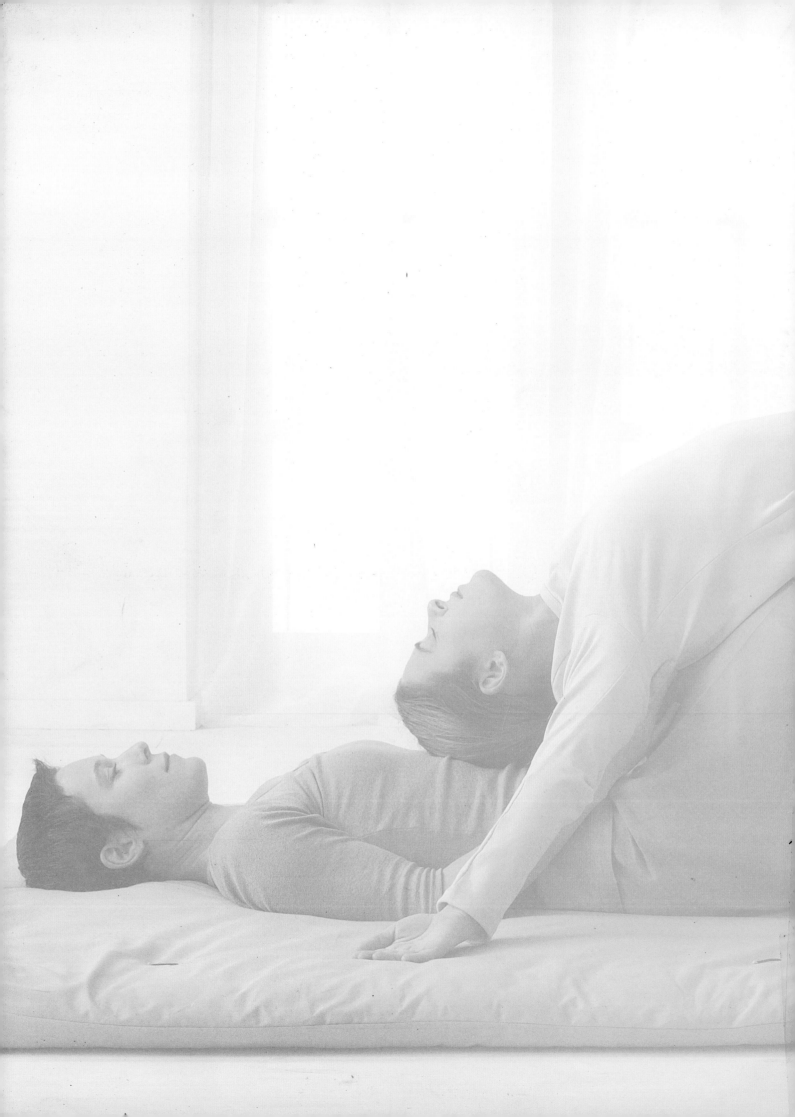